ADVANCE PRAISE FOR MAYO CLINIC CASES
IN NEUROIMMUNOLOGY

"Over the last thirty years, the field of neuroimmunology has exploded. We understand how to diagnose and treat an array of neuroimmunological diseases from inflammatory muscle disease to multiple sclerosis. We also can diagnose and treat disorders that were previously unrecognized, such as anti-MOG antibody demyelinating disease, or poorly understood, such as neuromyelitis optica. Dr. McKeon and his colleagues at the Mayo Clinic have been at the forefront of the expansion of our knowledge about neuroimmunology. *Mayo Clinic Cases in Neuroimmunology* is a highly engaging presentation of cases that reveal the current status of this important area of neurology. All neurologists need to keep up-to-date on this burgeoning field and there is no better way than learning from the cases presented by Dr. McKeon and colleagues."

—Dennis Bourdette, MD, FANA, FAAN,
Chair and Professor Emeritus, Department of Neurology,
Oregon Health & Science University

"Mayo Clinic Cases in Neuroimmunology is a fantastic way to learn how to approach patients with suspected autoimmune neurologic and neuroimmunoliogic conditions. The succinct, case-based format aides the readers in retention of the pertinent information to identify these diagnoses in their own clinical practice. Each case is unique mystery that keeps the readers engaged and eager for the next — I highly recommend this book to clinicians seeking a 'page-turner' style of learning to get up to speed on Neuroimmunology and Autoimmune Neurology."

Stacey L. Clardy MD PhD,
University of Utah and Salt Lake City VA,
Salt Lake City, UT

MAYO CLINIC CASES IN NEUROIMMUNOLOGY

EDITORS

Andrew McKeon, MB, BCh, MD

Consultant,
Departments of Laboratory Medicine & Pathology, and Neurology
Mayo Clinic, Rochester, Minnesota;
Professor of Laboratory Medicine & Pathology and of Neurology
Mayo Clinic College of Medicine and Science

B. Mark Keegan, MD

Chair, Division of Multiple Sclerosis & Autoimmune Neurology
Mayo Clinic, Rochester, Minnesota;
Professor of Neurology
Mayo Clinic College of Medicine and Science

W. Oliver Tobin, MB, BCh, BAO, PhD

Consultant, Department of Neurology
Mayo Clinic, Rochester, Minnesota;
Associate Professor of Neurology
Mayo Clinic College of Medicine and Science

MAYO CLINIC SCIENTIFIC PRESS   OXFORD UNIVERSITY PRESS

MAYO
CLINIC

The triple-shield Mayo logo and the words MAYO, MAYO CLINIC, and MAYO CLINIC SCIENTIFIC PRESS
are marks of Mayo Foundation for Medical Education and Research.

OXFORD
UNIVERSITY PRESS

Oxford University Press is a department of the University of Oxford. It furthers
the University's objective of excellence in research, scholarship, and education
by publishing worldwide. Oxford is a registered trade mark of Oxford University
Press in the UK and certain other countries.

Published in the United States of America by Oxford University Press
198 Madison Avenue, New York, NY 10016, United States of America.

Library of Congress Cataloging-in-Publication Data
Names: McKeon, Andrew (Neurologist) editor. | Keegan, Mark B., editor. | Tobin, Oliver W., editor.
Title: Mayo Clinic cases in neuroimmunology / [edited by] Andrew McKeon, B. Mark Keegan, W. Oliver Tobin
Other titles: Cases in neuroimmunology | Mayo Clinic scientific press (Series)
Description: New York, NY : Oxford University Press, [2022] |
Series: Mayo clinic scientific press series | Includes bibliographical references and index.
Identifiers: LCCN 2021033760 (print) | LCCN 2021033761 (ebook) |
ISBN 9780197583425 (paperback) | ISBN 9780197583449 (epub) | ISBN 9780197583456
Subjects: MESH: Autoimmune Diseases of the Nervous System—iagnosis |
Autoimmune Diseases of the Nervous System—therapy | Case Reports
Classification: LCC RC600 (print) | LCC RC600 (ebook) | NLM WL 140 |
DDC 616.97/8—dc23
LC record available at https://lccn.loc.gov/2021033760
LC ebook record available at https://lccn.loc.gov/2021033761

DOI: 10.1093/med/9780197583425.001.0001

In remembrance of our late Mayo Clinic neuroimmunology colleague and friend, Istvan Pirko, MD

FOREWORD

Investigators at Mayo Clinic have been at the forefront of the field of neuroimmunology for several decades. Researchers at Mayo Clinic discovered that neuromyelitis optica (NMO) is characterized by autoantibodies to the aquaporin-4 water channel, proving NMO to be distinct from multiple sclerosis. Subsequently, Mayo Clinic neurologists devised the diagnostic criteria for NMO spectrum disorder, fully defined its clinical course and neuroimaging characteristics, and identified eculizumab as an effective treatment for NMO. Investigators from Mayo Clinic also have been leaders in the identification of paraneoplastic disorders affecting the nervous system and have provided the clinical community with diagnostic tests for these diseases.

Building on the vast expertise available at Mayo Clinic, coeditors Andrew McKeon, B. Mark Keegan, and W. Oliver Tobin have assembled a stellar group of neurologists and neuroimmunologists to document 83 highly instructive, case-based scenarios drawn from actual cases seen by the authors. Despite the many different authors, all of the case histories have been written and formatted uniformly, which makes them easier to read. The senior authors for each case are well-known and respected clinician-investigators in the fields relevant to those cases. Most are recognized as the authors of some of the key papers on the corresponding topics.

The book is divided into 3 sections with the general topics of central nervous system (CNS) demyelinating disease, autoimmune neurologic disorders, and other inflammatory CNS disorders and neuroimmunologic mimics. Reading these case histories provides a truly enjoyable way to learn about the clinical diagnosis and treatment of a multitude of disorders in a rapidly expanding field. This collection of case studies, some with a frequently encountered diagnosis and others quite esoteric, was fun to read. Each case can be viewed as a mystery to be solved. Each case starts with a typical history and examination, then provides a diagnostic workup, including pertinent negative tests, and concludes with the correct diagnosis and best current treatment. The format allows the reader to follow each case as it unfolds and attempt to determine the diagnosis as would be done in practice. Associated suggested reading and a short quiz on each topic are also included to emphasize key educational points.

This compilation of instructional neuroimmunologic and neuroimmunologic-mimic case histories will surely be appreciated by general neurologists, midlevel neurology providers, and resident and fellow trainees interested in multiple sclerosis and related diseases and CNS autoimmunity. In addition, the *Questions and Answers* section makes this book a valuable adjunct for clinicians preparing for board examinations.

Congratulations to Doctors Andrew McKeon, B. Mark Keegan, and W. Oliver Tobin for assembling an outstanding group of contributing authors to provide up-to-date instruction on a wide range of neurologic diseases in such an enjoyable format.

Anne H. Cross, MD
Professor of Neurology and
Section Head, Neuroimmunology/Multiple Sclerosis
Washington University School of Medicine
St. Louis, Missouri USA

PREFACE

In the past 2 decades, diagnostics and therapeutics in neuroimmunology have rapidly evolved and increased in complexity. Diagnosis is assisted by various laboratory and advanced imaging techniques. Randomized clinical trials in multiple sclerosis (MS) and neuromyelitis optica (NMO), and smaller studies for rarer autoimmune diseases, have led to distinct immune molecule–targeted and mechanism-specific therapies. The fields of cerebrovascular medicine, neurooncology, and neuroinfectious diseases have not remained static either. All of these gains present a challenge, however, in that early and accurate neurologic diagnosis is more important than ever. In our experience, some diagnostic pitfalls lie in the interpretation of test results and images without reference to the nuances of the clinical history and examination. Although some things change (eg, technology), other things never change (eg, clinical common sense).

The 83 case-based chapters of *Mayo Clinic Cases in Neuroimmunology* are intended to provide a sampling of our clinical experiences across our Division of Multiple Sclerosis and Autoimmune Neurology at Mayo Clinic in Minnesota, Arizona, and Florida. These cases focus on key components of the history, examination and test findings, and differential diagnosis, although we also reference treatment approaches extensively throughout. To bring some form to this extensive repertoire of cases, we have divided the book into 3 sections covering central nervous system (CNS) demyelinating disease (MS, NMO, and limited forms of those disorders), autoimmune neurologic disorders (usually defined by immunoglobulin G antibody biomarkers), and others (CNS inflammatory disorders not fitting into the first 2 categories, along with neuroimmunologic mimics). We have illustrated the cases extensively with imaging and, where relevant, pathologic images and video material. The book will be useful to all clinicians who evaluate patients with neurologic disorders, both generalists and neuroimmunology subspecialists. The book will also be useful to medical students and resident and fellow trainees in neurology, medicine, and psychiatry. Board review–style questions are also provided.

We wish to thank Kenna Atherton, LeAnn Stee, Jane Craig, Ann Ihrke, and Alyssa B. Quiggle, PhD, for their conscientious help in editing and preparing the manuscript for publication. We also thank Collette Justin for her expert help in preparing the figures. We are indebted to our patients and also to our Department of Neurology colleagues outside our subspecialty division (several of whom have authored chapters herein), without whom we never would have encountered many of the patients described. Finally, we wish to express our humble gratitude to our respective partners, Jen, Jenny, and Mairead, and our children, for their enduring patience and love.

Andrew McKeon, MB, BCh, MD
B. Mark Keegan, MD
W. Oliver Tobin, MB, BCh, BAO, PhD

CONTENTS

SECTION III
OTHER INFLAMMATORY
CNS DISORDERS AND
NEUROIMMUNOLOGIC
MIMICS

SECTION IV
QUESTIONS AND ANSWERS

CONTRIBUTORS

David N. Abarbanel, MD
Resident in Neurology, Mayo Clinic School of Graduate Medical Education, Mayo Clinic College of Medicine and Science, Rochester, Minnesota

Marie D. Acierno, MD
Senior Associate Consultant, Department of Ophthalmology, Mayo Clinic, Scottsdale, Arizona; Assistant Professor of Ophthalmology, Mayo Clinic College of Medicine and Science

Samantha A. Banks, MD
Resident in Neurology, Mayo Clinic School of Graduate Medical Education, Mayo Clinic College of Medicine and Science, Rochester, Minnesota

Eduardo E. Benarroch, MD
Consultant, Department of Neurology, Mayo Clinic, Rochester, Minnesota; Professor of Neurology, Mayo Clinic College of Medicine and Science

M. Tariq Bhatti, MD
Senior Associate Consultant, Department of Ophthalmology, Mayo Clinic, Rochester, Minnesota; Professor of Neurology and of Ophthalmology, Mayo Clinic College of Medicine and Science

Silvia Bozzetti, MD
Department of Neuroscience, Biomedicine, and Movement Sciences, University of Verona, Verona, Italy

Jeffrey W. Britton, MD
Chair, Division of Epilepsy, Mayo Clinic, Rochester, Minnesota; Professor of Neurology, Mayo Clinic College of Medicine and Science, Rochester, Minnesota

Robert D. Brown Jr, MD, MPH
Chair, Division of Stroke and Cerebrovascular Diseases, Mayo Clinic, Rochester, Minnesota; Professor of Neurology, Mayo Clinic College of Medicine and Science, Rochester, Minnesota

Adrian Budhram, MD
Research Collaborator in Neurology, Mayo Clinic School of Graduate Medical Education, Mayo Clinic College of Medicine and Science, Rochester, Minnesota

Ivan D. Carabenciov, MD
Senior Associate Consultant, Department of Neurology, Mayo Clinic, Rochester, Minnesota

Jonathan L. Carter, MD
Consultant, Department of Neurology, Mayo Clinic, Scottsdale, Arizona; Associate Professor of Neurology, Mayo Clinic College of Medicine and Science

John J. Chen, MD, PhD
Consultant, Department of Ophthalmology, Mayo Clinic, Rochester, Minnesota; Associate Professor of Neurology and of Ophthalmology, Mayo Clinic College of Medicine and Science, Rochester, Minnesota

Maria Elena De Rui, MD
Infectious Diseases Section, Department of Diagnostic and Public Health, University of Verona, Verona, Italy

Michelle F. Devine, MD
Research Collaborator in Neurology, Mayo Clinic School of Graduate Medical Education, Mayo Clinic College of Medicine and Science, Rochester, Minnesota

Divyanshu Dubey, MBBS
Senior Associate Consultant, Department of Laboratory Medicine & Pathology, Mayo Clinic, Rochester, Minnesota; Assistant Professor of Laboratory Medicine & Pathology and of Neurology, Mayo Clinic College of Medicine and Science, Rochester, Minnesota

Jaclyn R. Duvall, MD
Fellow in Neurology, Mayo Clinic School of Graduate Medical Education, Mayo Clinic College of Medicine and Science, Rochester, Minnesota; now with Utica Park Headache Clinic, Tulsa, Oklahoma

P. James B. Dyck, MD
Consultant, Department of Neurology, Mayo Clinic, Rochester, Minnesota; Professor of Neurology, Mayo Clinic College of Medicine and Science

Eric R. Eggenberger, DO
Consultant, Department of Ophthalmology, Mayo Clinic, Jacksonville, Florida; Professor of Neurology and of Ophthalmology, Mayo Clinic College of Medicine and Science

Stephen W. English Jr, MD, MBA
Senior Associate Consultant, Department of Neurology, Mayo Clinic, Jacksonville, Florida

Floranne C. Ernste, MD
Consultant, Division of Rheumatology, Mayo Clinic, Rochester, Minnesota; Associate Professor of Medicine, Mayo Clinic College of Medicine and Science

John C. Feemster
Graduate Research Employment Program, Center for Sleep Medicine, Mayo Clinic, Rochester, Minnesota; Medical College of Wisconsin, Central-Wisconsin, Wausau, Wisconsin

Sergio Ferrari, MD
Department of Neuroscience, Biomedicine, and Movement Sciences, University of Verona, Verona, Italy

Eoin P. Flanagan, MB, BCh
Consultant, Department of Neurology, Mayo Clinic, Rochester, Minnesota; Associate Professor of Neurology, Mayo Clinic College of Medicine and Science

Ralitza H. Gavrilova, MD
Consultant, Departments of Clinical Genomics and Neurology, Mayo Clinic, Rochester, Minnesota; Associate Professor of Medical Genetics and of Neurology, Mayo Clinic College of Medicine and Science

Marie F. Grill, MD
Consultant, Department of Neurology, Mayo Clinic Hospital, Phoenix, Arizona; Assistant Professor of Neurology, Mayo Clinic College of Medicine and Science

Yong Guo, MD, PhD
Research Associate, Department of Neurology, Mayo Clinic, Rochester, Minnesota

Julie E. Hammack, MD
Consultant, Department of Neurology, Mayo Clinic, Jacksonville, Florida; Associate Professor of Neurology, Mayo Clinic College of Medicine and Science

Josephe Archie Honorat, MD, PhD
Research Fellow in Neurology, Mayo Clinic School of Graduate Medical Education, Mayo Clinic College of Medicine and Science, Rochester, Minnesota; now with SUNY Downstate Health Sciences University, Brooklyn, New York

Jiraporn Jitprapaikulsan, MD
Research Collaborator, Mayo Clinic School of Graduate Medical Education, Mayo Clinic College of Medicine and Science, Rochester, Minnesota; now with Siriraj Hospital, Bangkok Noi, Thailand

Alicja Kalinowska-Lyszczarz, MD, PhD
Research Collaborator in Neurology, Mayo Clinic School of Graduate Medical Education, Mayo Clinic College of Medicine and Science, Rochester, Minnesota

Orhun H. Kantarci, MD
Consultant, Department of Neurology, Mayo Clinic, Rochester, Minnesota; Professor of Neurology, Mayo Clinic College of Medicine and Science

Roman Kassa, MD, PhD
Fellow in Neurology, Mayo Clinic School of Graduate Medical Education, Mayo Clinic College of Medicine and Science, Rochester, Minnesota; now with University of Cincinnati College of Medicine, Cincinnati, Ohio

B. Mark Keegan, MD
Chair, Division of Multiple Sclerosis & Autoimmune Neurology, Mayo Clinic, Rochester, Minnesota; Professor of Neurology, Mayo Clinic College of Medicine and Science

James P. Klaas, MD
Consultant, Department of Neurology, Mayo Clinic, Rochester, Minnesota; Assistant Professor of Neurology, Mayo Clinic College of Medicine and Science

Christopher J. Klein, MD
Consultant, Department of Neurology, Mayo Clinic, Rochester, Minnesota; Professor of Neurology, Mayo Clinic College of Medicine and Science

Neeraj Kumar, MD
Consultant, Department of Neurology, Mayo Clinic, Rochester, Minnesota; Professor of Neurology, Mayo Clinic College of Medicine and Science

Amy C. Kunchok, MBBS
Research Collaborator, Mayo Clinic School of Graduate Medical Education and Assistant Professor of Neurology, Mayo Clinic College of Medicine and Science, Rochester, Minnesota

Vanda A. Lennon, MD, PhD
Consultant, Department of Laboratory Medicine & Pathology, Mayo Clinic, Rochester, Minnesota; Professor of Immunology and of Neurology, Mayo Clinic College of Medicine and Science

Teerin Liewluck, MD
Consultant, Department of Neurology, Mayo Clinic, Rochester, Minnesota; Associate Professor of Neurology, Mayo Clinic College of Medicine and Science

A. Sebastian Lopez Chiriboga, MD
Senior Associate Consultant, Department of Neurology, Mayo Clinic, Jacksonville, Florida; Assistant Professor of Neurology, Mayo Clinic College of Medicine and Science, Jacksonville, Florida

Claudia F. Lucchinetti, MD
Chair, Department of Neurology, Mayo Clinic, Rochester, Minnesota; Professor of Neurology, Mayo Clinic College of Medicine and Science

I. Vanessa Marin Collazo, MD
Consultant, Department of Neurology, Mayo Clinic, Jacksonville, Florida; Instructor in Neurology, Mayo Clinic College of Medicine and Science

Sara Mariotto, MD
Department of Neuroscience, Biomedicine, and Movement Sciences, University of Verona, Verona, Italy

Fulvia Mazzaferri, MD, PhD
Infectious Diseases Section, Department of Diagnostic and Public Health, University of Verona, Verona, Italy

Stuart J. McCarter, MD
Fellow in Neurology, Mayo Clinic School of Graduate Medical Education and Instructor in Neurology, Mayo Clinic College of Medicine and Science, Rochester, Minnesota

Andrew McKeon, MB, BCh, MD
Consultant, Departments of Laboratory Medicine & Pathology, and Neurology, Mayo Clinic, Rochester, Minnesota; Professor of Laboratory Medicine & Pathology and of Neurology, Mayo Clinic College of Medicine and Science

John R. Mills, PhD
Consultant, Department of Laboratory Medicine & Pathology, Mayo Clinic, Rochester, Minnesota; Assistant Professor of Laboratory Medicine & Pathology, Mayo Clinic College of Medicine and Science

Margherita Milone, MD, PhD
Consultant, Department of Neurology, Mayo Clinic, Rochester, Minnesota; Professor of Neurology, Mayo Clinic College of Medicine and Science

Bhavya Narapureddy, MBBS
Research Assistant, Department of Neurology, Mayo Clinic, Rochester, Minnesota; now with Upstate Medical University, Syracuse, New York

Marcus V. R. Pinto, MD, MS
Fellow in Neurology, Mayo Clinic School of Graduate Medical Education and Assistant Professor of Neurology, Mayo Clinic College of Medicine and Science, Rochester, Minnesota

Sean J. Pittock, MD
Consultant, Department of Neurology, Mayo Clinic, Rochester, Minnesota; Professor of Neurology, Mayo Clinic College of Medicine and Science

Michael W. Ruff, MD
Senior Associate Consultant, Department of Neurology, Mayo Clinic, Rochester, Minnesota; Assistant Professor of Neurology, Mayo Clinic College of Medicine and Science

Ruba S. Saadeh
Clinical Research Assistant, Department of Neurology, Mayo Clinic, Rochester, Minnesota

Catalina Sanchez Alvarez, MD
Fellow in Rheumatology, Mayo Clinic School of Graduate Medical Education, Mayo Clinic College of Medicine and Science, Jacksonville, Florida; now with University of Florida Health, Gainesville, Florida

Elia Sechi, MD
Senior Research Fellow in Neurology, Mayo Clinic School of Graduate Medical Education and Assistant Professor of Neurology, Mayo Clinic College of Medicine and Science, Rochester, Minnesota; now with the University of Sassari, Sassari, Italy

Shailee S. Shah, MD
Fellow in Neurology, Mayo Clinic School of Graduate Medical Education, Mayo Clinic College of Medicine and Science, Rochester, Minnesota

Shahar Shelly, MD
Fellow in Neurology, Mayo Clinic School of Graduate Medical Education, Mayo Clinic College of Medicine and Science, Rochester, Minnesota

Kamal Shouman, MD
Senior Associate Consultant, Department of Neurology, Mayo Clinic, Rochester, Minnesota; Assistant Professor of Neurology, Mayo Clinic College of Medicine and Science

Erik K. St. Louis, MD, MS
Chair, Division of Sleep Neurology and Consultant, Division of Pulmonary and Critical Care Medicine, Mayo Clinic, Rochester, Minnesota; Associate Professor of Neurology, Mayo Clinic College of Medicine and Science

Jerry W. Swanson, MD, MHPE
Consultant, Department of Neurology, Mayo Clinic, Rochester, Minnesota; Professor of Neurology, Mayo Clinic College of Medicine and Science

W. Oliver Tobin, MB, BCh, BAO, PhD
Consultant, Department of Neurology, Mayo Clinic, Rochester, Minnesota; Associate Professor of Neurology, Mayo Clinic College of Medicine and Science

Michel Toledano, MD
Consultant, Department of Neurology, Mayo Clinic, Rochester, Minnesota; Assistant Professor of Neurology, Mayo Clinic College of Medicine and Science

Jennifer A. Tracy, MD
Consultant, Department of Neurology, Mayo Clinic, Rochester, Minnesota; Assistant Professor of Neurology, Mayo Clinic College of Medicine and Science

Cristina Valencia-Sanchez, MD, PhD
Resident in Neurology, Mayo Clinic School of Graduate
Medical Education, Mayo Clinic College of Medicine and
Science, Rochester, Minnesota

Rocio Vazquez Do Campo, MD
Fellow in Neurology, Mayo Clinic School of Graduate
Medical Education, Mayo Clinic College of Medicine and
Science, Rochester, Minnesota; now with UAB Medicine,
Birmingham, Alabama

Kenneth J. Warrington, MD
Chair, Division of Rheumatology, Mayo Clinic, Rochester,
Minnesota; Professor of Medicine, Mayo Clinic College of
Medicine and Science

Lauren M. Webb
Medical Student, Mayo Clinic Alix School of Medicine,
Mayo Clinic College of Medicine and Science, Rochester,
Minnesota

Brian G. Weinshenker, MD
Consultant, Department of Neurology, Mayo Clinic,
Rochester, Minnesota; Professor of Neurology, Mayo Clinic
College of Medicine and Science

Maria Alice V. Willrich, PhD
Consultant, Department of Laboratory Medicine &
Pathology, Mayo Clinic, Rochester, Minnesota; Associate
Professor of Laboratory Medicine & Pathology, Mayo Clinic
College of Medicine and Science

Dean M. Wingerchuk, MD
Chair, Department of Neurology, Mayo Clinic, Scottsdale,
Arizona; Professor of Neurology, Mayo Clinic College of
Medicine and Science

Nicholas L. Zalewski, MD
Senior Associate Consultant, Department of Neurology,
Mayo Clinic, Scottsdale, Arizona; Assistant Professor of
Neurology, Mayo Clinic College of Medicine and Science

Anastasia Zekeridou, MD, PhD
Associate Consultant, Departments of Laboratory Medicine
& Pathology and Neurology, Mayo Clinic, Rochester,
Minnesota; Assistant Professor of Laboratory Medicine
& Pathology and of Neurology, Mayo Clinic College of
Medicine and Science

Burcu Zeydan, MD
Associate Consultant, Department of Radiology, Mayo
Clinic, Rochester, Minnesota; Assistant Professor of
Neurology and of Radiology, Mayo Clinic College of
Medicine and Science

Cecilia Zivelonghi, MD
Research Fellow in Neuroimmunology, Mayo Clinic School
of Graduate Medical Education, Mayo Clinic College of
Medicine and Science, Rochester, Minnesota; now with
University of Verona, Verona, Italy

SECTION I

CNS DEMYELINATING DISEASE

1

A WOMAN WITH SUBACUTE PAINFUL VISION LOSS

Jiraporn Jitprapaikulsan, MD, M. Tariq Bhatti, MD, Eric R. Eggenberger, DO,

Marie D. Acierno, MD, and John J. Chen, MD, PhD

CASE PRESENTATION

HISTORY AND EXAMINATION

A 51-year-old White woman sought care for vision loss 1 week after a nonspecific upper respiratory tract infection. She reported pain in both eyes exacerbated by eye movement, which lasted for several days, followed by bilateral vision loss to the level of counting fingers–only vision. Optic neuritis (ON) was diagnosed, and she was treated with 1 g intravenous methylprednisolone (IVMP) for 3 days. Her vision improved substantially, and the pain resolved during the corticosteroid treatment. However, 1 week later, she woke up with right eye pain and vision loss. She was again treated with 5 days of IVMP, with vision improvement nearly back to baseline. Two weeks later, she had recurrence of painful vision loss in both eyes. Visual acuity was hand motion in the right eye and 20/50 in the left eye, with a right relative afferent pupillary defect. Fundus photography showed bilateral optic disc edema (Figure 1.1A). Optical coherence tomography showed bilateral retinal nerve fiber layer thickening (Figure 1.1B). Extraocular eye movements were intact. Neurologic examination findings were normal. Possible causes of ON are compared in Table 1.1. A diagnosis of chronic relapsing inflammatory optic neuropathy (CRION) was made.

TESTING

Orbital magnetic resonance imaging (MRI) performed as part of her workup showed bilateral (right greater than left) optic nerve and perineural enhancement (Figures 1.1C and 1.1D). Findings of MRI of the brain and cervical and thoracic spine were unremarkable. Cerebrospinal fluid analysis showed 2 white blood cells/μL (87% lymphocytes); protein, 31 mg/dL; glucose, 63 mg/dL; no oligoclonal bands; normal immunoglobulin G (IgG) index; and negative paraneoplastic panel.

Tests for serum angiotensin-converting enzyme, antineutrophil cytoplasmic antibody, antinuclear antibody, Lyme disease, syphilis, tuberculosis, and aquaporin-4 (AQP4)-IgG antibodies were negative. Serum was definitively positive for myelin oligodendrocyte glycoprotein (MOG)-IgG antibodies at a titer of 1:1,000.

DIAGNOSIS

MOG-IgG–associated recurrent ON was diagnosed.

MANAGEMENT

After her diagnosis of recurrent corticosteroid-dependent ON associated with MOG-IgG positivity, the patient was treated with 5 days of IVMP. The eye pain resolved, and her vision returned to normal. Oral prednisone at a dosage of 50 mg/d and azathioprine 100 mg/d (divided dose) were started after infusion. The azathioprine dosage was increased to 150 mg/d (divided dose) after 1 week, and the prednisone dosage was gradually tapered over 6 months. At follow-up evaluation, the patient's visual acuity, color vision, and visual fields were normal in both eyes, but there was mild bilateral optic disc pallor. She has not had recurrent demyelinating episodes while on chronic immunotherapy.

DISCUSSION

ON is an inflammatory demyelination of the optic nerve manifesting as acute to subacute vision loss, classically associated with pain with eye movement. The nadir of visual impairment typically occurs within 1 week of onset. ON symptoms range from mild dyschromatopsia to no light perception. Physical examination typically reveals a relative afferent pupillary defect. Optic disc edema is present in one-third of patients. Treatment of typical acute ON consists of IVMP 1 g/d for 3 to 5 days, possibly with a short oral prednisone taper. Plasma exchange can be used in severe corticosteroid-refractory cases. The long-term prevention and prognosis depend on the cause of the ON.

The most common causes of ON in the developed world are idiopathic and multiple sclerosis (MS). Recently, serologic markers have been identified for ON and inflammatory central nervous system disorders such as neuromyelitis optica

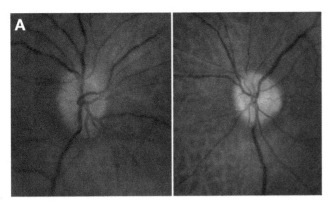

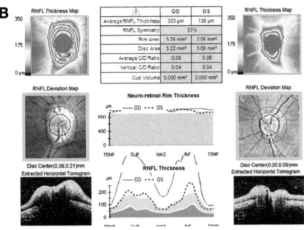

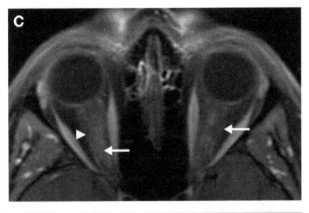

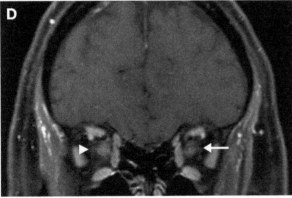

Figure 1.1 Imaging Findings for Case Patient.
A, Fundus photography shows bilateral optic disc edema. B, Optical coherence tomography indicates a peripapillary retinal nerve fiber layer thickness of 333 μm in the right eye and 136 μm in the left eye. C and D, Magnetic resonance imaging of the orbit in the axial (C) and coronal planes (D) shows bilateral optic nerve enhancement (white arrows) with extension to the optic nerve sheath and periorbital fat (arrowheads). C/D indicates cup-disc; RNFL, retinal nerve fiber layer.

spectrum disorders (NMOSD) and MOG-IgG–associated disorders. ON associated with MS (MS-ON), AQP4-IgG (AQP4-ON), and MOG-IgG (MOG-ON) are compared in Table 1.2. ON is the initial presentation of disease in one-fourth of patients with MS and occurs in up to three-fourths of patients during the disease course. The vision loss at nadir is often milder for MS-ON than MOG-ON and AQP4-ON. MRI of the orbits typically shows short segments of optic nerve enhancement. Cerebrospinal fluid oligoclonal bands and MS-like brain lesions on MRI are helpful for establishing the diagnosis of MS-ON. After an episode of ON, 50% of patients will have development of MS within 15 years—25% if no MS-like lesions are present on baseline brain MRI and 72% if MS-like lesions are present. Numerous disease-modifying therapies are available for MS. Overall, MS-ON is usually associated with a good visual outcome, with 92% of patients achieving 20/40 acuity or better.

The antibody responsible for NMOSD, AQP4-IgG, was discovered in 2004; this has not only improved diagnosis but also revolutionized our understanding of NMOSD. The phenotype of NMOSD has expanded beyond ON and transverse myelitis and now includes other demyelinating manifestations, such as area postrema syndrome (hiccups, nausea, or vomiting), acute brainstem syndrome, symptomatic narcolepsy or acute diencephalic clinical syndrome, and symptomatic cerebral syndrome with NMOSD-typical brain lesions. Patients with AQP4-ON typically have more severe vision loss than do patients with MS-ON. Orbital MRI typically shows a long segment of optic nerve enhancement that more often involves the optic chiasm than other forms of ON. AQP4-IgG positivity is associated with a high risk of relapse and poor visual outcomes, with a median visual acuity outcome of counting fingers. Because of the severity of episodes and poor recovery, early plasma exchange should be used for AQP4-ON in addition to corticosteroid therapy. All patients should also receive chronic immunotherapy. Rituximab, mycophenolate mofetil, and azathioprine have been used off-label to prevent symptomatic episodes in NMOSD. Eculizumab, satralizumab, and inebilizumab are US Food and Drug Administration–approved treatments for NMOSD.

This case highlights a classic presentation of MOG-ON, the newest biomarker of ON. The phenotype for MOG-IgG–associated disorder is diverse, but patients often have severe ON, which is corticosteroid responsive and often has a favorable outcome. Optic disc edema is present in up to 86% of patients, and up to 50% of cases can be bilateral. Patients with MOG-IgG–associated disorder can also have concurrent transverse myelitis and meet the criteria for seronegative NMOSD, or they can have development of brain lesions on MRI and encephalopathy consistent with acute disseminated encephalomyelitis. MOG-IgG is positive in 25% to 50% of cases that were previously designated *idiopathic CRION*. MRI of the orbits typically shows gadolinium enhancement involving more than half the optic nerve. Perineural enhancement is observed in half of patients with MOG-ON, which is a fairly specific sign of the disease. Recurrent demyelinating symptoms from

Table 1.1 | CAUSES OF OPTIC NEURITIS AND DIAGNOSTIC CLUES

CAUSE	CLUES
Multiple sclerosis–associated ON	Not corticosteroid dependent
	Commonly, abnormal brain and/or spinal cord MRI findings
AQP4-IgG–positive ON	Not corticosteroid dependent
	Often poor vision recovery
	Optic disc edema uncommon
Optic neuropathy associated with systemic inflammatory disease or infection	Systemic symptoms often present
	Typically, abnormal imaging or laboratory findings, such as abnormal chest CT for sarcoidosis
Idiopathic intracranial hypertension	Absence of optic nerve enhancement on MRI
	Presence of headache and other increased ICP features, but not eye pain
	Unlikely to cause profound vision loss unless severe or chronic papilledema
Leber hereditary optic neuropathy	Pseudo-optic disc edema
	Painless
	Rarely causes optic nerve enhancement on MRI
	Usually affects young males
	Not corticosteroid responsive or dependent

Abbreviations: AQP4-IgG, aquaporin-4–immunoglobulin G; CT, computed tomography; ICP, intracranial pressure; MRI, magnetic resonance imaging; ON, optic neuritis.

MOG-IgG–associated disorder tend to be ON rather than other central nervous system symptoms. The average visual acuity at nadir of MOG-ON is counting fingers, similar to AQP4-ON, but MOG-ON typically is associated with better recovery and, thus, better visual outcomes. After a MOG-ON episode, slow tapering of corticosteroids is recommended because many cases will demonstrate corticosteroid dependence. Chronic immunotherapy is recommended for relapsing disease, especially if permanent deficits are present. Off-label maintenance therapies include azathioprine, mycophenolate mofetil, rituximab, and intravenous immunoglobulin.

Table 1.2 | COMPARISON OF AQP4-ON, MOG-ON, AND MS-ON

CHARACTERISTIC	AQP4-ON	MOG-ON	MS-ON
Typical age of onset	40s	30s	20s
Sex distribution	Female>>Male	Female≈Male	Female>Male
Pain	++	+++	+++
Bilateral simultaneous ON	++	++	+
Visual acuity defect at nadir	Severe	Severe	Less severe
Risk of recurrent ON	+++	+++	++
CRION	Rare	++	Rare
Other symptoms/findings			
ADEM	Rare	++	Rare
Brainstem effects	+	++	+
Diencephalic symptoms	++	Rare	Rare
LETM	+++	++	Rare
Conus medullaris	+	+++	+
Other autoimmune conditions	+++	+	+
MRI optic nerve lesions	Long and posterior	Long and anterior	Typically short
MRI perineural enhancement	Rare	Common	Rare
Optic chiasm involvement	+++	+	Rare
Lesions on brain MRI	+	+	MS-like lesions
CSF OCB	Rare	Rare	+++
Rapid recovery	Rare	++	+
Spontaneous recovery	Rare	++	++
Corticosteroid dependent	Rare	++	Rare
Visual outcome	Poor	Good	Good

Abbreviations: +, infrequent; ++, frequent; +++, very frequent; ADEM, acute disseminated encephalomyelitis; AQP4-ON; aquaporin-4-IgG–positive ON; CRION, chronic relapsing inflammatory optic neuropathy; CSF, cerebrospinal fluid; IgG, immunoglobulin G; LETM, longitudinally extensive transverse myelitis; MOG-ON, myelin oligodendrocyte glycoprotein-IgG–positive ON; MRI, magnetic resonance imaging; MS-ON, multiple sclerosis–associated ON; OCB, oligoclonal bands; ON, optic neuritis.

KEY POINTS

- ON is an inflammatory condition of various causes, including MS, AQP4-IgG, and MOG-IgG.

- Serologic and radiologic tests are helpful for establishing the diagnosis.

- MOG-IgG–associated disorders can present with severe bilateral painful ON, which is corticosteroid responsive and has a favorable outcome compared with AQP4-IgG.

- High-dose corticosteroids are the mainstay of treatment of most episodes of ON. Plasma exchange is recommended for AQP4-ON and can be considered in cases of severe ON with poor recovery despite corticosteroid treatment.

- The type of long-term preventive medications used depends on the cause of ON.

RAPIDLY PROGRESSIVE NUMBNESS AND WEAKNESS AFTER SOFT-TISSUE ABSCESS

Elia Sechi, MD, and Dean M. Wingerchuk, MD

CASE PRESENTATION

HISTORY AND EXAMINATION

A previously healthy 45-year-old man had development of neck pain and swelling, followed 1 week later by fevers, chills, and night sweats. Cervical computed tomography showed a left-sided cervical soft-tissue abscess. The patient was initially treated with oral cephalexin for 10 days, without benefit. Fine-needle aspiration biopsy of the mass showed granulomatous inflammation and a heterogeneous lymphocyte population without evidence of malignancy. Cultures grew *Bordetella hinzii*, and his antibiotics were switched to amoxicillin/clavulanate and azithromycin. Follow-up aspiration and culture 2 weeks later again showed *Bordetella* species and pan-sensitive, coagulase-negative staphylococci. Meropenem and gentamicin were started. Ten days later, he had development of acute urinary retention requiring catheterization, numbness and weakness in the lower extremities, and numbness in the upper extremities. At symptom nadir 2 days later, he required the aid of a walker to ambulate. Lhermitte sign and erectile dysfunction were also present. The patient was admitted to the hospital.

TESTING

Spinal cord magnetic resonance imaging (MRI) showed a longitudinally extensive, nonenhancing, T2-hyperintense lesion predominantly affecting the ventral and lateral parenchyma of the cervical and thoracic spinal cord (Figure 2.1A, B, E, and F). Findings of brain MRI were unremarkable. Cerebrospinal fluid (CSF) examination showed a white blood cell count of 581 cells/µL (reference range, <5 cells/µL) with 42% neutrophils, 35% lymphocytes, and 22% monocytes, increased protein concentration (109 mg/dL; reference range, <45 mg/dL), and normal glucose concentration. No CSF-specific oligoclonal bands were detected, and the immunoglobulin G (IgG) index was normal. Extensive CSF investigations for infection were negative. Results of serum testing for aquaporin-4 (AQP4)-IgG antibodies, myelin

oligodendrocyte glycoprotein (MOG)-IgG antibodies, comprehensive autoimmune serologic studies, and paraneoplastic antibody panel were negative.

DIAGNOSIS

A diagnosis of postinfectious idiopathic transverse myelitis (ITM) was made.

MANAGEMENT

The patient was treated with intravenous (IV) immunoglobulin, IV methylprednisolone (500 mg/d for 5 days), and broad-spectrum antibiotics, with improvement of both the abscess and his neurologic symptoms. After discharge, he was able to walk unassisted. At follow-up evaluation 6 months after the initial evaluation, neurologic examination showed only mild weakness of the left iliopsoas muscle and brisk reflexes in the lower extremities. Repeated spinal cord MRI showed marked improvement of the previously identified abnormalities (Figure 2.1C, D, G, and H). Findings of whole-body ^{18}F-fludeoxyglucose–positron emission tomography (FDG-PET), performed to exclude subclinical inflammatory activity, were unremarkable.

DISCUSSION

Acute transverse myelopathies are a heterogeneous group of spinal cord disorders characterized by acute or subacute signs and symptoms of spinal cord dysfunction, typically a combination of sensory, motor, and autonomic manifestations. Underlying causes include vascular (eg, spinal cord infarction), infectious (eg, syphilis), neoplastic, postirradiation, traumatic, and inherited/metabolic (eg, vitamin B_{12} deficiency), and inflammatory processes.

Inflammatory myelopathies (myelitis) may affect any age or sex, although young women (aged 20-50 years) are overall more commonly affected. Multiple sclerosis (MS) is the most common cause of myelitis and generally manifests with short myelitis lesions (≤3 contiguous vertebral segments) on

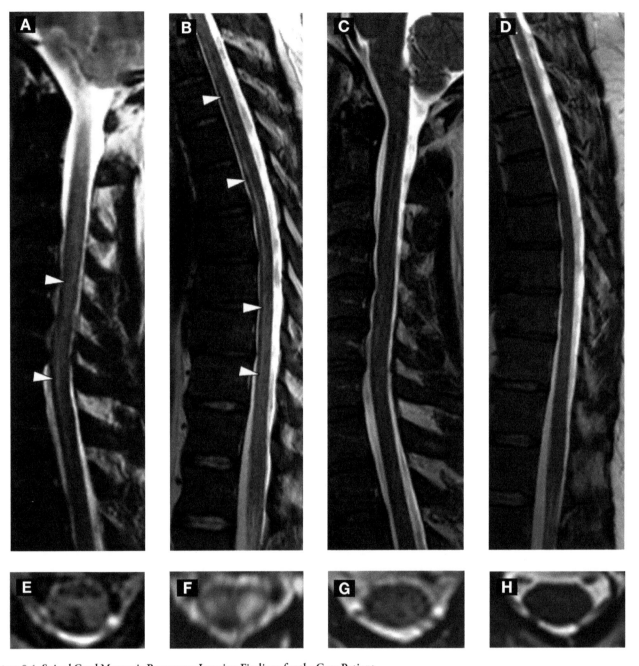

Figure 2.1 Spinal Cord Magnetic Resonance Imaging Findings for the Case Patient.
Sagittal (A-D) and axial (E-H) images. A,B,E,F, Acute T2-weighted sequences show a longitudinally extensive lesion (arrowheads), predominantly involving the ventrolateral regions of the cervical (A and E) and thoracic (B and F) spinal cord; the thoracic abnormalities are less clearly contiguous. This lesion did not demonstrate enhancement after gadolinium administration (not shown). C,D,G,H, At 6-month follow-up, images demonstrate nearly complete resolution of the cervical (C and G) and thoracic (D and H) cord abnormalities.

spinal cord MRI, which result in incomplete spinal cord dysfunction (*partial* transverse myelitis), and, rarely, paraplegia. Characteristic MS demyelinating lesions on brain MRI and CSF oligoclonal bands (approximately 90% of cases) are frequent accompaniments.

Other causes of myelitis include acute disseminated encephalomyelitis (typically accompanied by brain involvement), systemic inflammatory disorders (eg, sarcoidosis), and myelitis associated with specific central nervous system (CNS) autoantibodies. Among the latter, AQP4-IgG and MOG-IgG are typically associated with acute transverse

myelitis. In contrast with MS, both AQP4-IgG– and MOG-IgG–associated myelitis are generally longitudinally extensive (>3 contiguous vertebral segments), and CSF oligoclonal bands are usually not detected.

Predominant involvement of the ventral spinal cord parenchyma on MRI is also seen with anterior spinal artery–related cord infarction and some viral infections. In the case patient, however, extensive evaluation for infections was unrevealing, and the subacute presentation and marked CSF pleocytosis argued against cord infarction. Spinal cord sarcoidosis may also manifest with longitudinally extensive myelitis, but this is typically accompanied by dorsal subpial gadolinium enhancement on MRI, the clinical evolution is usually more gradual (weeks to months), and symptoms tend to recur after corticosteroid discontinuation. If neurosarcoidosis is suspected, whole-body FDG-PET (which was negative in this patient) may help identify occult foci of systemic inflammation to biopsy for diagnostic confirmation. The case patient also had no risk factors (eg, smoking history) for a paraneoplastic myelopathy, which is generally associated with symmetric involvement of the dorsal and/or lateral spinal cord column.

Despite extensive investigations, a substantial proportion of myelopathies are eventually labeled as *idiopathic*. The term ITM identifies a subgroup of acute transverse myelopathies of presumed inflammatory origin but for which a definite cause cannot be identified. Proposed diagnostic criteria aim to distinguish ITM from disease-associated myelopathies. According to these criteria, a definite ITM diagnosis requires 1) onset between 4 hours and 21 days (to distinguish from the hyperacute spinal cord infarction and more insidious inflammatory or metabolic myelopathies); 2) bilateral (although not necessarily symmetric) signs/symptoms of spinal cord dysfunction; 3) a clear sensory level on the trunk; 4) evidence suggestive of inflammation on MRI (eg, gadolinium enhancement of a spinal cord lesion) or in CSF (pleocytosis); and 5) exclusion of other candidate causes. The incidence and prevalence of ITM using these criteria are 8.6/1,000,000 and 7.9/100,000 person-years, respectively. However, these criteria are not 100% specific, and about 15% of patients initially diagnosed with ITM subsequently fulfill MS diagnostic criteria. Moreover, the clinical and MRI features of ITM are often heterogeneous (ranging from milder MS-like myelitis to severely disabling longitudinally extensive myelitis), suggesting different underlying causes.

ITM can be preceded by infections or vaccinations (postinfectious/postvaccination ITM). The infectious agent, often viral but sometimes bacterial, is thought to trigger an autoimmune CNS reaction in cases for which there is no evidence to support direct CNS infection. Although the mechanisms are not fully understood, it is postulated that antibodies targeting an antigen on the infecting agent or vaccine cross-react with a CNS antigen that has a similar conformation ("molecular mimicry"), which results in autoimmune CNS injury. However, infections may also trigger an acute clinical episode in a patient with an underlying disorder such as MS or who harbor AQP4-IgG or MOG-IgG antibodies; therefore, testing for these disorders is required even if there is a documented infection.

No clinical trials have established the optimal treatment strategies for ITM. A therapeutic trial with high-dose corticosteroids is usually initiated after diagnosis; rescue plasma exchange, IV immunoglobulin, and cyclophosphamide may also be used in severe or corticosteroid-refractory cases.

KEY POINTS

- Despite extensive investigations, a substantial proportion of acute inflammatory myelopathies remain idiopathic.

- Given the absence of specific biomarkers, ITM remains a diagnosis of exclusion. Gadolinium enhancement on spinal cord MRI or CSF pleocytosis supports an inflammatory cause but can be seen with other noninflammatory myelopathies.

- The clinical and MRI characteristics of ITM are heterogeneous and frequently overlap with those of other types of disease-associated myelitis (eg, MS myelitis, AQP4-IgG– and MOG-IgG–associated myelitis).

- Treatment with high-dose corticosteroids is standard; plasma exchange or IV immunoglobulin should be considered in severe or corticosteroid-refractory cases.

WEAKNESS WITH NECK FLEXION

Brian G. Weinshenker, MD

CASE PRESENTATION

HISTORY AND EXAMINATION

A 51-year-old woman sought care for difficulty "picking up" her right foot after walking for 30 minutes; with rest, the symptoms would subside. A few months later, she reported a "zinging" sensation in her right 4th and 5th fingers and down her right side with neck flexion. By the end of each day, she would have paresthesias of her feet, especially when exposed to heat. She had no symptoms referable to her bladder.

Her medical history was pertinent for type 2 diabetes that was treated with diet and oral agents, well-controlled hypertension, and long-standing asthma.

Examination showed mild bilateral finger extensor and interossei weakness, which increased substantially with neck flexion. Both legs were mildly spastic and had brisk deep tendon reflexes. The right plantar response was equivocal, whereas the left was flexor. Gait was normal, and she could walk heel-to-toe with minimal difficulty.

TESTING

Brain magnetic resonance imaging showed tiny nonspecific lesions not suggestive of demyelinating disease and a single T2 hyperintensity at the cervicomedullary junction that did not enhance with gadolinium administration (Figure 3.1). Cerebrospinal fluid analysis showed 10 oligoclonal bands on isoelectric focusing electrophoresis and a mildly increased immunoglobulin G index of 0.73. Electromyography was negative for indicators of chronic denervation or reinnervation.

The differential diagnosis for progressive myelopathy is extensive and beyond the scope of this description. However, the key items on the differential diagnosis in this case, especially considering her change in strength with neck flexion, are shown in Table 3.1.

Next, her change in finger strength during neck flexion was assessed with a device constructed to evaluate strength in this muscle group with a torque measurement cell. By this method, a 14% decrease in finger extension strength (averaged

over 4 trials) was observed during neck flexion compared with neck extension (Figure 3.2).

DIAGNOSIS

The patient was diagnosed with solitary sclerosis, an entity of still uncertain and unclassified nosology but suspected to be a form of central nervous system (CNS) demyelinating disease strongly related to multiple sclerosis (MS).

MANAGEMENT

Treatment was based on a diagnosis of "primary progressive MS," although the patient did not satisfy the criterion of dissemination in space. The patient was being treated with glatiramer acetate 40 mg 3 times weekly for a presumptive diagnosis of MS before evaluation at Mayo Clinic. After our evaluation, she was advised that no treatments at that time were efficacious to prevent deterioration in patients with primary progressive MS. Ocrelizumab has recently been approved for primary progressive MS and would have been discussed as a treatment option had it been approved for this indication at the time. However, the efficacy of ocrelizumab for this indication is relatively modest. The mainstay of treatment is physical medicine modalities, including principles of energy conservation and, when necessary, mobility aids, such as braces and canes.

DISCUSSION

The presentation of disease in this patient suggested a chronic myelopathy. Her symptoms did not develop acutely and manifested only after she walked a distance. Symptoms involving the upper and lower extremities and precipitation of Lhermitte sign with neck flexion also suggested a spinal cord lesion, typically a demyelinating lesion. However, a single spinal cord lesion present at the cervicomedullary junction, and lack of a history of prior events or other lesions in the spinal cord or brain that credibly supported evidence of "dissemination in space," precluded a convincing diagnosis of MS. Oligoclonal bands, however, are rarely detectable in

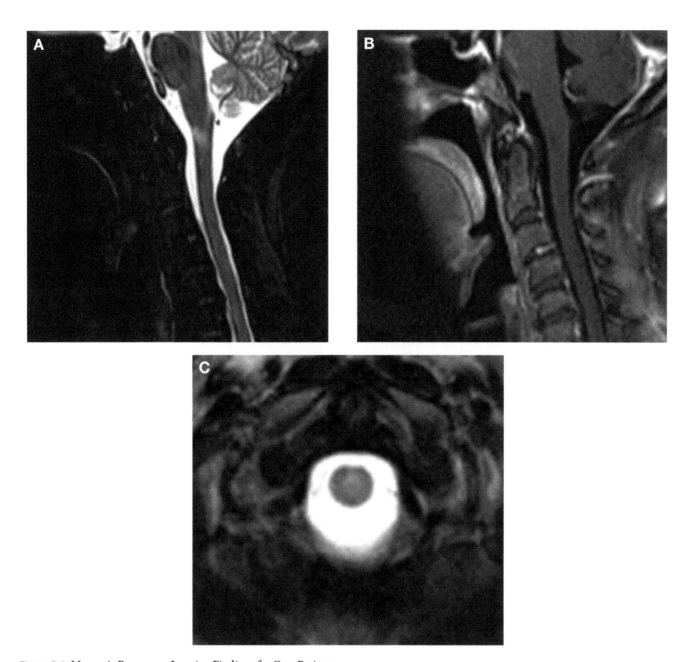

Figure 3.1 Magnetic Resonance Imaging Findings for Case Patient.
Images show sagittal short tau inversion recovery (A), sagittal T1 (B), and axial T2 sequences (C) at the level of the cervicomedullary junction. A focal area of T2 hyperintense, T1 hypointense, but nonenhancing signal abnormality is present in the ventral medulla, corresponding to the decussation of the medullary pyramids.

healthy persons. Occasionally, oligoclonal bands are detected in patients with CNS infections or paraneoplastic disorders that might be associated with myelopathy, such as HIV infection and tractopathies associated with amphiphysin or collapsin-response mediator protein 5 autoantibodies, which are in the differential diagnosis.

McArdle sign is a transient increase in upper motor neuron pattern weakness in patients with cervical cord demyelinating lesions. Dynamic weakness with neck flexion had been reported once before, in 1987, in a patient with advanced MS who was unable to walk down stairs with his neck flexed because this aggravated his impairment. Exaggerated weakness with neck flexion seems to be present in most patients

with MS who have myelopathy and is commonly present even in those without symptoms of myelopathy when demyelinating lesions are present in the spinal cord. Exaggerated weakness with neck flexion has even been detected in a patient with solitary sclerosis, as illustrated by this patient. McArdle sign, which is generally reliably evaluated at the bedside, may be a useful clinical clue to the cause of cryptogenic spinal cord lesions because of its high specificity for demyelinating disease. When the presence of this sign was evaluated quantitatively in a blinded study of patients at Mayo Clinic with various causes of myelopathy—including cord compression due to spondylosis, amyotrophic lateral sclerosis, or spinal cord tumors, among others—it was highly specific and

Table 3.1 | DIFFERENTIAL DIAGNOSIS OF PROGRESSIVE MYELOPATHY IN THE CASE PATIENT

POSSIBLE DIAGNOSIS	COMMENTS
MS	Lack of other symptoms suggesting remote events of demyelination and lack of convincing imaging changes on MRI of the head decreased but did not eliminate MS as a diagnostic possibility; patient did not satisfy MRI criteria for dissemination in space required for diagnosis of MS
Low-grade glioma	Oligoclonal bands in CSF would be unusual for glioma; lack of enhancement and mass effect are compatible
Amyotrophic lateral sclerosis/ primary lateral sclerosis	Lack of lower motor neuron or bulbar findings; negative EMG findings; spinal cord lesion credibly accounts for symptoms
Dynamic compression of the spinal cord	Symptoms typically worsen with extension of the spine when due to dynamic compression associated with cervical spondylosis; myelopathy may result from dynamic compression by tight posterior dural sac with neck flexion, the manifestations of which are nonprogressive atrophy of the arm, typically in a young person (Hirayama disease), features not seen in this patient

Abbreviations: CSF, cerebrospinal fluid; EMG, electromyography; MRI, magnetic resonance imaging; MS, multiple sclerosis.

moderately sensitive. With use of a cutoff determined by area under the receiver operating characteristic curve analysis, a 10% decrease in strength was entirely specific for a diagnosis of MS compared with cervical myelopathy of causes other than demyelinating disease.

Investigators at Mayo Clinic have proposed the term *solitary sclerosis* for progressive myelopathies associated with a single lesion suggestive of demyelinating disease. Solitary sclerosis lesions are often wedge-shaped, peripheral lesions typical of MS spinal cord lesions, often at the cervicomedullary junction. The pathologic basis of progression in those with progressive MS, which is usually dominated by symptoms of progressive myelopathy, is widely debated. Widespread pathologic findings in the CNS, which are underestimated by

conventional magnetic resonance imaging, are usually present in patients with progressive forms of MS; these findings include atrophy (especially of gray matter structures) and progressive decrease in neuronal markers (such as *N*-acetyl aspartate) on spectroscopy. Furthermore, progressive MS shows evidence of widespread cortical demyelination, which has also been correlated with progression and clinical features manifested by our patient. However, some clinicians believe that the presence of "critical" spinal cord lesions, manifested as focal cord atrophy, may actually determine the localization of symptoms and may be the key determinant of "progression," rather than brain lesions or diffuse CNS pathologic processes associated with MS, even though brain lesions and diffuse CNS pathologic findings may be present.

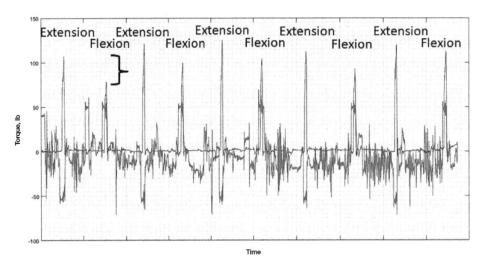

Figure 3.2 Measurement of McArdle Sign.
With a torque cell strength measurement device, the patient is tested with the neck alternately extended (downward deflection of the orange line) and flexed (upward deflection of the orange line) over approximately 15 minutes. The blue peaks represent force exerted by the patient against a bar which is used to flex the fingers at the metacarpophalangeal joint. The reduction in strength with neck flexion, highlighted by the bracket, is consistent, although variable in degree. This patient had an average of 14% reduction in strength with the neck flexed compared with extended, as averaged over the last 4 of 5 successive trials.

KEY POINTS

- Progressive myelopathy has a broad differential diagnosis.

- McArdle sign, a transient increase in upper motor neuron pattern weakness with neck flexion, best elicited in finger extensor muscles, is a helpful sign to confirm a suspected clinical diagnosis of demyelinating disease.

- Progressive myelopathy may be due to demyelinating disease, even in the presence of a single potentially causative lesion with appropriate imaging characteristics of a chronic demyelinating lesion (ie, solitary sclerosis). The key to diagnosis in this setting is the ability to correlate the symptoms and signs with the lesion. Solitary sclerosis lesions typically neither enhance with gadolinium nor progressively enlarge, unlike a tumor. An additional helpful clue is the frequent presence of oligoclonal bands.

NEW-ONSET RIGHT-SIDED NUMBNESS AND DOUBLE VISION

W. Oliver Tobin, MB, BCh, BAO, PhD

CASE PRESENTATION

HISTORY AND EXAMINATION

A 40-year-old right-handed man sought care for right hand numbness, right-sided facial numbness, and diplopia progressing to maximal severity over 10 days. At his worst he was unable to write. His symptoms remained maximal for 4 weeks. He was hospitalized and treated with 5 days of intravenous methylprednisolone. He improved to approximately 95% of normal over 4 weeks. He had residual mild right-sided facial and right leg numbness. His examination 6 months after symptom onset was normal.

TESTING

Complete blood cell count; kidney function; levels of liver enzymes, vitamin B$_{12}$, and folate; serologic tests for HIV, Lyme disease, and *Bartonella*; thyroid function; serum protein electrophoresis; and aquaporin-4 (AQP4)-immunoglobulin G (IgG) and myelin oligodendrocyte glycoprotein (MOG)-IgG antibodies were normal or negative. Antibodies to JC polyoma virus and varicella-zoster virus were positive, which indicated prior exposure to these viruses. Total 25-hydroxyvitamin D level was low at 8.2 ng/mL. Optical coherence tomography findings were normal. Magnetic resonance imaging (MRI) of the brain performed 3 months after the onset of symptoms demonstrated a T2-hyperintense lesion in the left midbrain peduncle extending into the upper pons, without gadolinium enhancement (Figure 4.1A and B). A small area of T2 hyperintensity was seen in the right frontal deep white matter. Follow-up brain MRI, performed 9 months after symptom onset, showed almost complete resolution of the left midbrain peduncle lesion with persistence of the right frontal deep white matter lesion (Figure 4.1C and D). MRI of the cervical and thoracic spine showed normal findings. Spinal fluid analysis showed 1 white blood cell/μL (reference range, 0-5/μL) with 95% lymphocytes,

protein 35 mg/dL (reference range, ≤35 mg/dL), 0 unique oligoclonal bands, and normal IgG index (0.54; reference range, ≤0.85).

DIAGNOSIS

A diagnosis of clinically isolated syndrome (CIS)–first episode of multiple sclerosis (MS) was made.

MANAGEMENT

After detailed discussion with the patient, he elected to commence disease-modifying therapy with fingolimod. He underwent routine monitoring with MRI of the brain and cervical and thoracic spine on an annual basis, without any further relapses at 5-year follow-up.

DISCUSSION

Patients with typical demyelinating syndromes—including optic neuritis, transverse myelitis, and internuclear ophthalmoplegia—may not always fulfill the diagnostic criteria for MS. After careful exclusion of other mimicking conditions, most notably AQP4-IgG– and MOG-IgG–associated disease, a diagnosis of CIS may be made.

The proportion of patients who fit into the CIS category has decreased with each iteration of the McDonald criteria for diagnosis of MS. Before the 2010 revisions, a history of multiple clinical episodes, or serial MRIs demonstrating new T2 lesions, were necessary to demonstrate dissemination in time. The 2010 revisions allowed for a diagnosis of MS to be made in the correct clinical scenario on the basis of a single MRI, when both enhancing and nonenhancing typical T2 lesions were seen. The most recent criteria (2017 revisions) allow for the presence of unique cerebrospinal fluid oligoclonal bands to be substituted for the presence of dissemination in time. The majority of patients included in the original trials of disease-modifying therapies in CIS would be classified as having MS if seen today.

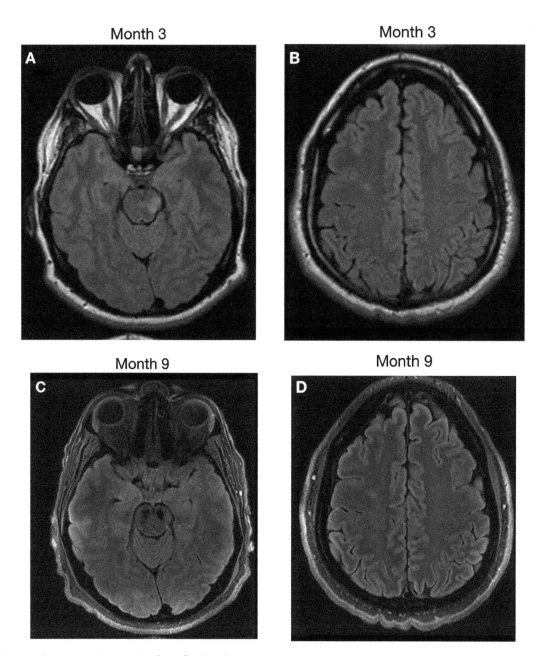

Figure 4.1 Magnetic Resonance Imaging Findings for Case Patient.
A and B, Fluid-attenuated inversion recovery brain images from 3 months after symptom onset demonstrate left-sided midbrain peduncle hyperintensity and a small, right, deep, white matter hyperintensity.
C and D, Follow-up imaging 9 months after symptom onset demonstrates almost complete resolution of the left midbrain peduncle lesion and persistence of the right frontal lesion, consistent with the typical evolution of a demyelinating event.

Nevertheless, early treatment of MS improves the overall outcome on a group basis. However, MS will develop in only 1 in 4 patients with optic neuritis as their only symptom of CIS over a 15-year follow-up. The diagnosis of CIS can be frustrating to patients, because it can sometimes imply that providers are unable to reach a diagnosis of MS. For this reason, we typically clarify the diagnosis of CIS as *clinically isolated syndrome–first episode of multiple sclerosis*.

Providers are recommended to discuss with patients the risks and benefits of commencing disease-modifying therapy, as opposed to serial MRI follow-up. If a conservative observational approach is used for a patient with CIS, early follow-up MRI is recommended. The purpose is to detect any development of highly active disease in the absence of disease-modifying therapy, which, if it occurs, typically does so within 6 to 8 months after the first MRI findings. Additional paraclinical testing such as optical coherence tomography or visual evoked potentials can be useful to identify other asymptomatic sites of demyelination, which may help in the decision-making process regarding disease-modifying therapy.

Finally, patients who have a single spinal episode, without unique oligoclonal bands in the cerebrospinal fluid, are typically diagnosed with CIS. These patients may have subsequent development of progressive neurologic dysfunction, consistent with secondary progressive MS, despite never fulfilling the diagnostic criteria for relapsing-remitting MS. Therefore, ongoing monitoring is recommended, just as in patients with a formal diagnosis of relapsing-remitting MS.

KEY POINTS

- CIS is essentially a first episode of MS.

- The definition of CIS has changed through each iteration of the MS diagnostic criteria.

- Exclusion of MS mimics, in particular AQP4-IgG– and MOG-IgG–associated diseases, is important to ensure correct treatment and monitoring.

PROGRESSIVE LEFT LOWER EXTREMITY WEAKNESS AND THORACIC SPINAL CORD LESION

B. Mark Keegan, MD

CASE PRESENTATION

HISTORY AND EXAMINATION

A 76-year-old man was seen for a neurologic evaluation with concerns of progressive left lower extremity weakness. He was well until age 39 years when it was noticed that he would drag his left lower extremity, with some limping. This progressively worsened over time, but very slowly. He was evaluated at age 40 years, at which time results of electromyography, brain computed tomography, and somatosensory evoked potentials were normal. He had progressive impairment and had to discontinue skiing at age 47 years. He was reevaluated at age 56 years and again 20 years later. He had 2 intervening lumbar spinal operations, the most recent being at age 68 years, and had a major motor vehicle accident with a pelvic fracture at age 67 years. He was documented to have new impairment in right ankle and distal lower extremity power after the operations and trauma. He began using a left-sided ankle-foot orthosis but used no other gait aid.

He had never had episodes of acute neurologic dysfunction with recovery. Specifically, he had no prior symptoms consistent with optic neuritis, painless binocular diplopia, Lhermitte sign, hemiparesis, hemisensory deficit, or prior symptoms of a sensory myelopathy with resolution. There was no family history of multiple sclerosis (MS). He had no other significant medical comorbid conditions.

On current neurologic examination, mental status and cranial nerve examination findings were normal, as was motor power in the face, neck, and bilateral upper extremities. He had moderate weakness of the left lower extremity in a pyramidal distribution, with mild right lower extremity lower motor neuron weakness of the tibialis anterior, foot inversion and eversion, and great toe extension. He had hyperreflexia on the left compared with the right, with an extensor plantar response on the left and a flexor plantar response on the right. Vibratory sense was moderately reduced at the toes bilaterally, but joint position sense and sensation in the hands were

intact. His gait indicated left lower extremity upper motor neuron–type impairment, right lower extremity lower motor neuron–type impairment, and difficulty getting up on his heels, left side greater than right side.

TESTING

Brain magnetic resonance imaging (MRI) revealed 2 prominent and stable T2-signal hyperintensities in the frontal cerebral white matter, with some periventricular T2 hyperintensity (Figure 5.1A) with associated T1 hypointensity, and no gadolinium-enhancing lesions or posterior fossa lesions. MRI findings of the cervical spine were normal. Sagittal and axial MRI of the thoracic spine showed an area of T2-signal abnormality without enhancement in the left hemicord at the T3 to T4 level (Figures 5.1B and 5.1C). The brain and spinal cord changes on MRI were identical to those observed on imaging from 7 years earlier and brain and cervical spine MRI changes from 20 years earlier. Cerebrospinal fluid was never examined. Optical coherence tomography findings were normal bilaterally. Nerve conduction studies and electromyography revealed a chronic right L5 radiculopathy without evidence of active denervation as the cause of the right lower motor neuron lower extremity weakness.

DIAGNOSIS

The possible diagnoses that were ruled out for this patient are shown in Table 5.1. He was diagnosed with progressive *paucisclerotic MS* with a primary progressive disease course.

MANAGEMENT

The use of ocrelizumab (anti-CD20) was considered initially. However, the exceedingly slow disease progression over many decades and the lack of new MRI lesions or gadolinium-enhancing lesions, as well as his age, were taken into consideration, and conservative rehabilitation management was recommended instead.

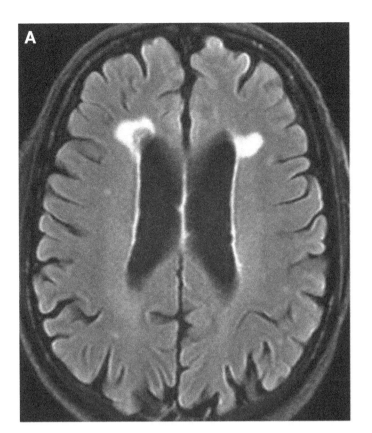

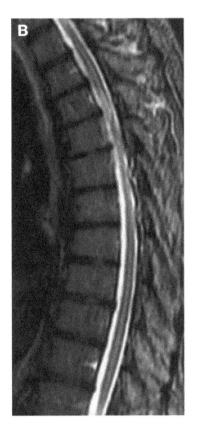

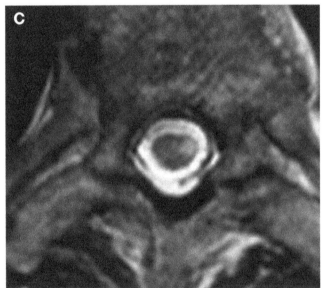

Figure 5.1 **Magnetic Resonance Imaging Sequences.**

A, Brain axial fluid-attenuated inversion recovery image shows limited demyelinating disease burden, with tandem nonenhancing lesions in left and right hemispheric white matter. B and C, Sagittal (B) and axial (C) thoracic spine images show the critical demyelinating lesion responsible for the patient's progressive left lower extremity weakness.

DISCUSSION

It is being increasingly recognized that the location of demyelinating disease lesions may be of crucial importance in the development of motor progression in MS. This is perhaps best evidenced by patients with progressive solitary sclerosis who have only 1 recognized demyelinating lesion within the central nervous system (CNS) and have progressive motor impairment that is directly anatomically attributable to that lesion location. Furthermore, some patients reportedly have exceedingly restricted CNS disease burden (as evidenced on MRI) but have motor progression that is still anatomically attributable to that particular lesion. These *critical demyelinating lesions* are also observed in patients with progressive unilateral hemiparetic impairment due to MS, in which unlimited lesion burden is allowable.

Table 5.1 OTHER DIAGNOSES CONSIDERED AND RULED OUT

DIAGNOSIS	PERTINENT NEGATIVES
Idiopathic transverse myelitis	Time to nadir of neurologic symptoms in transverse myelitis is within 20 days. It is not associated with progressive motor impairment
Nutritional myelopathy	Subacute combined degeneration of the cord is associated with bilateral and relatively symmetrical impairment
Spinal cord neoplasm	Neoplastic causes are associated with increasing mass effect and, often, gadolinium enhancement on MRI
Relapsing-remitting MS	There is no history to suggest any prior relapse with resolution, and progressive motor impairment is only associated with progressive forms of MS (primary progressive and secondary progressive MS)

Abbreviations: MRI, magnetic resonance imaging; MS, multiple sclerosis.

The patient in this case had insidiously progressive left lower extremity weakness that was entirely attributable to the left corticospinal tract lesion. He had no impairment due to CNS disease of the upper extremities or the right lower extremity, where the deficit was clearly related to the old lumbar radiculopathy that was lower motor neuron in nature, traumatic, and postsurgical related.

KEY POINTS

• Motor progression in some patients with highly restricted lesion burden (ie, ≤5 total CNS demyelinating lesions) on MRI (progressive pauciclerotic MS) is attributable to a critical demyelinating lesion, often in the spinal cord along corticospinal tracts.

• Most patients with progressive pauciclerotic MS have progressive motor impairment from onset (primary progressive disease), but some have progressive motor impairment after 1 or more clinical relapses with improvement (secondary progressive disease).

• Disease-modifying therapy for MS is of uncertain benefit in progressive pauciclerotic MS given the limited evidence of inflammation (ie, clinical relapses and highly restricted MRI lesion burden), which is the suspected main target of current disease-modifying therapy in MS.

PROGRESSIVE SPASTICITY WITH A SINGLE MAGNETIC RESONANCE IMAGING LESION

Samantha A. Banks, MD, and Eoin P. Flanagan, MB, BCh

CASE PRESENTATION

HISTORY AND EXAMINATION

A 59-year-old White man with a history of excised basal and squamous cell skin cancers was evaluated for gait difficulties. He reported walking troubles for the preceding 3 years. His ambulation worsened such that he was no longer able to work and had to retire 2 years previously. He had erectile dysfunction but no bowel or bladder dysfunction. He also reported fatigue. He began using a cane for ambulation 2 weeks before evaluation at our facility. He had been seen at an outside facility, but no diagnosis was forthcoming. He had been treated with empiric trials of high-dose intravenous methylprednisolone and intravenous immunoglobulin without benefit. He was also treated with baclofen and dalfampridine without benefit. His medications included vitamin D and sildenafil. He was a lifelong nonsmoker and had no family history of multiple sclerosis (MS). Neurologic examination at the time of our evaluation 3 years after onset was notable for a positive Hoffman sign on the right and mild weakness of the right triceps but preserved strength elsewhere. He had a spastic gait with moderate spasticity in both lower extremities, hyperreflexic patellar and ankle jerks bilaterally, and bilateral positive Babinski sign. The remainder of the examination was essentially normal.

TESTING

Magnetic resonance imaging (MRI) of the brain showed a single lesion at the cervicomedullary junction (Figure 6.1A) and medullary pyramids, more prominent on the right. There was also some accompanying atrophy that was also visible on cervical spine MRI (Figure 6.1B), without accompanying gadolinium enhancement. Results of cerebrospinal fluid analysis showed a normal white blood cell count, increased protein concentration (108 mg/dL; reference range, 0-35 mg/dL), and positive oligoclonal bands. Extensive laboratory evaluations for alternative causes of his symptoms, including tests for human T-lymphotropic virus

type 1, HIV, paraneoplastic autoantibodies, and levels of folate, vitamin B_{12}, methylmalonic acid, copper, and vitamin E were unrevealing.

DIAGNOSIS

The progressive nature of his symptoms, spinal fluid results, and lesion appearance were all consistent with a diagnosis of progressive solitary sclerosis.

MANAGEMENT

At the time this patient was seen, no immunomodulatory medications for progressive solitary sclerosis were approved, so no immunomodulatory medication was tried. Ongoing symptomatic management was recommended.

DISCUSSION

Progressive solitary sclerosis is a rare variant of MS in which patients have a single central nervous system demyelinating lesion and development of motor progression attributable to that lesion. Patients can initially have a clinical episode followed by progression or can have a progressive course without an initial relapse. The single lesion generally prevents these patients from fulfilling MS criteria because they lack dissemination in space. This often leads to difficulties in obtaining a diagnosis (such as in this case), and some have suggested that this variant of MS be incorporated into future MS diagnostic criteria.

Progressive motor impairment attributable to a characteristic MS-appearing lesion on MRI and the presence of oligoclonal bands or a positive family history of MS (although not occurring in this case) are clues to this disorder. The lesions are typically found along eloquent regions of the corticospinal tracts with 2 major locations accounting for the vast majority of lesions: 1) the medullary pyramids/anterior cervicomedullary junction, usually resulting in a progressive quadriparesis; and 2) the spinal cord lateral columns, usually resulting in a progressive face-sparing hemiparesis. The lesions

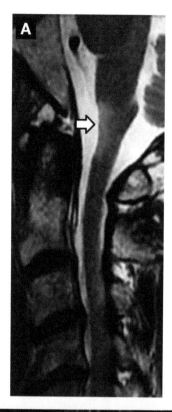

typically become focally atrophic over time, which helps distinguish them from neoplastic lesions that expand over time. The spinal cord T2-hyperintense lesions are short, extending less than 3 vertebral segments on sagittal images, and on axial sequences are usually restricted to the lateral columns.

These single *critical lesions* provide potential insight into the genesis of progression in MS by showing that motor progression can be attributable to a single lesion in an eloquent region. It was later shown that, in a subset of patients with more typical MS with 2 or more lesions that fulfill MS diagnostic criteria, the motor progression can also be attributable to a single lesion located in these regions (medullary pyramids or lateral columns). Most patients with MS have many lesions scattered throughout the brain and spinal cord, which makes it difficult to determine the contribution of individual lesions to motor progression. However, the low lesion burden and/or unilateral progression in some patients with MS allows the motor progression to be attributable to a single lesion. These critical lesions challenge the concept that motor progression in MS arises from a diffuse degenerative disorder and suggest that single lesions in eloquent locations may have a disproportionate effect on progression. Further studies are needed to determine their exact role in the genesis of motor progression.

KEY POINTS

- Progressive solitary sclerosis is a rare variant of MS in which patients have only 1 lesion and have development of progressive motor impairment attributable to that lesion.

- Patients with progressive solitary sclerosis generally do not fulfill MS diagnostic criteria because they lack dissemination in space.

- The lesion in progressive solitary sclerosis is typically located in the lateral column or medullary pyramids/anterior cervicomedullary junction.

- The progressive solitary sclerosis MRI lesion becomes focally atrophic over time.

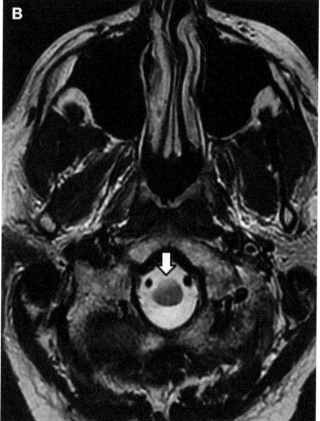

Figure 6.1 **Magnetic Resonance Imaging in Case Patient.**
A, A T2 hyperintensity is seen on a sagittal image at the cervicomedullary junction and extends to the medullary pyramids (arrow). B, On an axial image, the hyperintensity is slightly more prominent on the right side of the spinal cord (arrow).

FLUCTUATING VISION LOSS, SEIZURES, AND LEFT PARIETO-OCCIPITAL MASS

Alicja Kalinowska-Lyszczarz, MD, PhD, W. Oliver Tobin, MB, BCh, BAO, PhD,

Yong Guo, MD, PhD, and Claudia F. Lucchinetti, MD

CASE PRESENTATION

HISTORY AND EXAMINATION

A 35-year-old man sought care for progressive visual disturbance. Magnetic resonance imaging (MRI) of the brain showed a large, left-sided, parieto-occipital, contrast-enhancing lesion (Figure 7.1A). He was treated with dexamethasone with brief improvement in vision. Within 5 days he had progressive vision worsening. Two weeks after the onset of his symptoms, brain MRI showed a decrease in lesion size (Figure 7.1B), and corticosteroids were discontinued. Cerebrospinal fluid (CSF) analysis showed a normal white blood cell count and immunoglobulin G (IgG) index and absence of oligoclonal bands. Two months after symptom onset he was found to have alexia without agraphia, and follow-up MRI showed an increased size of the lesion, which now expanded into the right hemisphere (Figure 7.1C).

TESTING

Two months after disease onset, the patient underwent a left occipital brain biopsy, which demonstrated a macrophage-enriched active demyelinating lesion with relative axonal sparing (Figure 7.2). The next day, right arm weakness and aphasia developed, along with a fever of 38.5 °C. He was treated with dexamethasone. Electroencephalography indicated multiple seizures. Repeated CSF analysis showed a slightly increased white blood cell count (10 cells/μL; reference range, ≤5 cells/μL), increased protein level (98 mg/dL; reference range, ≤35 mg/dL), IgG index of 0.84 (reference range, ≤0.85), and the presence of 3 CSF-unique oligoclonal bands. He was treated with 5 days of intravenous methylprednisolone and levetiracetam, with improvement.

Four weeks after the brain biopsy, he became disoriented, which was associated with headache and blurred vision. Follow-up brain MRI showed a probable left parieto-occipital abscess/hemorrhage (Figure 7.1D). He was treated with empiric antibiotics. He was discharged 10 days later on an empiric antibiotic regimen of metronidazole, vancomycin, and cefepime, which was continued for 4 weeks.

After he was discharged, his visual field started to deteriorate, leaving him with a small wedge area of vision in the inferior left quadrant. Brain MRI findings were relatively stable (Figure 7.1E). Results of optical coherence tomography were normal, as were spine MRI findings. The patient underwent plasma exchange, followed by 6 monthly doses of cyclophosphamide. Findings on brain MRI obtained 11 months into the disease showed substantial improvement (Figure 7.1F).

Three and a half years later, the patient came to the emergency department with weakness of the left leg associated with reduced sensation. Brain MRI findings were unchanged from earlier images, but spinal MRI showed a new demyelinating contrast-enhancing lesion from T2 to T7. Serum was negative for aquaporin-4 (AQP4)-IgG and myelin oligodendrocyte glycoprotein (MOG)-IgG antibodies. He was treated with 5 days of intravenous methylprednisolone followed by 6 sessions of plasma exchange, with improvement.

DIAGNOSIS

A diagnosis of relapsing tumefactive demyelination was made.

MANAGEMENT

The patient was subsequently treated with ocrelizumab.

DISCUSSION

Tumefactive demyelinating lesions (TDLs) pose a diagnostic challenge, both clinically and radiologically, especially if they are the first manifestations of demyelinating disease. Typically, TDLs are large (>2 cm) and are associated with edema, mass effect, and variable patterns of contrast

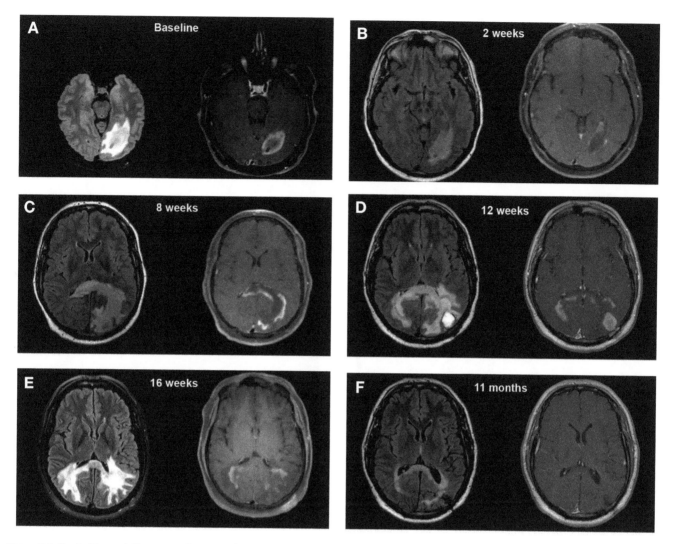

Figure 7.1 Brain Magnetic Resonance Imaging Showing Progression of Disease in the Case Patient.
In each panel, the left image is fluid-attenuated inversion recovery (FLAIR) and the right image is T1 postcontrast. A, At baseline, a large, left parieto-occipital lesion is seen, which enhanced on T1 postcontrast. B, At 2 weeks, both the size and enhancement of the lesion are decreased. C, At 8 weeks, lesion size is increased, with extension into the splenium. D, At 12 weeks (4 weeks after biopsy), images show a biopsy complication, which was interpreted as an abscess. E, At 16 weeks, imaging is relatively stable. F, At 11 months, after 6 monthly doses of cyclophosphamide, lesion size and enhancement show substantial improvement.

enhancement (ie, open ring pattern); this can make it difficult to distinguish them from neoplasms and may prompt biopsy. Other MRI clues to TDLs include a peripherally restricted diffusion pattern on diffusion-weighted imaging, the presence of rapid changes on diffusion-weighted imaging from sequential brain MRI scans, and the presence of a T2-weighted hypointense rim.

As in this case, the diagnosis is often based on histopathologic analysis of the lesion. Histopathologically, TDLs may still be confused with gliomas because of the presence of astrocytic mitoses and Creutzfeldt-Peters cells (reactive astrocytes with fragmented nuclear inclusions) but are distinguished by the presence of a prominent macrophage infiltrate and, typically, a clear lesion border (Figure 7.2). If biopsy is performed, histopathologic analysis should include stains for myelin, axons, and macrophages to carefully screen for possible demyelinating disease and prevent unnecessary radiotherapy.

TDLs are a relatively rare (1-2/1,000 multiple sclerosis [MS] cases) atypical form of central nervous system (CNS) demyelination. Some overlap is present between atypical forms of CNS demyelination. Baló concentric sclerosis, which is characterized by a concentric ring appearance on pathologic analysis and MRI, is the result of demyelinating areas alternating with relatively preserved myelin and can also be tumefactive. In both TDLs and Baló concentric sclerosis, the clinical presentation is often related to a cerebral tumor-like mass, with symptoms varying by location, which may deteriorate rapidly unless promptly treated. Despite atypical and sometimes aggressive onset, both conditions may have a favorable prognosis, with a longer interval to second episode and less-severe long-term motor disability, compared with patients with typical MS matched for disease duration over 10 years.

Importantly, not every case of tumefactive demyelination will evolve into clinically definite relapsing-remitting

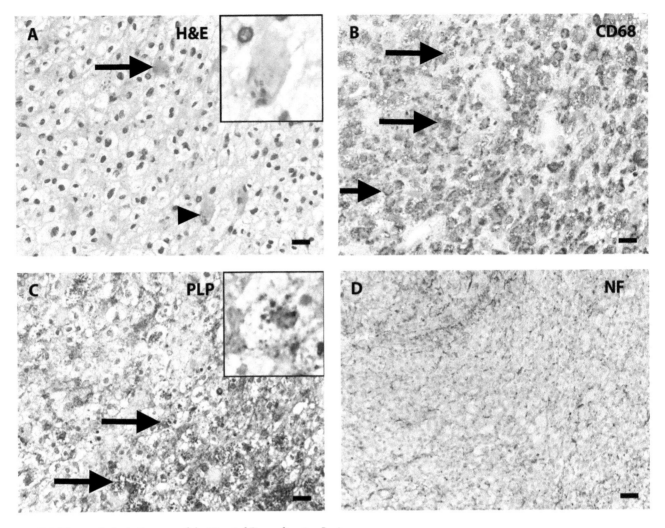

Figure 7.2 Histopathologic Features of the Biopsied Demyelinating Lesion.
A, The brain occipital lobe biopsy shows eosinophilic reactive astrocytes (arrow) and Creutzfeldt-Peters cells (arrowhead and inset [magnification ×400]) (hematoxylin-eosin [H&E]). B-D, Immunohistochemical staining. B, Anti-CD68 staining shows that the lesion is enriched with macrophages (arrows). C, With anti–myelin proteolipid protein (PLP) staining, focal myelin loss and myelin debris are seen within macrophages (arrows) suggesting active demyelination, and inset shows lipid-laden macrophages (magnification ×400). D, Anti-neurofilament (NF) staining shows that axons are relatively preserved. Scale bars=20 μm.

MS (RRMS). The clinical course associated with TDLs varies widely, from a highly aggressive, fulminant Marburg variant MS associated with substantial mortality rates, to classical RRMS after a tumefactive onset. Other patients will recover completely, never fulfilling McDonald criteria for MS-related dissemination in space and time. Cases with relapses and remissions from TDLs only (without classical MS plaques) have also been reported. Moreover, tumefactive demyelination has been associated with immunotherapies for MS such as fingolimod, in which TDLs developed after a classic RRMS course. TDLs have also been associated with neuromyelitis optica spectrum disorders, MOG-IgG–associated disease, Baló concentric sclerosis, and acute disseminated encephalomyelitis. In the case patient, the presence of a longitudinally extensive transverse myelitis would be atypical for classic RRMS, despite the presence of CSF-specific oligoclonal bands and the absence of AQP4-IgG and MOG-IgG

autoantibodies. This underlines the complexity in diagnostic classification and possible overlap between different CNS inflammatory diseases.

Importantly, in most cases of TDL, other CNS demyelinating lesions can be identified even on prebiopsy MRI on careful review. If possible, brain biopsy should be avoided because of the associated morbidity.

KEY POINTS

- TDLs are an atypical form of CNS demyelination that must be distinguished from neoplasms and may prompt diagnostic brain biopsy. Although aggressive treatment (plasma exchange, immunosuppression with the use of cyclophosphamide) may be required at onset, complete recovery and monophasic course are not uncommon, and long-term prognosis is often favorable.

- TDL characteristics on MRI include lesion size >2 cm, associated edema, mass effect, contrast enhancement (especially open ring pattern), peripherally restricted diffusion pattern, T2-weighted hypointense rims, or butterfly configuration involving corpus callosum.

- Despite atypical MRI findings at presentation, most TDLs are multifocal on MRI before biopsy. Whenever possible, brain biopsy should be avoided because of the associated morbidity.

- TDLs can be associated with prototypic MS, fulminant Marburg variant MS, Baló concentric sclerosis, neuromyelitis optica spectrum disorders, MOG-IgG–associated disease, and acute disseminated encephalomyelitis.

DIFFUSE PAIN AND ABNORMAL BRAIN MRI FINDINGS

Andrew McKeon, MB, BCh, MD

CASE PRESENTATION

HISTORY AND EXAMINATION

A 46-year-old woman with a remote history of classical migraine, but without symptoms for 2 decades, had development of pain behind her left eye followed by holocephalic headache, which resolved after 1 day. She subsequently began to have episodic headaches, 10 days per month, occurring in the early morning and usually relieved promptly by ibuprofen. Her sleep became disrupted. Irritability, cognitive symptoms, and fatigue then developed. Her headaches occurred daily, along with whole-body discomfort, predominantly affecting her limbs and low back. At night, she was kept awake by pain, particularly when changing position in bed.

She underwent polysomnography and was diagnosed with obstructive sleep apnea syndrome. Her sleep quality improved with continuous positive airway pressure therapy, but her daily headaches, cognitive symptoms, and limb pain persisted. Although she had no history of tick bites, rash, fever, or *Borrelia burgdorferi* test positivity, she was diagnosed with "seronegative Lyme disease." Fourteen days of doxycycline therapy was not accompanied by improvement in symptoms.

TESTING

After extensive laboratory evaluations and consultations with internal medicine and rheumatology specialists, the patient was diagnosed with fibromyalgia. Short trials of low doses of amitriptyline, nortriptyline, gabapentin, and pregabalin were undertaken, but these were poorly tolerated and discontinued in each instance. The patient was concerned that she may have multiple sclerosis, and she underwent magnetic resonance imaging (MRI) of the brain with and without contrast. The radiology report documented multiple, small areas of T2-signal change, and demyelinating disease was included in the radiologic differential diagnosis. The patient then sought a second opinion.

Evaluations at Mayo Clinic confirmed the patient history and normal neurologic and rheumatologic examination findings and supported evidence of diffuse myofascial limb and back pain and tenderness. She had 15 of 18 fibromyalgia-characteristic tender points on examination. Brain MRI images

were reviewed, which showed nonspecific T2-signal change in the deep white matter but no demyelinating disease–typical ovoid lesions of spinal cord, brainstem, cerebellum, juxtacortical regions, or corpus callosum (Figure 8.1). The nonspecific lesions

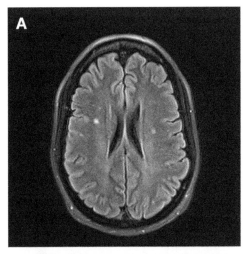
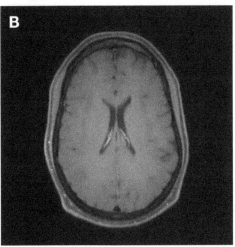

Figure 8.1 Brain Magnetic Resonance Imaging Findings for the Case Patient.
Axial, T2/fluid-attenuated inversion recovery (A) and T1 postgadolinium images (B) show numerous, small areas of T2 abnormality, nonspecific in shape and distribution (restricted to deep white matter) (A) that did not enhance (B).

Metabolic disorder
  Kidney failure
  Liver failure
  Respiratory failure
Endocrinopathy
  Hypothyroidism
  Hypoadrenalism
  Hypopituitarism
Neoplasia
  Dysproteinemias
  Metastatic bone disease
Vitamin/mineral deficiency
  Vitamin B_{12}
  Folate
  Iron
  Copper/vitamin E
Autoimmune disease
  Rheumatoid arthritis
  Systemic lupus erythematosus
  Mixed connective tissue disease
  Polymyositis
  Celiac disease
  Polymyalgia rheumatica
Seronegative arthropathies
  Osteoarthritis
  Psoriatic arthritis
  Chondrocalcinosis
  Hemochromatosis
Other causative or contributing factors
  Untreated sleep disorder
  Small-fiber neuropathy
  Depression, anxiety

did not demonstrate postgadolinium enhancement. Extensive workup for alternative differential diagnostic considerations for her pain was unremarkable (Box 8.1).

DIAGNOSIS

The patient was diagnosed with fibromyalgia with features of central sensitization, with brain MRI demonstrating nonspecific radiologic abnormalities.

MANAGEMENT

A detailed discussion about the biological concepts underlying fibromyalgia and central sensitization was undertaken with the patient. The concepts of changing from a diagnostic and acute treatment strategy to rehabilitative approaches were reviewed. Slowly progressive, incremental, physical reconditioning and cognitive behavioral retraining were recommended.

She was advised to complete a fibromyalgia and chronic fatigue treatment program, an 8-hour self-management program focusing on cognitive and behavioral approaches, stress management, sleep hygiene, balanced lifestyle, moderation, energy conservation, and graded exercise. No new medications were recommended given her previous poor tolerance.

DISCUSSION

The patient's atypical symptoms (pain only), normal examination findings, and brain MRI appearance assisted in excluding a diagnosis of demyelinating disease (multiple sclerosis). The radiologic findings, termed *white matter leukoaraiotic change* (or *leukoaraiosis*), are commonly encountered in healthy persons as they age, particularly in patients with migraine (eg, our case patient) or those with microvascular risk factors (eg, diabetes, tobacco use, hypertension, and hypercholesterolemia).

The more challenging aspect of this evaluation was the need to exclude diverse other causes of her symptoms and give the patient a clear diagnosis. Fibromyalgia is a symptom-based diagnosis described by body pain and tenderness. As for migraine, the diagnosis is based partly on the exclusion of other diagnoses and partly on positive findings. Fatigue, disrupted sleep, and altered mood are common contributing factors to and outcomes of fibromyalgia. In addition, some patients have amplification of neural signaling within the central nervous system, eliciting pain hypersensitivity. This phenomenon is known as *central sensitization*. Acral paresthesias, headache, ear pain, jaw pain, vibratory sensations, and amplified limb and axial pain are common. Cognitive symptoms, often referred to by patients as "brain fog," generally occur secondary to disrupted sleep and altered mood. Patients with long-standing symptoms may be wheelchair-bound at initial evaluation, anticipating an untreatable neurodegenerative diagnosis such as amyotrophic lateral sclerosis.

Tenderness to minor pressure in specific regions (trigger points) is typical but not required for diagnosis of fibromyalgia. Bedside cognitive examination typically shows inattention (poor number and word registration) but no true amnesia (preserved 5-minute recall). Poor effort or give-way weakness is common during the motor strength examination. Most other diagnoses are excludable by history and examination, although minor small-fiber sensory changes (decreased temperature sensation, in particular) may be found. Electromyography and nerve conduction studies exclude widespread neuropathy but are also poorly tolerated.

Fibromyalgia occasionally occurs as a secondary phenomenon, in the context of chronicity of any of the diagnoses in Box 8.1, or can occur without an identifiable cause. Undiagnosed and untreated, fibromyalgia can have serious disability outcomes. Treatment consists of extensive counseling regarding the diagnosis, neuropathic pain–directed medication, and rehabilitation. Opioids are ineffective and should be gradually tapered and discontinued. First-line medications effective for treatment of pain (but which also may improve sleep and mood) include tricyclic antidepressants (amitriptyline or nortriptyline, 25-75 mg at night) and gabapentin (300-3,600 mg/d, usually in 3 divided doses). Duloxetine and pregabalin are US Food and Drug Administration approved for treatment of fibromyalgia but are often used second line in practice. Rehabilitation consists of a graded exercise program and possibly 1 or more other interventions such as hydrotherapy, yoga, tai chi, and some oral supplements. In addition to exclusion of the diagnoses in Box 8.1, it is critical for the physician to also evaluate for, specialty refer, and treat, as appropriate, any contributory disorders, including depression, anxiety, and sleep disorders (restless legs or obstructive sleep apnea).

KEY POINTS

- Multifocal leukoaraiotic changes on MRI are common in the general population and are routinely misdiagnosed as representing demyelinating disease.

- Fibromyalgia is a common cause of diffuse pain and disability, but full functional restoration can occur with appropriate treatment.

- Exclusion of other causes of diffuse pain should precede assignment of a clear, positive fibromyalgia diagnosis.

- Fibromyalgia management consists of counseling, appropriate pain-directed medication, and a graded exercise program.

LESIONS FOUND BY CHANCE

Dean M. Wingerchuk, MD

CASE PRESENTATION

HISTORY AND EXAMINATION

A healthy 26-year-old woman with a history of episodic migraine without aura since age 12 years had a first-ever event of transient visual impairment. She reported to her neurologist that she "lost vision" for 15 minutes and described a "black blob" with a bright jagged border that moved across her binocular visual field and resolved without sequelae. Minutes later, one of her typical migraine headaches developed. Given the patient's history of typical episodic migraine, the new visual event's clinical characteristics were highly consistent with a migraine aura. Because of the new transient visual symptoms, the neurologist ordered brain magnetic resonance imaging (MRI), which showed several periventricular white matter lesions (Figure 9.1), including some that involved the corpus callosum and were oriented perpendicular to the septocallosal surface. One lesion enhanced after gadolinium administration. Subsequent review of the patient's neurologic history indicated no symptoms or clinical events other than migraine and the single visual event. Findings of neurologic examination were normal.

Although MRI excluded structural lesions that could have caused the visual event, they raised the possibility of multiple sclerosis (MS) because of the white matter lesion pattern. In patients with headaches in whom brain MRI reveals white matter lesions, the differential diagnosis includes disorders with several underlying causes including ischemia, inflammation, vasculitis, and demyelination, among others. Clinicoradiologic correlation is crucial. In patients with new-onset headaches, the white matter lesions may be etiologically relevant (eg, vasculitis). However, in most cases, the detected white matter lesions are either indirectly related or unrelated to the headache disorder. The lesion pattern is helpful in making this judgment. In patients with typical migraine, white matter lesions are most commonly punctate or small, subcortical, and nonspecific, resembling those seen with small-vessel cerebrovascular disease but more numerous than expected for age. In contrast, extensive and confluent subcortical lesions that involve the external and extreme capsules and the anterior temporal lobes suggest CADASIL syndrome (cerebral autosomal dominant arteriopathy with subcortical infarcts and leukoencephalopathy), and inquiring about a family history of migraine, early-onset stroke, and dementia is important.

In this case, the pattern of white matter lesions is strongly suggestive of a demyelinating process. The ovoid shape, moderate size, and periventricular location of the lesions are characteristics supporting that conclusion. Sagittal T2-weighted fluid-attenuated inversion recovery sequences are helpful in confirming involvement of the corpus callosum and demonstrating the Dawson finger lesion that extends radially and is perpendicular to the ventricular surface; this lesion is highly consistent with demyelination. These findings raised the possibility of MS, but that is a clinical diagnosis. In this situation, the patient should be reassessed with a focused history, seeking any prior evidence of symptoms consistent with a clinical demyelinating event. This should include inquiry about Lhermitte sign (paresthesias in the spine or limbs elicited by neck flexion), painful monocular vision loss (suggesting prior optic neuritis), or episodes lasting days to weeks that included sensory symptoms, weakness, gait disorder, or vertigo or other brainstem symptoms, either in isolation or in combination. In this case, the patient could not recall any such symptoms or events. She reported that she has a distant cousin with advanced MS.

TESTING

The patient was counseled about the MRI findings and expressed the desire to fully evaluate her risk of MS. Findings on MRI of the cervical and thoracic spine were normal. Lumbar puncture and cerebrospinal fluid (CSF) analysis showed 2 white blood cells/μL, normal glucose and protein concentrations, normal immunoglobulin G index, and no CSF-specific oligoclonal bands.

DIAGNOSIS

The patient was diagnosed with radiologically isolated syndrome (RIS).

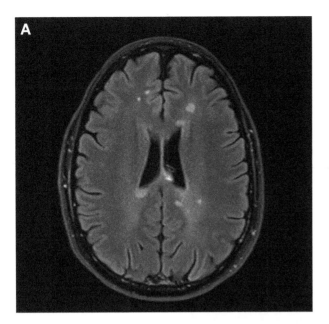
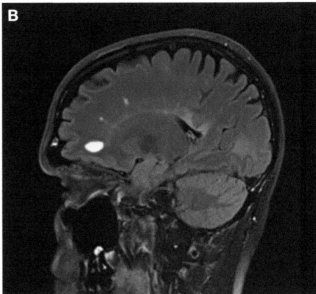
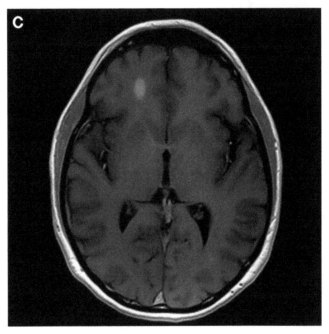

Figure 9.1 **Magnetic Resonance Imaging Findings for Case Patient.**
A and B, Axial (A) and sagittal (B) fluid-attenuated inversion recovery sequences show several periventricular lesions, including lesions oriented perpendicular to the lateral ventricular surface (B). C, A right anterior frontal lesion shows enhancement after gadolinium administration on T1-weighted axial imaging.

MANAGEMENT

The patient was counseled regarding the relevance of the MRI findings and risk of future development of MS. Follow-up brain MRI 4 months later showed resolution of gadolinium enhancement of the right frontal lesion and no new lesions. Clinical and MRI follow-up was recommended in 1 year, sooner if any neurologic symptoms of concern developed, and she was educated about the pattern and timing of symptom evolution with demyelinating events to assist her in distinguishing symptoms of concern from normal neurologic symptoms such as transient paresthesias. She was not prescribed a disease-modifying therapy (DMT) for MS.

DISCUSSION

This patient has RIS—incidentally found MRI lesions consistent with demyelination in a patient with no symptoms or signs suggestive of MS. Recent consensus recommendations for RIS diagnosis include demonstration of MRI lesion dissemination in space by detecting 1 or more T2-hyperintense lesions involving at least 2 of the following topographies: periventricular white matter, corticojuxtacortical, spinal cord, or infratentorial. Exclusionary factors are 1) clinical evidence of neurologic dysfunction suggestive of MS on the basis of historical symptoms and/or objective signs, and 2) MRI abnormalities explained by any other disease process, with particular attention to aging or vascular-related abnormalities, and those due to exposure to toxins or drugs.

People with RIS are at risk for development of clinical MS; approximately 30% to 50% will meet MS criteria by 5 years of follow-up. Factors that increase the risk of conversion (development of symptoms) include detection of spinal cord lesions at RIS presentation, younger age at RIS diagnosis (younger than 37 years), and male sex. Detection of CSF-specific oligoclonal bands or the presence of gadolinium-enhancing lesions may also increase the risk.

There is no established treatment for RIS. Two randomized placebo-controlled trials of existing MS DMTs (dimethyl fumarate and teriflunomide) are in progress and are assessing the primary outcome of time to first acute or progressive clinical neurologic event. Until treatments are established to be beneficial, most patients are counseled and followed up clinically and with annual brain MRI. DMT may be considered if clinical symptoms and signs consistent with MS develop.

Treatment may also be considered in patients with new asymptomatic MRI lesions that are compatible with demyelination, especially if they have abnormal neurologic examination findings (eg, extensor plantar responses or other long tract signs) or an unusually high burden of white matter lesions, but this remains of uncertain benefit.

KEY POINTS

- RIS is used to describe incidentally found MRI lesions consistent with demyelination in a patient with no symptoms or signs suggestive of MS.

- Clinical MS will develop in some people with RIS; detection of spinal cord lesions and younger age are risk factors.

- There is no established treatment for RIS, but clinical and MRI surveillance is recommended.

ENCEPHALOPATHY AND QUADRIPARESIS AFTER AN UPPER RESPIRATORY TRACT INFECTION

A. Sebastian Lopez Chiriboga, MD

CASE PRESENTATION

HISTORY AND EXAMINATION

A 23-year-old woman with no pertinent medical history sought care at the emergency department after having difficulties with ambulation, with bilateral leg weakness and incoordination. Her coworkers reported that she was acting erratically during the previous 24 hours. Two weeks before the onset of the neurologic symptoms, the patient had a fever, productive cough, and generalized myalgias and was diagnosed with influenza type B based on a positive nasopharyngeal swab. The family history was noncontributory, and the patient did not use illicit drugs or have relevant occupational exposures.

After the patient was admitted to the hospital, her clinical condition continued to deteriorate, with worsening encephalopathy, progressing to a comatose state requiring admission to the intensive care unit for airway protection. Bilateral arm weakness and urinary retention also developed. Her vital signs were normal except for increased temperature (38 °C); neurologic examination was limited because of the encephalopathy, but bilateral extensor plantar responses were noted. Diagnoses considered at the time are shown in Table 10.1.

TESTING

Brain magnetic resonance imaging (MRI) demonstrated large confluent white matter hyperintensities, without restricted diffusion or enhancement, and a longitudinally extensive lesion in the cervical spine extending from C3 to C7 (Figure 10.1A). Cerebrospinal fluid (CSF) analysis revealed increased protein concentration (86 mg/dL; reference range, 15-45 mg/dL), glucose level of 42 mg/dL, red blood cell count of 2/µL, and white blood cell count of 84/µL (reference range, 0-5 leukocytes/µL) with 78% lymphocytes. Results of cytologic analysis and flow cytometry were normal. Results of CSF bacterial culture, Lyme disease screen, VDRL test, varicella-zoster virus testing, herpes simplex virus testing, and Epstein-Barr virus polymerase chain reaction were negative.

Laboratory analysis showed normal complete blood cell count; normal liver, kidney, and thyroid function; and normal vitamin B_{12} level. Testing for HIV, syphilis, antinuclear antibody, extractable nuclear antigens, anticardiolipin antibody, anti-dsDNA, antineutrophil cytoplasmic antibodies, angiotensin-converting enzyme, tuberculosis, neural autoantibodies, and urine toxicology were negative. Erythrocyte

---

Table 10.1 | **DIFFERENTIAL DIAGNOSIS**

CATEGORY	CONDITIONS
CNS infection	Broad spectrum of bacterial or viral infections; common causes include herpes viruses, enteroviruses, Lyme disease, HIV, progressive multifocal leukoencephalopathy, syphilis, toxoplasmosis, West Nile virus
Inflammatory disease	First episode of MS, antiphospholipid antibody syndrome, Behçet syndrome, Bickerstaff brainstem encephalitis, chronic lymphocytic inflammation with pontine perivascular enhancement responsive to corticosteroids, hemorrhagic leukoencephalitis, immune reconstitution inflammatory syndrome, lupus cerebritis, neuromyelitis optica spectrum disorders, primary CNS vasculitis
Granulomatous disease	Neurosarcoidosis, granulomatosis with polyangiitis (formerly Wegener granulomatosis)
Malignant process	Lymphoma and other lymphoproliferative disorders, high-grade glioma
Leukodystrophy	Metachromatic leukodystrophy, X-linked adrenoleukodystrophy, Alexander disease
Miscellaneous	Nutritional deficiencies (vitamin B_{12}, folate, thiamine), mitochondrial disease (MELAS, Leber hereditary optic neuropathy), inborn errors of metabolism, toxic metabolic disorders (posterior reversible encephalopathy syndrome, heavy metal toxicity)

Abbreviations: CNS, central nervous system; MELAS, mitochondrial encephalopathy, lactic acidosis, and stroke-like episodes; MS, multiple sclerosis.

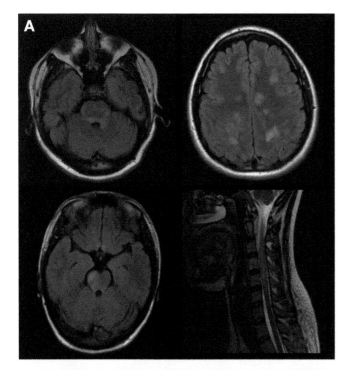

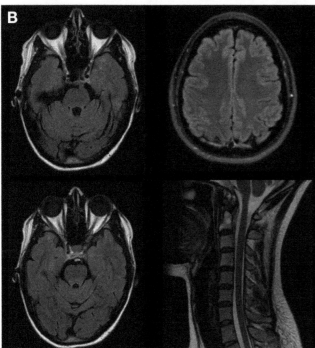

Figure 10.1 **Magnetic Resonance Imaging (MRI) Findings for Case Patient.**

A, T2-axial MRI of the head and sagittal MRI of the cervical spine demonstrates multiple T2 hyperintense lesions affecting the cerebellar peduncles, brainstem, and the subcortical white matter bilaterally and a longitudinally extensive lesion from C3 to C7. B, Repeated imaging 4 months after symptom onset shows complete resolution of the T2 hyperintense lesions.

(From Lopez-Chiriboga AS, Majed M, Fryer J, Dubey D, McKeon A, Flanagan EP, et al. Association of MOG-IgG serostatus with relapse after acute disseminated encephalomyelitis and proposed diagnostic criteria for MOG-IgG–associated disorders. JAMA Neurol. 2018;75[11]:1355-63; used with permission.)

sedimentation rate and C-reactive protein level were mildly increased. Immunoglobulin G1 (IgG1) antibodies against myelin oligodendrocyte glycoprotein (MOG) were detected in the serum on a live cell-based flow cytometric assay but were not detected in CSF (testing for the IgG1 subtype gives better disease specificity than testing for IgG in general).

DIAGNOSIS

On the basis of the preceding infection, imaging findings, and negative infectious investigations, there was a high suspicion for a diagnosis of acute disseminated encephalomyelitis (ADEM).

MANAGEMENT

Because of the suspicion for ADEM and before the confirmation of seropositivity for MOG-IgG1, the patient was treated with 1,000 mg of intravenous methylprednisolone for 5 days and also 7 courses of plasma exchange. After administration of immunotherapy, the encephalopathy improved substantially, which allowed for extubation and improvement of her quadriplegia and urinary retention. The patient was discharged from the hospital on oral prednisone therapy, and the dose was tapered until discontinuation after 3 months. MRI 4 months after the initial event showed complete resolution of the diffuse T2 hyperintense lesions (Figure 10.1B). MOG-IgG1 was undetectable in serum 8 months after her initial event. The patient has had no further episodes as of the last follow-up (5 years after the initial event).

DISCUSSION

ADEM is a monophasic idiopathic inflammatory demyelinating disease that predominantly affects the white matter of the brain and spinal cord. ADEM typically follows an infection or, rarely, immunization. The clinical presentation is subacute and is characterized by multifocal neurologic deficits including encephalopathy (the level of consciousness ranges from lethargy to coma), seizures (focal or multifocal, with or without secondary generalization), and various degrees of motor deficits. Imaging findings demonstrate multifocal T2 hyperintensities that affect the deep and subcortical white matter diffusely and are usually bilateral and asymmetric. The basal ganglia, thalamus, and brainstem are often involved, and contrast enhancement is uncommon. The CSF shows inflammatory changes in most cases, with lymphocytic pleocytosis and increased protein levels. In contrast to multiple sclerosis (MS), oligoclonal bands are rare.

Histologically, ADEM is characterized by perivenular demyelination with associated lymphocytic and macrophage infiltrates that form confluent plaques with indistinct margins.

ADEM is more common in children and young adults and, by definition, is self-limited. Therefore, sequential MRI is required to confirm the diagnosis of ADEM, because relapses or the appearance of new MRI lesions are suggestive of an alternative diagnosis, particularly other demyelinating disorders such as multiphasic ADEM, MOG-IgG1–associated disorders, or MS. Figure 10.2 shows a proposed therapeutic approach for the treatment of the first episode of MOG-IgG1–associated disorders.

The differential diagnosis of ADEM is broad, and central nervous system infections must be ruled out. ADEM must

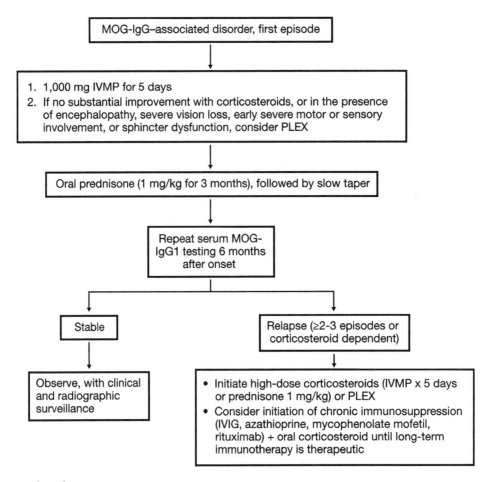

Figure 10.2 **Treatment Algorithm.**
Proposed therapeutic approach (class IV evidence based) for myelin oligodendrocyte glycoprotein (MOG)-immunoglobulin G1 (IgG1)–associated disorders. IVIG indicates intravenous immunoglobulin; IVMP, intravenous methylprednisolone; PLEX, plasma exchange.

be distinguished from the first episode of MS, particularly in children, but this can be clinically challenging. In recent years, the identification of MOG-IgG1 using cell-based assays has helped confirm the diagnosis of ADEM and allows for distinction from MS. The identification of MOG-IgG1 can also assist in the longitudinal follow-up of these patients. MOG-IgG1 is found in approximately 40% of pediatric and adult patients with ADEM. Transient seropositivity is a good prognosticator and highly associated with a monophasic clinical course. Conversely, persistent MOG-IgG1 seropositivity increases the risk of further relapses, typically in the form of recurrent optic neuritis and, less likely, myelitis or recurrent episodes of encephalitis.

No randomized clinical trials have been performed for the treatment of ADEM or MOG-IgG1–associated disorders. The current recommended treatment of ADEM includes supportive care and administration of high-dose intravenous methylprednisolone, followed by or in conjunction with plasmapheresis. Corticosteroid treatment is typically continued by transitioning to oral prednisone with gradual tapering over 12 weeks to reduce the risk of relapses. Most patients improve, but adults tend to have worse outcomes, with full recovery seen in approximately 50% of patients. Cognitive impairment, seizures, motor deficits, and neurogenic bladder

are common long-term neurologic sequelae. The ideal timing of retesting for MOG-IgG1 is unclear. We typically retest for serum MOG-IgG1 at 6 months because it can help with decision making regarding long-term immunotherapy. Follow-up of patients with an initial diagnosis of ADEM is important because patients can have an ADEM-like presentation as the first episode of a chronic demyelinating disease.

KEY POINTS

- ADEM is a self-limited, immune-mediated, inflammatory demyelinating disorder that predominantly affects the white matter of the brain and spinal cord.

- ADEM usually follows an infection or immunization. It presents with multifocal neurologic deficits, such as altered mental status and motor, sensory, and systemic symptoms including headache, malaise, and fever.

- Detection of MOG-IgG1 supports the diagnosis of ADEM and may assist in prognostication.

- Monophasic ADEM may evolve over as long as 3 months. Symptoms that appear during tapering of glucocorticoid therapy are considered to be part of the same episode.

SEVERE MONOCULAR VISION LOSS FOLLOWED BY GAIT DIFFICULTY

Brian G. Weinshenker, MD

CASE PRESENTATION

HISTORY AND EXAMINATION

A 56-year-old woman sought care for painless vision loss over 24 hours in the superior field of her right eye, which progressed to total vision loss. Intravenous corticosteroids were administered over 5 days, and she recovered well. Approximately 6 months later, paresthesias and sensory loss of her legs developed, which was sufficiently severe that she was unable to walk. She had severe impairment of vibration sense and lesser impairment of position sense, as well as proximal weakness of both legs. She recovered but had persistent burning dysesthesias of the legs. Diagnoses considered at the time are shown in Table 11.1.

TESTING

Magnetic resonance imaging (MRI) of the orbits at the onset of symptoms showed gadolinium enhancement extending from the middle of the orbit posteriorly, almost to the level of the optic chiasm (Figure 11.1A). MRI of the brain 8 months later showed nonspecific T2 hyperintensities that were not suggestive of multiple sclerosis (MS) (Figure 11.1B). MRI of the spine at the time of acute myelitis revealed a long spinal cord lesion extending from the lower cervical cord to the conus which was central and homogeneous on T2 images (Figure 11.1C) and exhibited patchy gadolinium enhancement (Figure 11.1D). Cerebrospinal fluid analysis showed 37 leukocytes/μL with lymphocyte predominance and negative tests for oligoclonal bands. On serologic analysis, she was positive for aquaporin-4 (AQP4)-immunoglobulin G (IgG) antibodies by enzyme-linked immunosorbent assay.

DIAGNOSIS

The patient was diagnosed with neuromyelitis optica (NMO) spectrum disorder (NMOSD), AQP4-IgG seropositive.

Table 11.1 | DIFFERENTIAL DIAGNOSIS FOR CASE PATIENT

DIAGNOSIS	DIAGNOSTIC CONSIDERATIONS
MS	Severe vision loss and inability to walk are uncommon during myelitis and ON episodes in MS. MRI findings in the brain suggestive of MS and oligoclonal bands in CSF were absent
Systemic lupus erythematosus	May be associated with optic neuropathy and myelitis, but systemic symptoms suggestive of lupus, such as rash, arthritis, and fever, were absent. In most patients with ON or myelitis in the context of systemic lupus erythematosus, patients also are seropositive for AQP4-IgG
Paraneoplastic disorder	Paraneoplastic disorders with antibodies to collapsin-response mediator protein 5 may be associated with optic neuropathy and myelopathy. Occasionally, AQP4-IgG NMOSD may occur with tumors that may express AQP4, but tumor association occurs in less than 5% of cases
Sarcoidosis	Sarcoidosis may cause ON and myelopathy, but the onset is typically more insidious and recovers more slowly after corticosteroids. Systemic symptoms, such as fever, weight loss, or cough, are often present. There were no typical symptoms of neurosarcoidosis in this case: meningitis, facial palsy, or hypothalamic involvement

Abbreviations: AQP4-IgG, aquaporin-4 immunoglobulin G; CSF, cerebrospinal fluid; MRI, magnetic resonance imaging; MS, multiple sclerosis; NMOSD, neuromyelitis optica spectrum disorder; ON, optic neuritis.

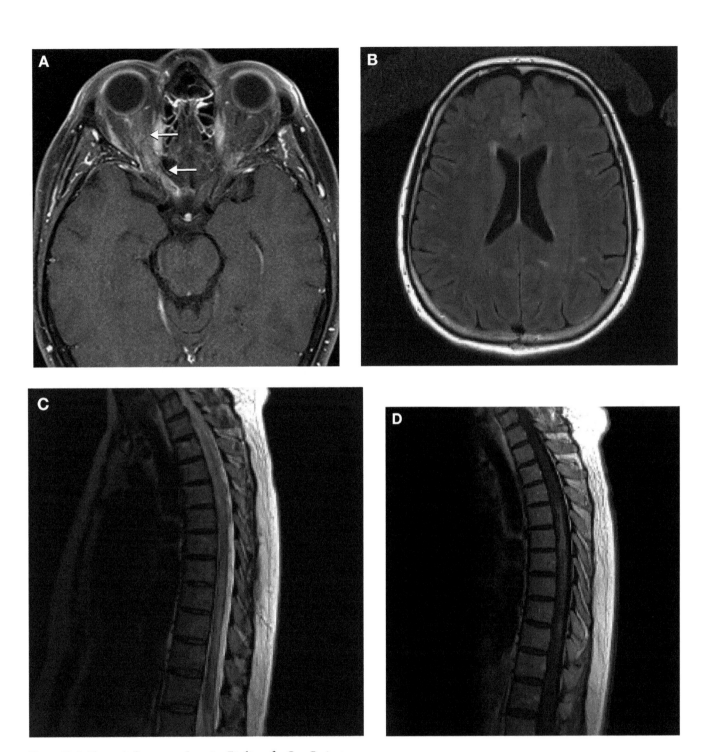

Figure 11.1 Magnetic Resonance Imaging Findings for Case Patient.
A, Axial T1 images after gadolinium administration show a long lesion of the right optic nerve (arrows). B, Axial fluid-attenuated inversion recovery images of the brain show nonspecific white matter lesions that are not suggestive of multiple sclerosis. C, Sagittal T2 image of the thoracic spine shows a central homogeneous T2 hyperintense lesion spanning the length of the thoracic cord. D, Sagittal T1 images after gadolinium administration show patchy enhancement of the lesion visible in panel C.

MANAGEMENT

The patient was started on rituximab treatment. After 2 years, she decided to discontinue treatment because she was concerned about potential adverse effects, even though she had had no problems while taking the medication. Six months after discontinuing rituximab, severe weakness of her right leg developed, which improved with intravenous corticosteroids.

Over the next 2 months, she had 3 further discrete episodes consisting, sequentially, of left optic neuritis (ON), right ON, and an additional myelitis. Rituximab therapy was restarted, 2 doses of 1 g each, but she had 1 further episode of myelitis 2 weeks after receiving rituximab. Six months later, her visual acuity in the right eye was only counting fingers, and she had a flaccid paraplegia with areflexia of the lower extremities and total loss of sensory function below T4.

DISCUSSION

The term NMO came into use in the early 20th century as an approximate translation of the French term *neuromyelite optique aigue*, coined by Eugene Devic. The disease was often referred to as Devic disease because of his report of a patient in 1894 who had development of myelitis and bilateral ON in quick succession and died within months. This report, and the literature review by Devic's student Gault published as a thesis, suggested that this condition might be a unique form of inflammatory disease of the central nervous system. Devic mused but did not speculate about why the optic nerve and spinal cord were uniquely targeted. On the basis of that case, it was widely believed that the condition was monophasic and that a diagnosis could not be made if relapses occurred.

Several groups suggested that this illness might have a wider spectrum than first appreciated, and some unique characteristics were identified. Diagnostic criteria were first proposed by neurologists at Mayo Clinic in 1999, who reported several clinical, MRI, and cerebrospinal fluid characteristics, in various combinations of major and minor criteria, that distinguish NMO from MS. These unique characteristics included long spinal cord lesions, normal brain MRI findings at initial presentation, and prominent cerebrospinal fluid pleocytosis during episodes, among others. Shortly thereafter, Lennon and Weinshenker collaborated to demonstrate that an indirect immunofluorescence pattern of staining on a substrate of rodent brain was highly specific for NMO. In 2005, Lennon established the identity of the target autoantigen AQP4, a brain water channel that is expressed widely in the brain and central nervous system to varying degrees but is also expressed on a few organs outside the brain. This complement-activating antibody has since been shown to have pathogenic potential in vitro and in vivo.

NMOSD is more frequently diagnosed since 1) the original criteria for diagnosis, bilateral ON and myelitis, were liberalized to include unilateral ON or myelitis, and 2) AQP4-IgG autoantibody was recognized to increase the sensitivity and specificity of the diagnosis. ON and myelitis account for 90% of clinical episodes that occur in patients with NMOSD. These episodes vary in severity but are more severe as a group than those that occur in MS. In the spinal cord, myelitis episodes are associated with lesions that extend over 3 or more vertebral segments in 85% of instances and typically affect the central spinal cord. Other clinical manifestations now recognized to be phenomena of the disease, in part because of their association with AQP4-IgG, include 1) intractable nausea and vomiting, reflecting inflammation of the area postrema (although such events are relatively less common, occurring in about 20% of patients with this disease), and 2) various hypothalamic and thalamic syndromes, including eating disorders, symptomatic types of narcolepsy, and others. Encephalopathy may accompany inflammation in the corpus callosum, large tumefactive lesions, and, rarely, posterior reversible encephalopathy syndrome. The latter seems to occur at increased frequency in NMOSD, possibly because of functional interference with water channels of the brain.

Supportive investigations include MRI, which reveals long spinal cord lesions during episodes and occasionally long optic nerve lesions that may involve the optic chiasm and either relatively normal brain imaging or lesions that are typical of those that occur in NMOSD. An international panel recommended that a confident diagnosis could be made in those seropositive for AQP4-IgG, even after a single compatible clinical presentation. NMOSD was proposed as the official umbrella term for all clinical presentations of the disease, regardless of whether the patient was seropositive and whether ON or myelitis occurred.

Recently, it has been recognized that some patients who are seronegative for AQP4-IgG have detectable IgG antibodies to myelin oligodendrocyte glycoprotein (MOG). There are clinical and radiologic differences between these patients and those who are AQP4-IgG seropositive and MOG-IgG seronegative, although there is substantial overlap. Both conditions seem to relapse in a high proportion of cases, although the exact proportion of patients with MOG-IgG who have relapse is unclear. MOG-IgG–associated disease has greater predilection for the optic nerve than the spinal cord, and episodes tend to be associated with less severe sequelae. Patients with MOG-IgG may also have other clinical manifestations, including encephalitis with seizures, acute disseminated encephalomyelitis, and recurrent ON, which may not qualify for a diagnosis of NMOSD.

Treatment of NMOSD requires high-dose corticosteroids for acute relapses and rapid rescue with plasma exchange for those who do not respond promptly to corticosteroids. Long-term treatment involves 1 of several immunosuppressive agents to reduce the frequency and severity of episodes. Several agents seem effective, and the optimum treatment remains undefined. Azathioprine, mycophenolate mofetil, long-term low-dose prednisone, and rituximab are the most widely used treatments. Recently, phase 3 clinical trials have shown positive results for 3 agents: eculizumab, a C5 complement inhibitor; inebilizumab, an anti-CD19 monoclonal antibody directed to B cells; and sartralizumab, an interleukin 1 receptor antagonist. These medications have been approved by the US Food and Drug Administration for treatment of AQP4-IgG–seropositive NMOSD. Many MS immunomodulators are apparently ineffective or potentially harmful, including interferon beta, glatiramer acetate, natalizumab, and alemtuzumab.

On the basis of retrospective studies, 80% of episodes of NMO can be averted with rituximab or other currently used immunosuppressive agents, and episodes that do occur are likely milder than those in untreated patients. If not treated, however, episodes are severe and disabling, often occurring in clusters, as illustrated by the case patient. Permanent blindness and paraparesis are common complications in untreated patients, also as exemplified by the case patient. Some patients may die as a result of respiratory failure associated with upper cervical myelitis.

KEY POINTS

- NMOSD is a relapsing disease, dominated by episodes of ON and myelitis, which is distinct from MS and does not respond to many MS disease-modifying treatments.

- NMOSD has more clinical manifestations than previously appreciated and includes syndromes that target periependymal structures in the brainstem, most distinctively and commonly the area postrema, manifested by intractable nausea and vomiting.

- AQP4-IgG and MOG-IgG are 2 biomarkers that are present in 70% and 15%, respectively, of those with NMOSD. MOG-IgG is associated with other clinical syndromes including recurrent ON and acute disseminated encephalomyelitis. ON associated with MOG-IgG generally resolves more favorably than ON associated with AQP4-IgG.

- Patients with NMOSD, especially those with AQP4-IgG, require long-term immunosuppression to prevent recurrent episodes. Withdrawal of treatment may be associated with severe sequential relapses of ON, myelitis, and occasionally brainstem or brain syndromes. Patients with MOG-IgG who have recurrent episodes require similar immunosuppressive treatment.

MULTIPLE SCLEROSIS AND COGNITIVE IMPAIRMENT[a]

Cristina Valencia-Sanchez, MD, PhD, and Jonathan L. Carter, MD

CASE PRESENTATION

HISTORY AND EXAMINATION

A 60-year-old woman with a history of multiple sclerosis (MS) was evaluated for cognitive concerns. At age 30 years she had an episode of optic neuritis, followed by an episode of bilateral lower extremity numbness at age 35 years. In the following years, she had at least 6 further MS relapses, the last one approximately 3 years before the current presentation. She was initially treated with interferon, but she did not tolerate it. She had been taking glatiramer acetate for the past 3 years. She had noticed progressive deterioration of her gait for the past 3 years, having to use a cane on occasion.

In the past year, she reported short-term memory difficulties, and she was advised not to drive because of these cognitive concerns. She became depressed owing to the loss of her ability to do activities that she enjoyed, such as going to sing in choir. Her husband had noticed that she seemed more apathetic and fatigued than before and that she had no interest in other activities she used to enjoy, such as going for walks. The patient also reported interrupted sleep because of pain in her legs.

Her examination showed disinhibition and mild pseudobulbar affect. Her Kokmen Short Test of Mental Status score was 35 of 38 (missing 1 point for calculation, 1 point for construction, and 1 point for delayed recall). She had spastic dysarthria, mild pyramidal weakness and spasticity of the lower extremities, and proprioception and vibration impairment in her lower extremities. Her gait was spastic paraparetic. Diagnoses considered as the cause of her cognitive symptoms are shown in Table 12.1.

TESTING

Magnetic resonance imaging (MRI) of the brain showed multiple demyelinating lesions (Figure 12.1), and MRI of the cervical spine showed 1 small demyelinating lesion at C6. Vitamin B_{12} level and thyroid function were normal.

Comprehensive neuropsychological testing showed multidomain cognitive impairment, mainly impairment of speed of information processing, spatial discrimination skills, and attention/concentration.

DIAGNOSIS

The patient's MS phenotype was consistent with secondary progressive MS. Her cognitive impairment profile, mainly affecting information processing speed and disinhibition suggestive of frontal dysfunction, was consistent with MS.

MANAGEMENT

The patient began a cognitive rehabilitation program, and learning and memory aids (eg, lists, repetition, increased structure) were recommended. Lifestyle changes were also recommended, including weight loss and physical exercise. She was given recommendations for sleep hygiene and began taking gabapentin for neuropathic pain and restless legs.

She was referred to a psychiatrist for management of depressive symptoms and anxiety. She continued treatment

Table 12.1 | **DIAGNOSES CONSIDERED AS THE CAUSE OF COGNITIVE IMPAIRMENT**

POSSIBLE DIAGNOSIS	COMMENT
Coexistence of Alzheimer disease or other neurodegenerative disorder	No presentation as "cortical" dementia (no severe amnesia, aphasia, apraxia, or agnosia)
Vitamin B_{12} deficiency, hypothyroidism	Normal laboratory findings
Mood disorder	Contributing factor
Sleep disturbance due to pain, sleep apnea	Contributing factor
Effects of polypharmacy	Contributing factor

[a] Portions previously published in Tobin WO. Management of multiple sclerosis symptoms and comorbidities. Continuum (Minneap Minn). 2019 Jun;25(3):753–72 and Kalb R, Beier M, Benedict RH, Charvet L, Costello K, Feinstein A, et al. Recommendations for cognitive screening and management in multiple sclerosis care. Mult Scler. 2018 Nov;24(13):1665-80. Epub 2018 Oct 10; used with permission.

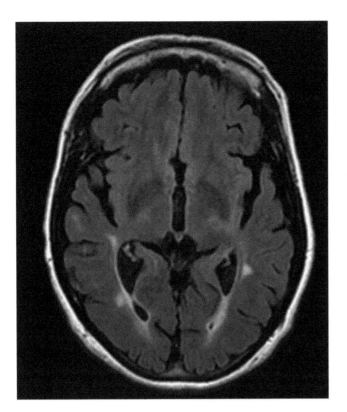
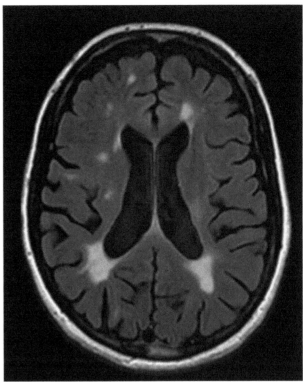
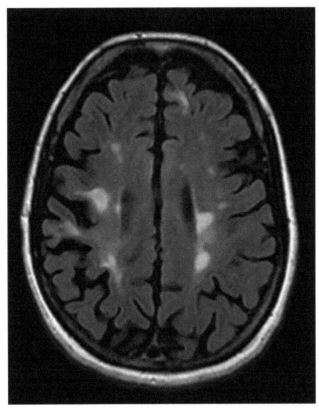

Figure 12.1 **Brain Magnetic Resonance Imaging Findings for Case Patient.**
Axial fluid-attenuated inversion recovery sequences at 3 different levels show multiple periventricular and juxtacortical T2 hyperintensities consistent with demyelination and mild generalized brain volume loss.

with venlafaxine and clonazepam, and she initiated cognitive behavior therapy.

Glatiramer acetate was discontinued because of the transition of the MS from a relapsing-remitting disease to a secondary progressive course without relapses.

The patient's cognitive concerns improved with changes to her sleep habits, better pain management, physical activity, communication with her husband and family, and social engagement in her community (participating in a choir and volunteering). She was referred for a road test and passed, although her driver's license was restricted to daylight hours within 10 miles of her house and off freeways. Findings of follow-up neuropsychological testing 4 and 5 years later were stable.

DISCUSSION

Cognitive impairment is common in patients with MS. The prevalence in adults ranges from 34% to 65%. It may occur in patients with all MS phenotypes, including clinically isolated and radiologically isolated syndromes, although cognitive impairment is more prevalent and severe in progressive MS. Cognitive impairment is highly variable in severity and progression, and it may occur in the absence of Expanded Disability Status Scale progression, which is largely a measure of ambulatory ability. Cognitive impairment at the time of diagnosis predicts overall disability progression.

Slowed cognitive processing speed and episodic memory decline are the most common cognitive deficits in MS, with additional difficulties in executive function, verbal fluency, and visuospatial analysis.

Although not used for the case patient, the Symbol Digit Modalities Test (SDMT) is a valid measure of cognitive processing speed, recommended for baseline screening and annual reassessment of cognitive impairment in people with MS. If results of an initial SDMT are positive, comprehensive neuropsychological testing is recommended. A 4-point or 10% decrease on SDMT at follow-up is also considered a significant decrease that would require further assessment. Neuropsychological testing may identify areas of cognitive deficit and factors that could be affecting cognition such as cognitive reserve, mood disorders, fatigue, medical comorbid conditions, and polypharmacy. Early cognitive screening could identify patients at risk for job loss, deficits that may interfere with driving safely, and difficulties with self-care, treatment adherence, and medical decision-making.

Cognitive dysfunction in MS may be confounded by other factors such as depression, fatigue, and sleep disruption. These factors have variable effects on both objective and self-reported cognitive performance. Depression and anxiety are associated with worse visual-spatial memory, processing speed, and executive functioning. Sleep disorders such as obstructive sleep apnea are associated with reduced visual and verbal memory, executive function, attention, processing speed, and working memory.

In addition, patients with MS who are older than 65 years may also have Alzheimer disease pathologic changes, in a similar proportion to that in the general population. In cases with diagnostic uncertainty about the cognitive changes, additional testing such as evaluation for cerebrospinal fluid biomarkers (amyloid-β and tau), ^{18}F-fludeoxyglucose–positron emission tomography (PET), and amyloid-β PET may help distinguish between MS and a coexistent neurodegenerative process.

To date, clinical trials of symptomatic treatments, such as acetylcholinesterase inhibitors and memantine, have not demonstrated significant benefit for cognitive impairment in MS. Recommended treatment modalities to improve cognition include cognitive rehabilitation, compensatory strategies (eg, memory aids), exercise programs, and frequent social contact. Adequate management of comorbid conditions that may affect cognition (such as depression, fatigue, sleep problems, and medications) may improve cognitive performance.

KEY POINTS

- Cognitive impairment is common in MS and is a cause of substantial disability.

- The SDMT is recommended at baseline and annual reassessment to evaluate progression of cognitive impairment.

- There is no evidence to recommend pharmacologic symptomatic therapy for cognitive impairment in MS. Management strategies include cognitive rehabilitation, physical exercise, and management of comorbid conditions that may affect cognition.

NEW-ONSET GAIT DIFFICULTY WITH KAPPA FREE LIGHT CHAINS IN CEREBROSPINAL FLUID

Maria Alice V. Willrich, PhD, and Ruba S. Saadeh

CASE PRESENTATION

HISTORY AND EXAMINATION

A 49-year-old woman sought care for a 9-month history of gait difficulty. She noticed that she was dragging her right foot when walking and could not walk more than 3 blocks because of right leg weakness. These symptoms developed within hours and progressed to a maximum intensity within 2 days. Her symptoms subsequently started to improve with no intervention, and her function returned to 75% of normal within 3 weeks. At that time, she could walk one quarter of a mile before noticing that her right foot was dragging. Three months later, a symmetrical tingling sensation developed in both feet and legs to the knees. Physical examination showed right-sided weakness of hip flexion and foot dorsiflexion and symmetrical hyperreflexia at the knees and ankles. The plantar response was extensor on the right and mute on the left. There was decreased vibratory sensation to the ankle on the right and to the toes on the left. She walked with a spastic, ataxic right hemiparetic gait. Ophthalmologic examination was normal.

TESTING

Magnetic resonance imaging (MRI) of the brain showed multiple foci of T2 hyperintensity throughout the white matter in both cerebral and cerebellar hemispheres, predominantly in a periventricular distribution. Several small enhancing lesions and mild generalized cerebral volume loss were seen. The appearance and distribution were consistent with a demyelinating process such as multiple sclerosis (MS). MRI of the cervical and thoracic spine showed multiple small T2 hyperintensities, including 1 enhancing lesion in the cervical spinal cord. Findings of cerebrospinal fluid (CSF) analysis are shown in Table 13.1. Oligoclonal bands (OCB) were positive, with 11 unique bands in the CSF. The concentration of CSF kappa free light chains was increased, at 0.314 mg/dL (reference range, <0.100 mg/dL).

DIAGNOSIS

The patient was diagnosed with relapsing-remitting MS.

MANAGEMENT

Given that the patient had active disease, a 5-day course of intravenous corticosteroids was started, after which she noted clinical improvement. The decision was made to begin disease-modifying therapy, so her JC polyoma virus antibody status was assessed to help determine the appropriate medication regimen. Because she was found to be positive for JC polyoma virus antibodies, she was started on ocrelizumab infusion as opposed to natalizumab. She received the first dose divided in 2 infusions 2 weeks apart, followed by full-dose infusions once every 6 months. At her last follow-up 2 years after initial evaluation, the patient has been stable with no new clinical MS episodes and stable MRI disease burden with no new lesions.

Table 13.1 **CSF ANALYSIS RESULTS FOR THE CASE PATIENT**

MEASURE	RESULT	REFERENCE VALUE
OCB		
CSF	11 Bands[a]	≤1 band in CSF not
Serum	0 Bands	present in serum
IgG/albumin		
CSF	0.35	≤0.21
Serum	0.12	≤0.40
IgG index	2.92	<0.85
Synthesis rate, CSF	16.32 mg/24 h	≤12 mg/24 h
Kappa free light chains, CSF	0.314 mg/dL	<0.100 mg/dL

Abbreviations: CSF, cerebrospinal fluid; IgG, immunoglobulin G; OCB, oligoclonal bands.

[a] Eleven unique bands in CSF that are not present in serum represents a positive result.

VARIABLE (CUTOFF FOR POSITIVE TEST)	N	AUC (95% CI)	SENSITIVITY, % (95% CI)	SPECIFICITY, % (95% CI)	PPV, %	NPV, %	LR+	LR–	DIAGNOSTIC ODDS RATIO
OCB (≥4)	683	0.781 (0.729-0.833)	63.2 (52.7-72.6)	93.0 (90.7-94.8)	56.7	94.5	9.0	0.4	22.8
OCB (≥3)	683	0.803 (0.753-0.853)	70.1 (59.8-78.7)	90.4 (87.8-92.5)	51.7	95.4	7.3	0.3	22.1
OCB (≥2)	683	0.806 (0.757-0.854)	73.6 (63.5-81.7)	87.6 (84.7-90.0)	46.4	95.8	5.9	0.3	19.7
cKFLC (≥0.10 mg/dL)	692	0.766 (0.714-0.817)	67.0 (56.6-75.9)	86.1 (83.1-88.6)	41.3	94.7	4.8	0.4	12.6
OCB (≥4) and cKFLC (≥0.06 mg/dL)	681	0.767 (0.714-0.820)	59.8 (49.3-69.5)	93.6 (91.3-95.3)	57.8	94.1	9.3	0.4	21.8
OCB (≥4) or cKFLC (≥0.06 mg/dL)	684	0.758 (0.709-0.807)	73.9 (63.9-81.9)	77.7 (74.2-80.9)	32.8	95.3	3.3	0.3	9.9
CSF index[b] (≥0.61)	673	0.667 (0.615-0.718)	36.8 (27.4-47.3)	96.6 (94.8-97.8)	61.5	91.1	10.8	0.67	16.5
OCB (≥4) and CSF index (≥0.61)	671	0.737 (0.683-0.790)	52.9 (42.5-63.0)	94.5 (92.3-96.1)	59	93.1	9.6	0.5	19.3
OCB (≥4) or CSF index (≥0.61)	674	0.769 (0.719-0.819)	72.4 (62.2-80.7)	81.4 (78.1-84.3)	36.6	95.2	3.9	0.3	11.5

Abbreviations: AUC, area under the receiver operating characteristic curve; cKFLC, CSF kappa free light chains; CSF, cerebrospinal fluid; LR+, positive likelihood ratio; LR–, negative likelihood ratio; MS, multiple sclerosis; NPV, negative predictive value; OCB, oligoclonal bands; PPV, positive predictive value.

[a] From a retrospective cohort of 683 patients at Mayo Clinic, 88 of whom had a confirmed diagnosis of MS.

[b] Calculation of synthesis of intrathecal immunoglobulin G using a ratio between CSF and serum total immunoglobulin G and albumin.

DISCUSSION

The diagnosis of MS incorporates clinical, imaging, and laboratory evidence. The 2017 revised McDonald criteria state that a finding of CSF-specific OCB can replace the criterion for dissemination in time to make a diagnosis of definitive MS. The standard test for OCB is performed using isoelectric focusing electrophoresis and takes more than 3 hours to complete. In a retrospective cohort of 683 patients analyzed in 2018, of which 88 had demyelinating disease, the Mayo Clinic OCB test had a clinical sensitivity of 74% and clinical specificity of 88% when the presence of 2 unique CSF bands was used as a cutoff for positive. However, laboratories can define their own cutoffs for the number of positive OCB, which may make interpretation difficult when results show between 2 and 4 bands. The case patient had 11 unique CSF bands. The number of bands is not correlated with disease severity or prognosis.

Other CSF tests are frequently ordered in conjunction with OCB testing, such as the CSF immunoglobulin G index. The test also yields measurements of immunoglobulin G and albumin in both serum and CSF, from which synthesis rate may be calculated. The formulas for this calculation are not standardized across different laboratories, and the test does not add to clinical sensitivity or specificity for an MS diagnosis (Table 13.2).

A more recently developed test, which measures kappa immunoglobulin free light chains, appears to be a suitable alternative to OCB testing, with quantitative results reported within 20 minutes, at lower cost, and without the need for a paired serum specimen. In a cohort of 683 patients, a CSF concentration of kappa immunoglobulin free light chains of 0.100 mg/dL or higher had a sensitivity of 67% and specificity of 86% for detection of MS. The OCB and kappa immunoglobulin free light chain tests had comparable performance, with no significant differences between them ($P=.08$).

KEY POINTS

- The McDonald criteria for MS were revised in 2017 and now incorporate the detection of unique CSF OCB into the criteria for diagnosis of relapsing-remitting MS. Their presence may substitute for the dissemination in time criterion.

- The test for OCB with a cutoff of 2 unique CSF bands has a clinical sensitivity of approximately 74% and clinical specificity of 88% for detection of MS and requires a paired serum specimen for analysis.

- Other quantitative CSF tests are frequently ordered in combination with OCB testing. The CSF kappa free light chain concentration is a comparable marker to OCB, with a sensitivity of 67% and specificity of 86% for detection of MS.

A GIRL WITH BACK PAIN, PARESTHESIAS, AND PAINFUL VISION LOSS

Cecilia Zivelonghi, MD, and Andrew McKeon, MB, BCh, MD

CASE PRESENTATION

HISTORY AND EXAMINATION

A 12-year-old girl sought care for subacute onset of cramping back pain, along with paresthesias in her lower limbs up to the waistline, both hands, upper back, and chest, followed by rapidly progressive (over a few hours) painful vision loss affecting initially the right eye with subsequent involvement of the left eye. She underwent neuroophthalmologic evaluation and was diagnosed with bilateral optic neuritis. A positive Lhermitte sign was also present.

Brain magnetic resonance imaging (MRI) showed T2 hyperintensity and mild swelling of both optic nerves with chiasmatic involvement and a single small focus of nonenhancing T2-signal abnormality in the left frontal lobe. Spinal cord MRI showed a longitudinal, T2-hyperintense, central lesion extending from the foramen magnum through the T4 spinal level, associated with diffuse patchy enhancement after gadolinium administration. Cerebrospinal fluid (CSF) analysis was remarkable for slightly increased protein concentration (52 mg/dL; reference range, ≤35 mg/dL). She was treated with intravenous methylprednisolone (500 mg every 12 hours for 3 days, followed by oral tapering over 2 weeks) with gradual improvement of vision in the left eye, although the right eye remained severely impaired.

One month later, the patient had development of left-sided hemiparesis and ataxia, rapidly followed by worsening encephalopathy and ultimately coma. CSF analysis showed neutrophil-predominant leukocytosis (69 white blood cells/μL; reference range, ≤5/μL), protein value of 295 mg/dL, normal immunoglobulin G (IgG) index, and no oligoclonal bands. Brain MRI showed extensive, bihemispheric, white matter changes and multiple cerebellar lesions. Because of further clinical worsening with decreased pupillary reaction, decreased heart rate, and systemic hypertension suggestive of increased intracranial pressure, a cerebral white matter biopsy was performed, which showed changes consistent with demyelination.

The patient was diagnosed with probable acute disseminated encephalomyelitis (ADEM) and treated with intravenous immunoglobulin and corticosteroids (intravenous methylprednisolone and dexamethasone), with improvement. She subsequently had 5 additional relapses characterized by myelitis (always longitudinally extensive), optic neuritis, and 1 episode of intractable nausea and vomiting. She was diagnosed with multiple sclerosis (MS) and started on interferon beta, without benefit. Four of these relapses occurred while she was receiving interferon beta therapy.

Two years after the patient's first episode, her family sought a second opinion for their daughter. Despite numerous episodes, she was still able to walk without aid, although she had a broad-based gait. She was blind in the right eye, and visual acuity was markedly decreased in the left eye.

The first diagnostic consideration in this child with encephalopathy and extensive central nervous system (CNS) demyelination was ADEM. However, a monophasic course is typical of ADEM, and a relapsing course with recurrent optic neuritis and myelitis should prompt other considerations. Other processes considered for this patient were myelin oligodendrocyte glycoprotein (MOG) antibody–associated demyelinating disorder, MS (because of the relapsing course), γ-aminobutyric acid$_A$ receptor autoimmunity, and neuromyelitis optica spectrum disorders (NMOSD), or aquaporin-4 (AQP4) autoimmunity, which was the main consideration.

A careful review of the previously performed MRI showed several new lesions appearing over time, often contrast enhancing, concurrent with clinical relapses and leading to progressive accumulation of lesions in the brain and spinal cord. The lesions showed only limited resolution after

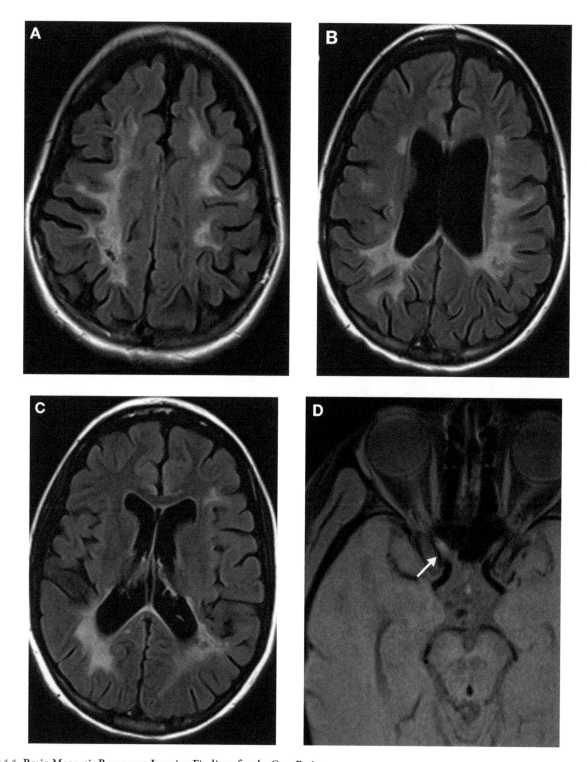

Figure 14.1 Brain Magnetic Resonance Imaging Findings for the Case Patient.
A-C, Axial, fluid-attenuated inversion recovery images at 3 levels show bilateral confluent white matter lesions. D, Axial, T1, postgadolinium image demonstrates focal enhancement of the right optic nerve (arrow).

therapy, and after 2 years of illness, marked cerebral atrophy was already evident. On the last brain MRI, T2-hyperintense confluent lesions were evident in both cerebral hemispheres, with increasing areas of cystic degeneration prominent in frontal lobes and corpus callosum (Figure 14.1). The spinal cord showed diffuse T2-signal abnormalities from foramen magnum to the level of T6, without gadolinium enhancement (Figure 14.2).

TESTING

The patient was tested for AQP4-IgG autoantibodies, which were positive in both serum and CSF.

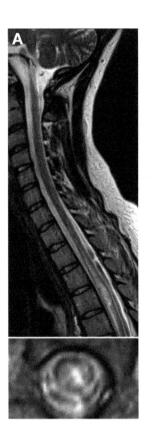
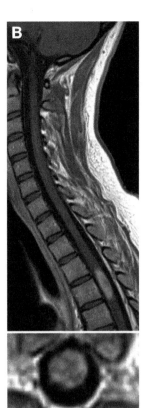

Figure 14.2 **Spinal Cord Magnetic Resonance Imaging Findings for the Case Patient.**

A, T2-weighted images show a well-demarcated, longitudinally extensive lesion from T2 to T5 (top, sagittal) and the same lesion at the T4 level involving gray matter (bottom, axial). B, T1 postgadolinium images show a ringlike pattern of enhancement at the T4 level in sagittal (top) and axial (bottom) views.

DIAGNOSIS

A diagnosis of AQP4-IgG–positive neuromyelitis optica (NMO) was made.

MANAGEMENT

The patient was treated with rituximab (anti-CD20 monoclonal antibody) and became episode-free, with no further accumulation of disability.

DISCUSSION

The discovery of AQP4-IgG in 2004 has permitted the distinction of NMOSD from other inflammatory CNS disorders. AQP4-IgG represents a highly specific biomarker for NMO (almost 100% using molecular-based techniques), with sensitivity of approximately 80%. According to the most recent diagnostic criteria published in 2015, a diagnosis of NMOSD can also be made for patients who are AQP4-IgG seronegative by any testing method, regardless of assay sensitivity, provided that more stringent clinical and radiologic requirements are met. Serial testing is recommended for these patients because late seroconversion has been described up to 4 years after the first episode.

Optic neuritis in patients with NMO, compared with MS, is severe, is more frequently bilateral, shows incomplete recovery after treatment, and tends to involve the posterior pathway, with typical involvement of the optic chiasm. Transverse myelitis in NMO is characterized by severe bilateral motor impairment and sensory loss, tonic spasms, and Lhermitte sign. Spinal cord MRI typically shows longitudinally extensive lesions (by definition involving more than 3 consecutive vertebral segments); in pediatric patients, more than 10 vertebral segments may be affected. This sign is less specific in children than in adults with NMO, however, because longitudinal spinal lesions are also common in myelitis of pediatric MS. Lesions that extend through the foramen magnum and into the medulla are suggestive of NMO. Axial MRI generally shows central spinal cord T2 hyperintensity with prominent involvement of gray matter. Gadolinium enhancement can be patchy or ringlike.

Brain disorders are more common in pediatric AQP4 autoimmunity than among affected adults and may initially mimic ADEM or MS. Area postrema syndrome, with intractable nausea, vomiting, and hiccups, occurs as the initial manifestation in 12% of patients with CNS AQP4 autoimmunity and is due to inflammation of the floor of the fourth ventricle, which is enriched with AQP4. Other clinicoradiologic syndromes include brainstem encephalitis; diencephalic, thalamic, or hypothalamic disorders; and cerebral syndromes.

In the differential diagnosis of encephalopathy and extensive CNS demyelination, MOG antibody–associated demyelinating disorder should be considered, especially in children, because encephalitis and optic neuritis are the most common presentations. Other manifestations include transverse longitudinally extensive myelitis (often involving conus-cauda segment) and meningoencephalitis. MOG-IgG–associated disorder follows a monophasic course in 50% of cases. Serial testing for MOG-IgG may help predict relapsing course in patients with a persistently high IgG titer. Unlike in our case patient, episodes of MOG autoimmunity, although often relapsing, are generally accompanied by recovery or near-recovery between episodes.

MS was also considered in the case patient because of the relapsing course. Several elements of this patient's case, however, were atypical for MS: 1) the persistent absence of oligoclonal bands in the CSF with normal IgG index; 2) the severity of clinical episodes with poor recovery; 3) the recurrence of longitudinally extensive transverse myelitis; 4) bilateral or sequential optic neuritis and episodes while receiving MS disease-modifying treatment; and 5) marked CSF pleocytosis with more than 50 white blood cells/μL with predominance of neutrophils.

γ-Aminobutyric acid$_A$ receptor autoimmunity should also be considered in the differential diagnosis of a suspected autoimmune encephalopathy with white matter lesions in children. However, in addition to encephalopathy, patients generally experience drug-resistant seizures, whereas myelitis and optic neuritis do not occur.

NMOSD (AQP4 autoimmunity) typically presents with recurrent, severe episodes of longitudinally extensive transverse myelitis and optic neuritis with often simultaneous (or sequential) involvement of both optic nerves. Encephalopathy and other brain symptoms are common in children. CSF testing typically shows an absence of oligoclonal bands (which are found only in 30% of patients) and pleocytosis (100-200 cells/μL), generally lymphocytic (about 75%), although predominance of neutrophils or eosinophils may also be seen.

It is essential to distinguish between AQP4 autoimmunity and other inflammatory diseases of the CNS, especially MS and MOG-IgG–associated disorder, because of the distinct therapeutic and prognostic profiles. Preventive therapy for MS may be ineffective or even harmful for patients with AQP4-IgG autoimmunity. After the diagnosis is established, even after 1 clinical episode with a positive AQP4 antibody test, long-term immunosuppression is strongly recommended to prevent long-term disability owing to the high risk of relapses with incomplete recovery. Of note, long-term disability, in general, is significantly higher for pediatric AQP4 autoimmunity than for MS, ADEM, and MOG autoimmunity. Disability accumulation tends to be stepwise and episode related—hence, the importance of preventing episodes with long-term immunosuppression.

For acute episodes, it is recommended to start intravenous methylprednisolone at a dose of 20 to 30 mg/kg (no more than 1 g) for 5 days, followed by 5 to 7 cycles of plasma exchange if no improvement is seen or in case of worsening. Long-term immunosuppressive treatment options include the US Food and Drug Administration–approved treatments (as of 2019-2020) eculizumab (anti-C5 complement cascade inhibitor), inebilizumab (anti-CD19 B-cell and plasmablast suppressor), and satralizumab (anti-interleukin-6 receptor), as well as trusted options such as rituximab, azathioprine, and mycophenolate mofetil.

KEY POINTS

- The presence of AQP4-IgG helps distinguish NMOSD from other inflammatory CNS disorders of childhood.

- The spectrum of pediatric NMO includes optic neuritis, myelitis, and encephalitides.

- Long-term immunosuppression is required for patients with AQP4-IgG–positive NMO, including after 1 clinical episode.

A SEPTUAGENARIAN WITH PROGRESSIVE HEMIPARESIS

Roman Kassa, MD, and B. Mark Keegan, MD

CASE PRESENTATION

HISTORY AND EXAMINATION

A 78-year-old man with no pertinent medical history sought care for an 18-month history of progressive right lower extremity weakness, gait impairment, and falls. He had started to use a cane 6 months after symptom onset and eventually required a scooter for mobility. Six months before seeking care, he noticed development of right upper extremity weakness. He had symptoms of neurogenic bladder dysfunction with urinary frequency and reduced bladder emptying. On neurologic examination, he had a hemiparetic gait. He had normal higher cognitive function and cranial nerve function. Motor examination showed decreased bulk of the right hand muscles with no fasciculations, mild spasticity of the right leg, and right hemiparesis with an upper motor neuron pattern. Deep tendon reflexes were brisk throughout his limbs, and he had an extensor plantar reflex (Babinski sign) on the right side. He had impaired vibratory sense at the toes, with otherwise normal sensory and coordination examinations. Diagnoses considered at the time are shown in Table 15.1.

TESTING

Serologic studies were negative for syphilis, screening for human T-lymphotropic virus 1 or 2 antibody was negative, and he had normal levels of vitamin B_{12} and ceruloplasmin. Postvoid residual urine volume was less than 50 mL, and urinalysis showed no evidence of urinary tract infection. Electrophysiologic studies with nerve conduction studies and needle electromyography showed no evidence of motor neuron disease, chronic right C8 radiculopathy, or sensory axonal peripheral neuropathy. Magnetic resonance imaging (MRI) of the brain showed ovoid periventricular and punctate subcortical and deep white matter T2 hyperintense foci (Figure 15.1A). Some of these had corresponding T1 hypointensity (Figure 15.1B). MRI of the cervical spine showed 1 eccentrically located T2 hyperintense lesion over the right lateral aspect of C2 (Figure 15.2A and 15.2B). None of the lesions were enhancing (Figure 15.2C). MRI of the thoracic spinal cord showed no signal changes.

Table 15.1 **DIFFERENTIAL DIAGNOSIS FOR CASE PATIENT**

POSSIBLE DIAGNOSIS	HELPFUL TESTS AND FINDINGS
Compressive myelopathy	Neuroimaging of the spinal cord to assess for compressive cause
Subacute combined degeneration	Sensory ataxia, serum vitamin B_{12} level, pernicious anemia evaluation (methylmalonic acid and gastrin), neuroimaging of the spinal cord to assess for dorsal column signal abnormality
Copper deficiency	Previous bariatric surgery, sensory ataxia, serum copper, ceruloplasmin, neuroimaging of the brain and spinal cord to assess for dorsal column signal abnormality
Motor neuron disease	Examination findings of upper and/or lower motor neuron dysfunction, fasciculations, fibrillations on needle electromyography
HTLV-1/2–associated myelopathy	Serum and CSF antibody testing
Arteriovenous dural fistula	Fluctuating weakness, stepwise progression, spinal catheter angiography to assess for fistula

Abbreviations: CSF, cerebrospinal fluid; HTLV-1/2, human T-lymphotropic virus 1 or 2.

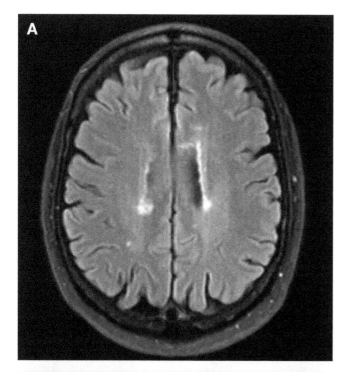

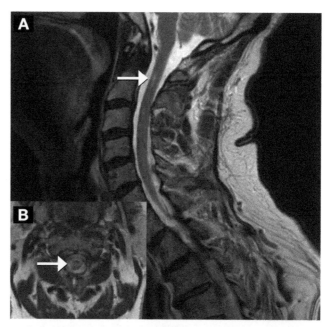

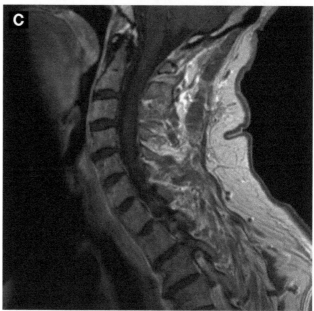

Figure 15.2 **Magnetic Resonance Imaging of the Cervical Spine.**
A and B, T2 sagittal (A) and axial (B) images show 1 eccentrically located T2 hyperintense lesion over the right lateral aspect of C2 (arrows). C, On T1 axial, postgadolinium imaging, none of the lesions demonstrated enhancement.

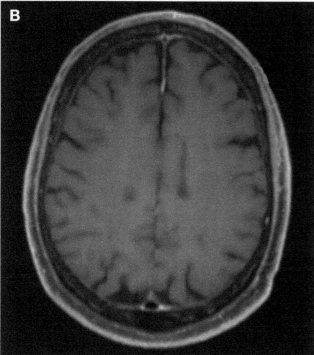

Figure 15.1 **Brain Magnetic Resonance Imaging Findings for Case Patient.**
A, T2 axial image demonstrates ovoid periventricular and punctate subcortical and deep white matter T2 hyperintense foci. B, On T1 axial imaging, some of the foci in panel A had corresponding T1 hypointensity.

Cerebrospinal fluid analysis showed no pleocytosis, an increased protein concentration of 66 mg/dL (reference range, ≤35 mg/dL), and 4 unique oligoclonal bands. Neural antibody testing for paraneoplastic disorders was negative.

DIAGNOSIS

A diagnosis of primary progressive multiple sclerosis (MS), very late onset, was made.

MANAGEMENT

With any diagnosis of late-onset MS (LOMS), a decision about whether MS disease-modifying agents are indicated should be carefully considered. Our older patient had a progressive disease course, and neuroimaging studies did not reveal evidence of active disease. Based on this, a decision was made to monitor him clinically and radiologically. Management of spasticity with regular daily stretching exercises was discussed with him.

In general, a multidisciplinary team approach is often needed in patients with MS to adequately address various symptoms. He was referred to specialists in physical medicine and rehabilitation with regard to strengthening and stretching exercises, balance training, assessment of current gait aids, and occupational therapy approaches to his dominant hand weakness. For symptoms of neurogenic bladder, the patient was referred for urologic consultation, and oxybutynin, an anticholinergic drug, was recommended.

DISCUSSION

A first clinical manifestation of MS can occur at a later-than-typical age. Most studies consider an onset at age 50 years or older to be LOMS, whereas first symptoms occurring at age 60 years or older are commonly referred to as *very late–onset MS* (VLOMS). In patients with onset at adolescence and young adulthood, a female-to-male ratio of 3.25:1 has been reported. In contrast, a decrease of this ratio in patients with LOMS approaching 1:1 to 1.4:1 has been described. Various population-based studies have reported a wide range of prevalence of 1.1% to 12% for LOMS and a much lower prevalence of 0.3% to 1.33% for VLOMS.

Initial motor symptoms and spinal cord lesions are more common in patients with VLOMS compared with typical MS, with optic neuritis substantially less frequent. Moreover, an increased risk of progressive disease and resultant disability has been reported. This appears to be independent of the duration of disease and number of relapses. Diagnostic challenges in VLOMS include, at times, confounding signal changes on brain MRI due to underlying comorbid conditions leading to small vessel disease.

With aging, marked functional and quantitative changes in the adaptive and innate immune system have been described. The use of disease-modifying agents in this context has been associated with a slightly increased risk of cancer and opportunistic infections. Infection risks include progressive multifocal leukoencephalopathy with use of natalizumab, fingolimod, and dimethyl fumarate, as well as cryptococcal meningitis with fingolimod.

KEY POINTS

- MS can present with first clinical symptoms after age 50 years.

- LOMS and VLOMS commonly present with motor symptoms, less often with optic neuritis.

- LOMS and VLOMS are more likely than young-onset MS to have a balanced sex ratio, less-complete recovery from clinical episodes, and progressive disease.

- In these older patients, the decision to initiate disease-modifying therapy should include consideration of the increased risk of opportunistic infections and attenuated tumor surveillance.

RECURRENT DEMYELINATING EPISODES

I. Vanessa Marin Collazo, MD

CASE PRESENTATION

HISTORY AND EXAMINATION

A 28-year-old woman with a history of migraine, type 2 diabetes, irritable bowel syndrome, and mild anxiety sought care for right monocular painful vision loss presenting over 3 days. Two years earlier, she had had back paresthesias for 1 week which were triggered by flexion of the neck suggestive of Lhermitte sign. She also reported intermittent bilateral arm paresthesias for 2 years. She had almost daily headaches, treated with naproxen daily. She reported no bladder, bowel, or sexual dysfunction or episodes of vertigo, diplopia, or unexplained nausea, vomiting, or hiccups.

Findings on neurologic examination, including visual acuity, color vision, pupillary response to light, eye movements, tone, power, coordination, reflexes, and sensation, were normal.

TESTING

Magnetic resonance imaging (MRI) of the brain revealed multifocal T2 fluid-attenuated inversion recovery white matter hyperintensities throughout the brainstem, cerebellum, and bilateral periventricular, subcortical, and juxtacortical areas (Figure 16.1A-D). MRI of the cervical and thoracic spinal cord showed intramedullary cord signal T2 hyperintensities peripherally located at C1 and on the left side at C3-C4 (Figure 16.1E and F). Thoracic spinal cord signal was unremarkable. Cerebrospinal fluid evaluation was not performed.

Results of testing for HIV antibodies, antinuclear antibody, antibodies to extractable nuclear antigens, complete blood cell count, kidney function, tuberculosis, and serum levels of vitamin B_{12}, thyrotropin, and liver enzymes were all normal or negative. Total serum 25-hydroxyvitamin D level was 54 ng/mL.

DIAGNOSIS

The patient was diagnosed with relapsing-remitting multiple sclerosis (MS) with activity on the basis of her clinical presentation and MRI findings.

MANAGEMENT

She received comprehensive education about the disease and the role of disease-modifying therapy (DMT) to decrease the risk of further clinical and radiographic activity. After discussion of the risks and benefits of the various agents, the patient started treatment with dimethyl fumarate 240 mg orally, twice per day (480 mg/d). Oral vitamin D_3 supplementation was recommended at 2,000 IU/d. Healthy lifestyle changes, including maintaining a healthy diet, normal weight range, regular exercise, and sleep hygiene were recommended.

DISCUSSION

DMTs for relapsing-remitting MS are primarily used to reduce the occurrence of clinical relapses and the appearance of new T2 or enhancing lesions on MRI of the brain and spine. Long-term treatment with DMT is associated with lower morbidity and mortality rates. Currently, over 20 medications are approved by the US Food and Drug Administration to treat relapsing-remitting MS.

Considerations when starting DMT include the medication's efficacy, safety profile, formulation, and dosing and the patient's pregnancy considerations, comorbid conditions, age, disability status, and preferences. A summary of the adverse effect profile of commonly used medications is shown in Table 16.1.

The medications with the greatest efficacy are the infusion medications, including natalizumab, ocrelizumab, and alemtuzumab. Alemtuzumab has US Food and Drug Administration approval to be used only after 2 other agents have been shown to be ineffective. Therefore, if efficacy is the priority, ocrelizumab or natalizumab should be considered first-line.

Patients should be tested for antibodies to JC polyoma virus before starting natalizumab. The risk of progressive multifocal leukoencephalopathy (PML) with natalizumab is increased in patients who are positive for JC polyoma virus antibodies. Fingolimod tends to be the best tolerated of the oral medications but is associated with macular edema in patients with a history of diabetes or uveitis and requires first-dose cardiac monitoring because of bradycardia. A few cases

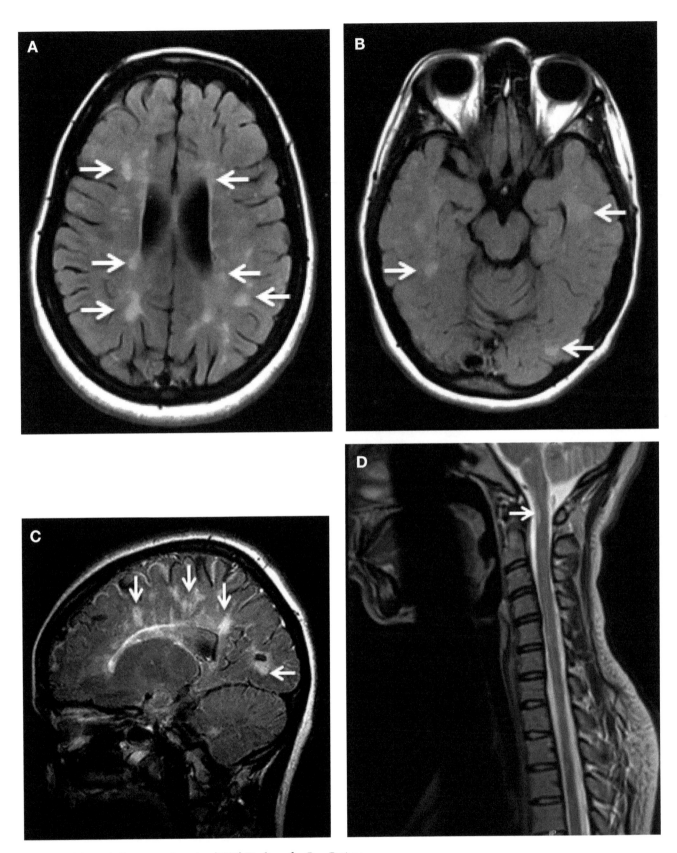

Figure 16.1 **Magnetic Resonance Imaging (MRI) Findings for Case Patient.**
A-C, Axial and sagittal MRI views of the brain show multifocal T2 fluid-attenuated inversion recovery hyperintensities throughout the brainstem, left side of the cerebellum, and right-sided predominant temporal and bilateral periventricular, subcortical, and juxtacortical areas (arrows). D-G, Axial and sagittal MRI of the cervical and thoracic spinal cord demonstrates intramedullary cord signal T2 hyperintensities eccentrically located on the right at ventral C1 (D and E) and left-sided at C3-C4 (F) (arrows). Thoracic spinal cord signal was unremarkable (G).

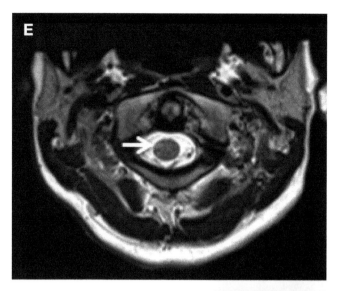

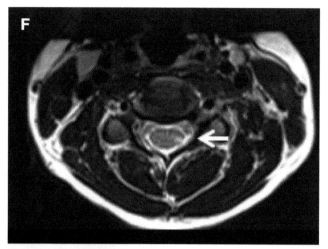

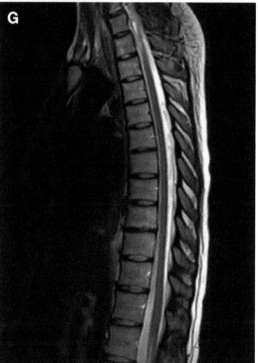

Figure 16.1 **Continued**

of PML have been associated with each of the oral medications. If the patient intends to become pregnant soon after starting DMT, her options would be to remain off therapy until pregnancy is completed or to start a DMT that is known to be safe during pregnancy. Teriflunomide should be avoided in patients who have the potential to become pregnant. The only relapse-preventing DMTs known to be safe during pregnancy are glatiramer acetate and interferon beta.

If ease of use is a priority, oral medications should be considered, including fingolimod, dimethyl fumarate, and teriflunomide. Of these medications, fingolimod is likely to be more effective than dimethyl fumarate. Teriflunomide has a similar efficacy to interferon medications, which is lower than that of fingolimod and dimethyl fumarate.

If long-term safety is the primary consideration, use of the injectable medications, including glatiramer acetate and interferon medications, should be considered. These medications have the longest safety profile, with interferon beta medications being on the market since 1993. These medications require self-injection, however, and have the lowest efficacy of the available DMTs. They have not been associated with PML.

Table 16.1 | COMMON ADVERSE EFFECTS OF MULTIPLE SCLEROSIS DMTS

DMT	FORMULATION	COMMON ADVERSE REACTIONS	OTHER CONSIDERATIONS
Interferon beta	Injectable	Flulike symptoms (myalgias, chills, headache, and fatigue), injection-site reactions, liver toxicity, thyroid disorder, lymphopenia	Variable dosing frequencies, depending on the agent
Glatiramer acetate	Injectable	Injection-site reactions, lipoatrophy, postinjection reactions with palpitations, flushing, diaphoresis, shortness of breath, chest pain	No drug monitoring required
Teriflunomide	Oral	Hair thinning/loss, hypertension, peripheral neuropathy, headache, nausea, diarrhea, liver toxicity, lymphopenia Highly teratogenic	Accelerated elimination protocol with activated charcoal is required if there is a suspicion of drug-induced liver injury, pregnancy, or a desire to conceive
Dimethyl fumarate	Oral	Flushing, abdominal pain, nausea, diarrhea, liver toxicity, lymphopenia, PML	Flushing and abdominal pain can be treated with concurrent aspirin use
Fingolimod	Oral	Bradycardia with first dose, macular edema, headache, herpes and cryptococcal infection, PML, cutaneous cancers, lymphopenia, liver toxicity, rebound after stopping medication	Macular edema is more common in patients with diabetes or uveitis
Siponimod	Oral	Bradycardia with first dose, macular edema, headache, herpes and cryptococcal infection, PML, cutaneous cancers, lymphopenia, liver toxicity	
Natalizumab	IV	Infusion-related reactions, liver toxicity, melanoma, lymphoma, herpes, fungal, and bacterial infections, PML, rebound after stopping medication	Requires regular tests for JC polyoma virus antibodies and MRI monitoring
Ocrelizumab	IV	Infusion-related reactions, herpes infection, PML, reactivation of hepatitis B, cancers	
Cladribine	Oral	Lymphopenia, PML, rash, hepatitis B and C activation, alopecia, cancers	Cancer risk is much higher than with other DMTs
Alemtuzumab	IV	Infusion-related reactions, anaphylaxis, autoimmunity, cancers, herpes and listeria infections	Substantial risk of treatment-related autoimmune disorders, including a 30% risk of autoimmune thyroid disease

Abbreviations: DMT, disease-modifying therapy; IV, intravenous; MRI, magnetic resonance imaging; PML, progressive multifocal leukoencephalopathy.

KEY POINTS

- DMTs for MS reduce the risk of both relapses and new T2 lesions on MRI of the brain and spine.

- Treatment efficacy, safety profile, formulation, dosing, pregnancy, comorbid conditions, age, disability status, and patient preference should be considered when initiating DMT for MS.

BREAKTHROUGH DISEASE WHILE ON MULTIPLE SCLEROSIS IMMUNOMODULATORY THERAPY

Jonathan L. Carter, MD

CASE PRESENTATION

HISTORY AND EXAMINATION

A 36-year-old woman with a history of relapsing-remitting multiple sclerosis (MS) was evaluated for new MS symptoms accompanied by new, enhancing, white matter lesions on brain magnetic resonance imaging (MRI). Her MS presented with Lhermitte sign when she was 24 years old, but she did not undergo MRI at that time. She had onset of bilateral lower extremity and left upper extremity tingling at age 26 years. MRI and cerebrospinal fluid examination at the time were supportive of the diagnosis of MS, and disease-modifying therapy was recommended by her neurologist but declined by the patient. She initiated therapy with dimethyl fumarate at age 30 years after several further relapses. She did well initially on this medication without symptoms of a new MS relapse, but surveillance MRI showed new gadolinium-enhancing lesions on brain MRI on each of 3 consecutive yearly scans.

She had an episode of possible mild optic neuritis while taking dimethyl fumarate 1 year before the current visit. At the current visit, she reported new worsening of lower extremity numbness, weakness, and imbalance. Brain MRI showed 1 new enhancing lesion. Neurologic examination showed hyperreflexia in lower extremities, patchy decreased pinprick from knees distally, reduced vibration sense in the toes, and difficulty with tandem gait.

In considering the differential diagnosis, several factors were appreciated. The patient had new or worsening neurologic deficits lasting at least 24 hours, which were not explained by concurrent illness or fever, hence meeting the operational definitions for an MS relapse. This was further confirmed by new disease activity on MRI. Given these factors, it is unlikely that another disease process would explain her clinical picture. However, patients with MS can have transient worsening of neurologic symptoms with heat exposure, fever, infection, or other concurrent medical conditions (termed *pseudorelapse*). This is more common in patients with progressive MS with more severe neurologic deficits than in this case. Pseudorelapses usually last less than 24 hours and do not become progressively more severe over a period of days, unlike true MS relapses. They usually improve rapidly once the triggering factor is corrected. New MS relapses can also be triggered by infections, especially viral infections, and may require treatment if deficits persist beyond treatment of the infectious trigger.

TESTING

Urine culture and sensitivity tests were performed to rule out occult urinary tract infection; results of this testing were negative. MRI of the brain concurrently showed new enhancing white matter lesions (Figure 17.1).

DIAGNOSIS

The patient was diagnosed with clinical and radiographic breakthrough disease activity while receiving therapy for MS.

MANAGEMENT

New relapses of MS can be treated with high-dose corticosteroids (methylprednisolone 500-1,000 mg/d), oral or intravenous, for 3 to 5 days. Although such treatment has been shown to speed recovery from MS relapses, currently there is no convincing evidence that treatment enhances recovery 1 year after the relapse. Plasmapheresis can be used for treatment of severe, corticosteroid-refractory relapses, and this intervention has been shown to reduce long-term disability resulting from a relapse. Importantly, breakthrough disease activity while on therapy, whether symptomatic or asymptomatic, has been associated with an increased risk of disability progression over the long term, especially when this involves new spinal cord lesions.

The patient was treated with 5 days of intravenous methylprednisolone for her relapse. After discussion with the patient, it was decided to transition therapy from dimethyl fumarate to ocrelizumab infusions for her breakthrough disease

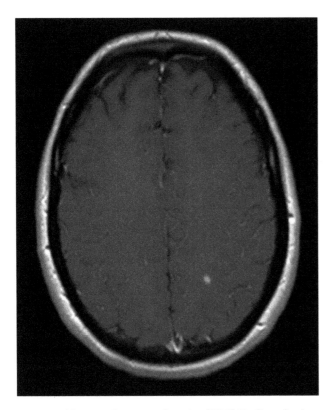

Figure 17.1 **Magnetic Resonance Imaging (MRI) Findings for the Case Patient.**
MRI of the brain in a patient taking dimethyl fumarate for multiple sclerosis shows a new gadolinium-enhancing lesion in the left parietal white matter.

activity. This decision was further supported by the patient's concerns that she might be entering an early progressive phase of the disease.

DISCUSSION

In patients with spinal-predominant MS, or with symptoms potentially indicating new spinal cord involvement, it may be necessary to include spinal cord imaging to assess for new disease activity. Whether routine spinal cord imaging in addition to brain imaging should be done for surveillance purposes is controversial. When possible, MRI should be performed with and without contrast unless there is a contraindication to contrast. Testing for occult infection or other medical conditions may be indicated if there is the possibility of a pseudorelapse.

Several publications have attempted to define objective measures of treatment failure in MS, but most have not been validated prospectively. The concept of *NEDA* (no evidence of disease activity) has been borrowed from the rheumatology literature and proposed as a target for MS therapy. Various definitions of NEDA exist, but the most commonly used term, *NEDA-3*, is defined as 1) no clinical relapses, 2) no clinical evidence of disease progression, and 3) no new or enlarging T2/fluid-attenuated inversion recovery (FLAIR) or gadolinium-enhancing white matter lesions

on MRI. *NEDA-4* includes measures of brain atrophy along with the above.

Rates of achieving NEDA with current MS therapies vary widely, and none of the available MS therapies have been reported to exceed a rate of 70% NEDA over a 2-year treatment period. NEDA is usually determined post hoc from pivotal clinical trials of MS disease-modifying therapies, with varying definitions of NEDA. To date, NEDA has not been a primary outcome measure for any MS clinical trials, so it has not been validated as a reliable, sensitive, primary outcome measure. Although the idea of "treat to target" is appealing for MS therapies, the current reality is that NEDA is most likely an unrealistic target for current therapies, especially for long-term treatment beyond the duration of typical clinical trials. Because *therapy failure* is more likely to be determined on the basis of new MRI activity (vs new clinical activity), some MS experts have proposed accepting the goal of *minimal evidence of disease activity*, with tolerance for a few new, small, T2/FLAIR-hyperintense lesions during therapy as long as there are no enhancing lesions and the patient is clinically stable. The frequency of optimal MRI surveillance during active treatment is also not clearly defined, but many clinicians use yearly scans as a convenient benchmark for monitoring therapy.

The decision of when to escalate MS therapy and which therapy to escalate to is complex and best reached in a shared decision-making model with the patient, considering their lifestyle, comorbid conditions, and risk tolerance for adverse events. Predictors of individual response to any MS therapy are lacking; there are no biomarkers or MRI signatures to help the clinician choose a therapy. In addition, relatively few MS trials have directly compared therapies in a head-to-head fashion, and most of these have compared older injectable therapies (eg, interferon beta, glatiramer acetate) with newer therapies. Combination therapy has not been adequately studied in MS and is currently cost prohibitive given the expense of individual MS disease-modifying therapies. Guidelines for escalating therapy in patients with early progressive disease are even less clearly defined than for relapsing MS.

KEY POINTS

- Patients with MS taking most current MS disease-modifying therapies still can have MRI activity and, less frequently, clinical disease activity.

- The threshold for determining both the occurrence of treatment failure during current therapy and when therapy should be switched is controversial for patients with relapsing forms of MS and undefined for patients with progressive forms of MS.

- The decision of when to switch therapy and which therapy to choose is best reached with shared decision making and considering the patient's unique characteristics.

HIGHLY ACTIVE MULTIPLE SCLEROSIS

Roman Kassa, MD, and W. Oliver Tobin, MB, BCh, BAO, PhD

CASE PRESENTATION

HISTORY AND EXAMINATION

A 16-year-old girl was evaluated for symptoms of thoracic myelitis with sensory loss below T12, gait difficulty, constipation, and incomplete bladder emptying. She had had 2 previous events. The first, at age 14 years, was thoracic myelitis with a T4 to T5 bandlike area of sensory loss, bilateral leg weakness, and Lhermitte sign, which resolved over 3 months. The second, at age 15 years, was light-headedness, episodic vomiting, and imbalance, which resolved after 6 weeks. Because of cognitive difficulties and problems keeping up with schoolwork since age 14 years, she had dropped out of school. She had a history of depression and polysubstance use disorders (tobacco, alcohol, and illicit drugs). On evaluation, she had a flat affect, normal cranial nerve function, and normal motor examination

findings. Deep tendon reflexes were symmetric, and plantar responses were flexor. She had a sensory level at T12 with diminished vibratory sense distal to the knees and normal coordination and gait. Diagnoses considered at the time are shown in Table 18.1.

TESTING

At initial evaluation at age 16 years, she had normal or negative findings for complete blood cell count, erythrocyte sedimentation rate, Lyme disease serologic testing, HIV, antinuclear antigen, extractable nuclear antigen, antineutrophil cytoplasmic antibody, antiphospholipid antibodies, and levels of liver enzymes, vitamin B_{12}, and folate. Magnetic resonance imaging of the brain, cervical spine, and thoracic spine showed a high burden of disease, with multiple enhancing lesions indicative of highly active disease (Figure 18.1, A-C, F-H). Spinal fluid analysis showed 16 white blood cells/μL (reference

Table 18.1 | DIFFERENTIAL DIAGNOSIS FOR CASE PATIENT

POSSIBLE DIAGNOSIS	CLINICAL & RADIOLOGIC FEATURES	TESTING FINDINGS
Multiple sclerosis	Subacute symptom onset, at least 24-hour duration, and no infection; examination findings consistent with optic neuropathy, internuclear ophthalmoplegia, or myelopathy; dissemination in space, dissemination in time	Unique CSF oligoclonal bands; optical coherence tomography demonstrating asymmetric thinning of the retinal nerve fiber layer; visual evoked potentials
Acute disseminated encephalomyelitis	Mostly pediatric age group; often monophasic, with preceding illness or vaccination; multifocal white matter, basal ganglia, thalamic, spinal cord lesions	±Serum MOG-IgG antibodies; CSF lymphocytic pleocytosis; absent oligoclonal bands
Neuromyelitis optica	African American/Asian/Latin American; optic neuritis with posterior optic pathway and chiasm involvement; longitudinally extensive myelitis; area postrema syndrome; other brainstem, diencephalic, or cerebral involvement; ± systemic autoimmunity	Serum AQP4-IgG antibodies (by cell-based assay); CSF WBC count >50/μL, neutrophil predominant; absence of oligoclonal bands; optical coherence tomography demonstrating severe unilateral or bilateral retinal nerve fiber layer thinning
MOG-IgG–associated disease	Optic neuritis; longitudinally extensive myelitis; brainstem lesions; encephalitis; anterior optic pathway involvement; perineural optic nerve sheath enhancement	Serum MOG-IgG antibodies; optical coherence tomography demonstrating unilateral or bilateral macular edema acutely, or retinal nerve fiber layer thinning in the chronic phase after an episode

Abbreviations: ±, with or without; APQ4-IgG, aquaporin-4 immunoglobulin G; CSF, cerebrospinal fluid; MOG-IgG, myelin oligodendrocyte glycoprotein immunoglobulin G; WBC, white blood cell.

range, 0-5/μL) with 95% lymphocytes; protein, 70 mg/dL (reference range, ≤35 mg/dL); 7 unique oligoclonal bands; and immunoglobulin G index, 0.87 (reference range, ≤0.85). Neurocognitive testing showed normal scores overall, and psychiatric evaluation indicated major depressive disorder.

DIAGNOSIS

She was given a diagnosis of relapsing-remitting multiple sclerosis (MS), highly active.

MANAGEMENT

On initial evaluation for thoracic myelitis when the patient was 16 years old, intravenous methylprednisolone 1,000 mg daily for 5 days was given, with resolution of bladder and bowel symptoms and 75% recovery of sensory loss. High-dose interferon beta-1a was then initiated. The patient underwent counseling for polysubstance use disorders and started pharmacologic antidepressant therapy and counseling with a mental health provider. In light of radiologic evidence of ongoing disease activity and adverse effects, interferon therapy was discontinued. Natalizumab was recommended. The patient was then lost to follow-up for 12 years, during which time she received short-term intravenous corticosteroids, glatiramer acetate, interferon beta-1b, and 3 doses of natalizumab.

At age 28 years, she came to Mayo Clinic with worsening left hemiparesis of 1 month's duration. She reported having had multiple relapses in the intervening years and slow cognitive decline. Neurologic examination showed word-finding difficulty, gaze-evoked horizontal nystagmus, moderate left-sided spastic hemiparesis in a pyramidal distribution, brisk reflexes with an extensor plantar response on the left, sensory ataxia in the left leg, and a hemiparetic gait. Neuroimaging findings at the time are shown in Figure 18.1 (D, E, I, and J). Intravenous methylprednisolone 1,000 mg/d for 5 days was given, with minimal improvement. She then received 7 sessions of plasmapheresis with about 50% recovery of power. The patient was seropositive for antibodies to JC polyoma virus.

Despite the increased risk of progressive multifocal leukoencephalopathy, natalizumab was reinitiated considering the even higher risk of long-term disability due to continued active disease (highly active MS [HAMS]). She switched to a different care provider, and her therapy was transitioned to teriflunomide. Six months later, at age 30 years, she returned to Mayo Clinic with new right leg weakness and received high-dose intravenous corticosteroids for 5 days, followed by rituximab infusion. On follow-up neuroimaging, breakthrough disease activity was noted, and her therapy was switched to alemtuzumab.

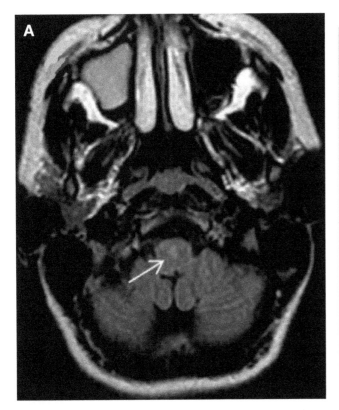
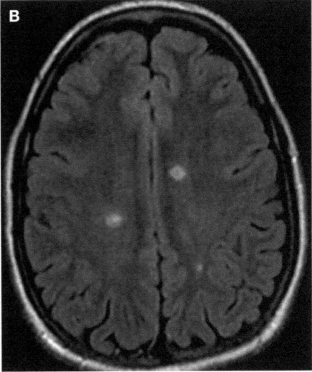

Figure 18.1 **Magnetic Resonance Imaging.**
Axial images of brain (T2, A, B, D, and E; T1 postgadolinium, F, G, I, and J) and spine (sagittal, C; axial, H) are shown. At initial presentation at age 16 years (panels A, B, C, F, G, and H), multiple enhancing lesions (arrows) and brainstem and spinal cord involvement (arrows) were observed. At follow-up at age 28 years (panels D, E, I, and J), imaging showed a high lesion burden (arrows) with cortical atrophy and ongoing gadolinium enhancement of lesions, indicating ongoing disease activity.

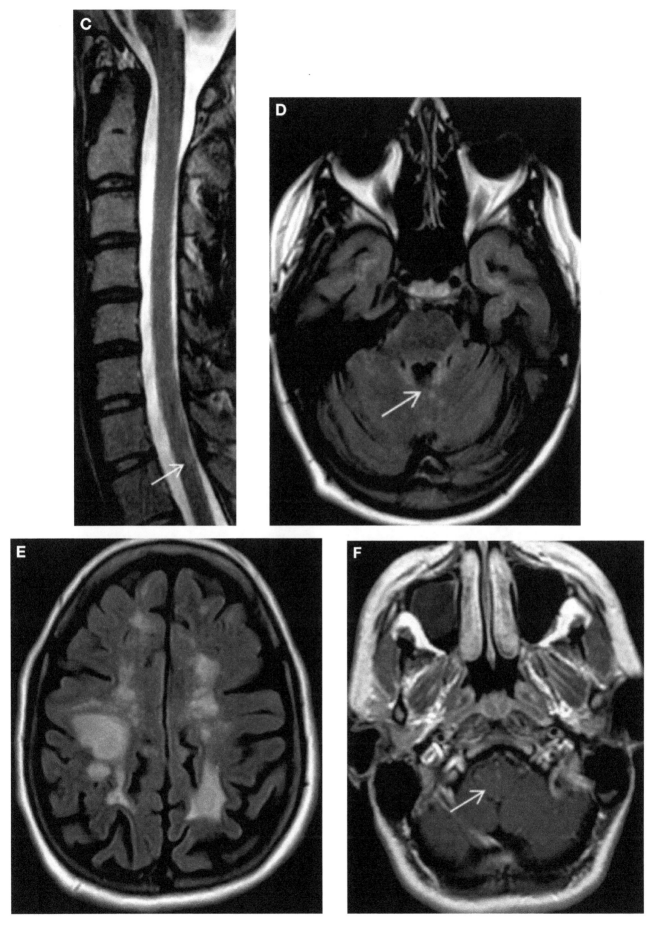

Figure 18.1 Continued

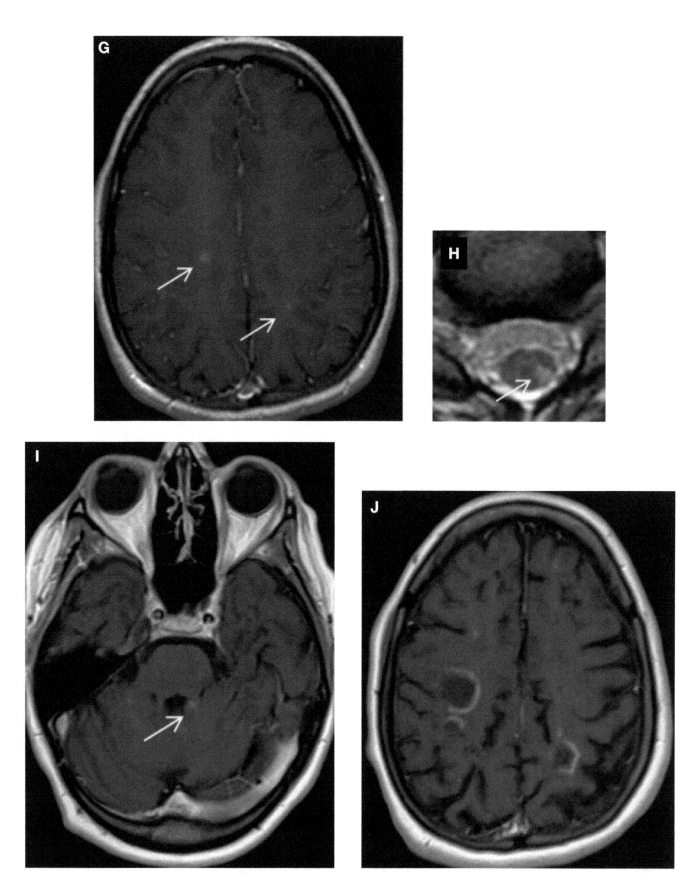

Figure 18.1 Continued

DISCUSSION

HAMS is characterized by frequent clinical episodes, with or without high disease activity on neuroimaging as evidenced by multiple enhancing lesions or interval new lesion formation, and disability accrual. It includes a spectrum of patients with clinical and radiologic evidence of ongoing disease activity who have no response to adequate treatment with MS disease-modifying therapy. There is no consensus definition of HAMS at present. In some studies, the criteria used to characterize HAMS have included at least 2 clinical relapses in the previous year, with at least 1 gadolinium-enhancing lesion on baseline magnetic resonance imaging, or inadequate response to disease-modifying therapy with 1 clinical episode in the previous year and radiologic evidence of disease activity. Various treatment algorithms have been proposed, but an individualized approach is often required. Considering that irreversible axonal damage and loss occur early in the course of relapsing-remitting MS, in this subgroup of patients with rapid accumulation of neurologic injury, early identification and institution of highly efficacious MS agents is warranted. Factors associated with poor prognosis include male sex; African American or Latin American ethnicity; age older than 40 years; clinical episode with motor, cerebellar, sphincter, or cognitive involvement; incomplete recovery from clinical episodes; short interepisode interval; and frequent relapses in the first 2 to 5 years.

The treatment approach for relapsing-remitting MS, in general, is controversial. Some advocate for a traditional escalation approach guided by clinical course, whereas others favor early aggressive treatment. To address this question, two randomized clinical trials (TREAT MS, NCT03500328 and DELIVER-MS, NCT03535298) are under way as of 2021. In patients with HAMS, considering the narrower window for effective treatment, early aggressive treatment is generally recommended. Natalizumab, ocrelizumab, alemtuzumab, and fingolimod are often used. The presence of JC polyoma virus antibodies in serum may dissuade a provider from using natalizumab in patients with HAMS. However, the risk of progressive multifocal encephalopathy within the first 2 years of treatment with natalizumab is less than 1 in 1,000 for all patients who have not previously received immunosuppressant medications, regardless of JC polyoma virus antibody status. The American Academy of Neurology practice guidelines from April 2018 give level B recommendations for treating HAMS with alemtuzumab, natalizumab, or fingolimod after careful consideration of the benefits vs risks for each patient. Off-label use of rituximab and cyclophosphamide may also be considered. In refractory cases, immunoablative therapy with very high doses of cyclophosphamide, followed by autologous hematopoietic stem cell transplant, may be explored.

In the case patient, considering the high disease activity on initial diagnosis and her premorbid history of depression, interferon beta-1a would not be an ideal first-line agent. Her medication intolerance and noncompliance, risk-averseness, cognitive deficits likely affecting health care decisions, and psychosocial issues were all barriers to optimal care. High-potency medications were required to control her clinical episodes, and she was stable when treated with either natalizumab or alemtuzumab, despite the risk of JC polyoma virus infection.

KEY POINTS

- Patients with HAMS require treatment with potent disease-modifying therapies and initial short follow-up intervals to monitor response.

- Poor prognostic factors include male sex; African American or Latin American ethnicity; age >40 years; clinical episode with motor, cerebellar, sphincter, or cognitive involvement; incomplete recovery from episodes; short interepisode interval; and frequent relapses in the first 2-5 years.

PROGRESSIVE GAIT DIFFICULTIES

I. Vanessa Marin Collazo, MD

CASE PRESENTATION

HISTORY AND EXAMINATION

A 58-year-old, right-handed man with a medical history of nephrolithiasis, essential hypertension, and type 2 diabetes sought care for a 6-year history of gait impairment. Initially, he noted subtle left foot and ankle weakness with associated falls that progressed over time. Orthopedic evaluations led to concern for left ankle ligamentous tears, for which he had surgery, with mild stabilization of symptoms. Two to 3 years later he again noted progressive left leg weakness and new arm weakness prompting the use of a cane to prevent falls. Subsequently, progressive pain developed on the soles of his feet in addition to edema with erythematous discoloration around the left ankle and foot. He reported 3 days of painless, unilateral, intermittent, mild visual blurriness in the past that had resolved spontaneously. He reported no past episodes of vertigo, diplopia, unexplained nausea, vomiting, or hiccups. He also disclosed no bladder, bowel, or sexual dysfunction.

On neurologic examination, pupillary response to light, eye movements, color vision, and visual acuity were normal in both eyes. He was found to have mild upper motor neuron pattern weakness in the left arm and leg, most pronounced in the left hand finger extensor and left hip flexion and abduction. Left patellar reflex was brisk, and there was an extensor Babinski sign on the left. There was mild reduction in pinprick sensation in both feet. His gait was spastic with left leg circumduction. Vibration sensation was normal, and Romberg sign was absent. Diagnoses considered at the time are shown in Box 19.1.

TESTING

Electromyography and nerve conduction studies were unremarkable. Magnetic resonance imaging (MRI) of the brain (Figure 19.1A) showed left-sided predominant periventricular and subcortical T2 fluid-attenuated inversion recovery hyperintensities. MRI of the cervical and thoracic spinal cord (Figure 19.1B and 19.1C) showed intramedullary cord T2 signal hyperintensities, eccentrically located on the left at C3,

C5, and C6, on the right at C7 to T1, and centrally at T4/T5 and T8/T9.

Cerebrospinal fluid analysis showed 37 red blood cells/μL (reference range, <5/μL), 4 white blood cells/μL (reference range, <5/μL), protein concentration of 66 mg/dL (reference range, 15-65 mg/dL), glucose value of 82 mg/dL (60% of plasma concentration), 9 unique oligoclonal bands (reference range, <2 bands), immunoglobulin G index, 1.14 (reference range, <0.85), and negative paraneoplastic autoantibodies.

Serum findings for vitamin B_{12}, copper, human T-lymphotropic virus, HIV, zinc, antinuclear antibodies, antibodies to extractable nuclear antigens, thyrotropin, liver enzymes, complete blood cell count, kidney function, and serum protein electrophoresis were normal. Total serum 25-hydroxyvitamin D level was 25 ng/mL (reference range, 25-80 ng/mL).

DIAGNOSIS

A diagnosis of primary progressive multiple sclerosis (MS) was made. The patient met the 2017 McDonald criteria for primary progressive MS (PPMS) by showing at least 1 year of disability progression; 1 or more T2

Box 19.1 | Differential Diagnosis for Progressive Myelopathy in the Case Patient

Multiple sclerosis (primary progressive and secondary progressive multiple sclerosis)

Compressive myelopathy

Subacute combined spine degeneration due to vitamin B_{12} deficiency

Copper deficiency myelopathy

Human T-lymphotropic virus myelopathy

HIV myelopathy

Spinal cord tumor

Spinal dural arteriovenous fistula

Amyotrophic lateral sclerosis

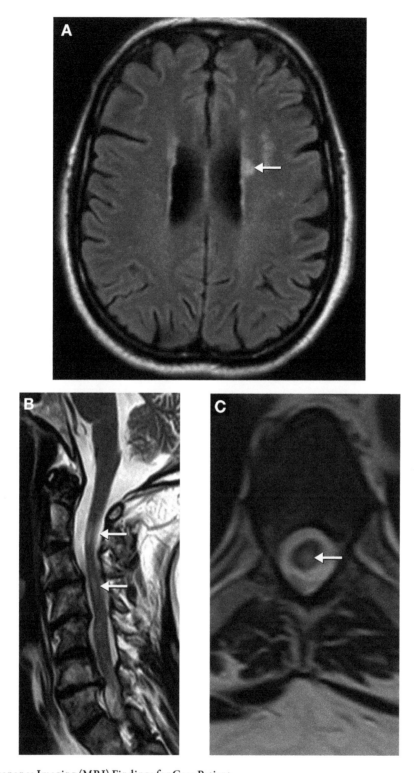

Figure 19.1 **Magnetic Resonance Imaging (MRI) Findings for Case Patient.**
A, Axial brain MRI shows T2 fluid-attenuated inversion recovery hyperintensities, including an ovoid periventricular lesion (arrow), typical of multiple sclerosis. B and C, MRI of the cervical spine shows multiple intramedullary cord T2 signal hyperintensities in sagittal view (B, arrows) and a centrally located intramedullary cord T2 signal hyperintensity at T4/T5 in axial view (C, arrow).

hyperintensities characteristic of MS in 1 or more of the following brain regions: periventricular, cortical, juxtacortical, and infratentorial; 2 or more T2 hyperintense lesions in the spinal cord; and the presence of cerebrospinal fluid–specific oligoclonal bands.

MANAGEMENT

After the diagnosis was confirmed and comprehensive education about the disease and the role of disease-modifying therapy (DMT) was discussed with the patient, he was started on ocrelizumab, every 6 months. Gabapentin was started at 300 mg/d and titrated up to 600 mg twice a day (1,200 mg/d) for management of painful foot paresthesias. Vitamin D$_3$ supplementation was started at 2,000 IU/d. Dalfampridine to aid in walking speed was offered, but the patient declined. Physical therapy was also initiated. Healthy lifestyle changes, including a healthy diet, healthy weight range, regular exercise, and sleep hygiene, were recommended.

DISCUSSION

MS is a chronic immune-mediated demyelinating disease of the central nervous system and is the leading cause of disability in the young population. Approximately 1 million people in the United States currently have MS. The usual age of disease onset is between 20 and 40 years. The clinical course is divided into 3 major types, including relapsing-remitting MS (RRMS), PPMS, and secondary progressive MS (SPMS). PPMS accounts for 10% to 15% of all cases of MS, with usual symptom onset in the 5th or 6th decade of life.

There is no cure for MS, but different DMTs for RRMS and 1 option for both SPMS and PPMS are available. The role of DMTs in RRMS is mainly to reduce the risk of relapse and accumulation of new T2 MRI lesions of the brain and spine, although their role in decreasing accumulation of disability and brain atrophy has been studied. The role of DMTs in PPMS and SPMS currently is to slow down the disability accumulation over time, in addition to reducing the risk of accumulation of T2 MRI lesions and brain atrophy. At present, ocrelizumab is the only available DMT approved for PPMS. Ocrelizumab is a humanized monoclonal antibody that selectively targets CD20, a cell-surface antigen that is expressed on pre-B cells, mature B cells, and memory B cells but not on lymphoid stem cells and plasma cells. Clinical trial results have shown a modest benefit; the percentage of patients with 12-week confirmed disability progression was 32.9% with ocrelizumab vs 39.3% with placebo (hazard ratio, 0.76; 95% CI, 0.59-0.98; P=.03).

Patients with progressive MS can also benefit from nonpharmacologic and pharmacologic management of common symptoms, including gait impairment, neurogenic bladder, neurogenic bowel, spasticity, and neuropathic pain. Gait impairment is one of the most ubiquitous and disabling features of MS. Dalfampridine, a potassium channel blocker, at a dose of 10 mg twice a day (20 mg/d), is reportedly effective in up to 40% of patients for improving walking speed. Functional electrical stimulation can improve walking in those with foot drop by stimulating the peroneal nerve and activating dorsiflexion and eversion of the ankle. Neurogenic bladder management depends on the type of bladder dysfunction. Intermittent self-catheterization is the first-line management in those with high residual urine volume in the bladder (>100 mL). Medications with anticholinergic effects (such as oxybutynin, solifenacin, tolterodine, and imipramine) and mirabegron (a β$_3$-adrenergic receptor agonist) are options for those with spastic bladder or with low residual urine volume (<100 mL). Pharmacologic alternatives for spasticity include baclofen, tizanidine, cyclobenzaprine, and onabotulinum toxin A. For spasticity, baclofen can be administered orally or via intrathecal pump in those with refractory symptoms or who are intolerant to high doses. Oral tizanidine is an alternative. Gabapentin, pregabalin, venlafaxine, duloxetine, amitriptyline, and nortriptyline are options for treating painful and nonpainful dysesthesias.

Regardless of the type of MS, a multidisciplinary team approach to disease management is recommended. MS has been associated with multiple symptoms that may or may not be direct sequelae of the disease, which require further symptomatic management. Health care providers involved in management of MS are diverse and include specialists in primary care, neurology, MS nursing, neuroradiology, neuro-ophthalmology, physical medicine and rehabilitation, physical therapy, occupational therapy, psychiatry, psychology, sleep medicine, urology, gastroenterology, and social work.

KEY POINTS

- PPMS accounts for 10% to 20% of all cases of MS.

- There is no cure for PPMS, but ocrelizumab, a humanized monoclonal antibody that selectively targets CD20, can potentially slow down disability accumulation.

- Dalfampridine can help increase walking speed but should be avoided if the patient has a history of seizure or kidney dysfunction.

- Early involvement of a multidisciplinary team with expertise in demyelinating diseases of the central nervous system is optimal for management of MS and its complications.

PROGRESSIVE CEREBELLAR ATAXIA AFTER NATALIZUMAB TREATMENT

Michel Toledano, MD

CASE PRESENTATION

HISTORY AND EXAMINATION

A 47-year-old woman with a history of relapsing-remitting multiple sclerosis (MS) receiving natalizumab therapy sought a second opinion regarding a recent diagnosis of secondary progressive disease.

She was first diagnosed with MS 8 years earlier. She was initially treated with interferon beta-1a, but her therapy was eventually switched to natalizumab 6 years later because of breakthrough disease and increased lesion burden in her spinal cord. After this intensification of disease-modifying therapy (DMT), her disease stabilized. While taking natalizumab, she was monitored for the development of antibodies to JC polyoma virus (JCV). Nine months before our evaluation, anti-JCV antibodies became positive, with an increased index of 1.1. Given sustained remission, she was continued on natalizumab with increased surveillance and a plan to switch to a different DMT after 24 months.

Five months later she noted subacute onset of slurred speech and right upper extremity incoordination. Findings of repeated magnetic resonance imaging (MRI) of the brain and spine with gadolinium were interpreted as largely unchanged from prior imaging, although right cerebellar atrophy was noted (Figure 20.1). Over the next 4 months she continued to have clinical decline, and her Expanded Disability Status Scale (EDSS) score increased from 4.5 to 7.5. There were no new bladder or bowel symptoms. She reported no fever, night sweats, anorexia, or weight loss. She was up to date on her cancer screening and had never smoked tobacco.

On examination she had moderate ataxic dysarthria and right greater than left appendicular ataxia. She relied on a wheelchair for transportation and required 1-person assist to stand. Reflexes were brisk with bilateral Babinski sign.

This patient with relapsing-remitting MS on natalizumab had a new subacute progressive cerebellar syndrome without radiographic evidence of disease activity. In the setting of prolonged natalizumab exposure, several diagnoses were considered for this patient (Table 20.1). Infection, particularly JCV central nervous system (CNS) infection, was a key diagnostic consideration.

TESTING

Repeated MRI showed worsening cerebellar atrophy, right sided greater than left sided, and evolving T2 hyperintensity in the brainstem without enhancement or mass effect (Figure 20.1). No new demyelinating lesions were noted. Autoimmune encephalopathy panels in serum and cerebrospinal fluid (CSF) were within normal limits. CSF analysis demonstrated a mildly increased protein level, normal blood cell count, and 7 unique CSF oligoclonal bands. Gram stain and bacterial cultures were negative. Polymerase chain reaction (PCR) testing for enterovirus, varicella-zoster virus, and *Tropheryma whipplei* were negative. JCV PCR was positive.

DIAGNOSIS

The patient was diagnosed with JCV granule cell neuronopathy (GCN).

MANAGEMENT

Natalizumab was discontinued, and she was treated with 4 of 5 planned cycles of plasma exchange every other day. After her 4th cycle, worsening symptoms developed. MRI showed gadolinium enhancement in the brainstem (Figure 20.2) supportive of immune reconstitution inflammatory syndrome (IRIS). She received 3 days of high-dose intravenous methylprednisolone followed by a prednisone taper. Her disability progression stabilized, and her EDSS score was 6.5.

DISCUSSION

JCV CNS infection, 1 of several infections reported among treated patients with MS (Table 20.2), occurs almost exclusively in immunosuppressed patients, including those receiving DMT for MS. In addition to causing progressive

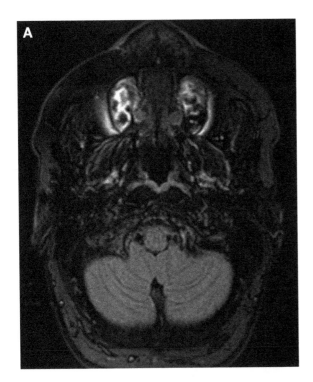
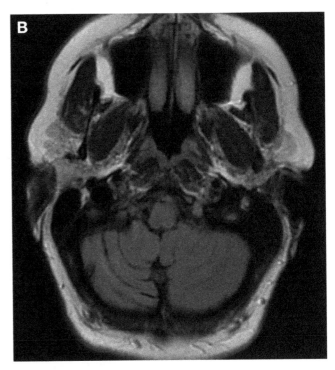
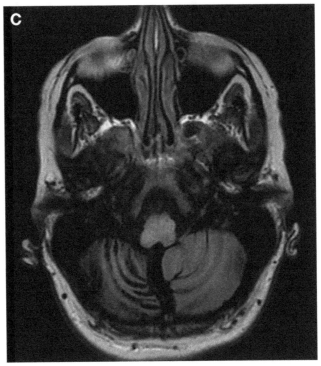

Figure 20.1 **T2 Axial Brain Magnetic Resonance Images.**
A, Before onset of ataxia, imaging demonstrates normal size of cerebellar folia and absence of demyelinating plaques in cerebellum or visualized portion of brainstem. B, Shortly after onset of symptoms there is evidence of cerebellar atrophy, right greater than left. C, Four months later there is progression of right-greater-than-left cerebellar atrophy, along with T2 fluid-attenuated inversion recovery signal change in the brainstem.

multifocal leukoencephalopathy (PML), which is a lytic infection of oligodendrocytes, JCV can also infect the cerebellar granule cell neurons, leading to progressive cerebellar degeneration. GCN, the term for this entity, has been associated with sequence variations in the C-terminus of the *VP1* capsid gene believed to make JCV tropic to the granule cell.

Although GCN usually develops in isolation, it can also occur together with PML.

Natalizumab, a recombinant monoclonal antibody against the α_4 subunit of integrin molecules (which inhibits ingress of T lymphocytes into the CNS), is a highly effective DMT for relapsing-remitting MS. However, its use is

Table 20.1 | DIFFERENTIAL DIAGNOSIS FOR THE CASE PATIENT

POSSIBLE DIAGNOSIS	MITIGATING FACTORS
Immune-mediated process	
MS relapse/natalizumab-neutralizing antibodies	No new lesions on scan to account for presentation
	Progressive course without stabilization
Secondary progressive MS	Progression more rapid than expected with progressive disease
	Progressive asymmetric spastic paraparesis more common than cerebellar syndrome
Paraneoplastic cerebellar degeneration	Absent systemic symptoms
Purkinje cell antibody (type 1 or 2)	Up to date on cancer screening
Purkinje cell antibody (anti-Tr)	
Metabotropic glutamate receptor type 1 antibody	
Anti–glutamic acid decarboxylase 65 antibody-associated cerebellar ataxia	Tends to be more slowly progressive
	Symmetric cerebellar atrophy more common
Celiac disease	Absent gastrointestinal tract manifestations
Infectious process	
Viral	
JCV	Brain MRI does not demonstrate classic white matter lesions of progressive multifocal leukoencephalopathy
VZV	VZV-associated cerebellitis more common in children than adults
	Subacute progressive course
	Absence of fever
	Absent zoster rash
Enterovirus (enterovirus 71)	More common in children
	No fever or headache
Bacterial	
Listeria monocytogenes	No fever
	No brainstem findings
Tropheryma whipplei	More common in middle-aged men
	No gastrointestinal tract or other systemic symptoms
Metabolic process	
Vitamin deficiency (B_{12} or E); copper deficiency	No history of bariatric surgery
	No macrocytic anemia
	No substantial proprioceptive or vibratory sensory loss
Degenerative/genetic syndrome	
Multiple system atrophy	No autonomic symptoms
	Median age of onset, mid 50s
	MRI does not demonstrate "hot cross bun" sign
Spinocerebellar ataxia	Rapid progression
	Late onset
	No family history
Friedreich ataxia	Late onset
	Preserved reflexes
	No cardiomyopathy

Abbreviations: JCV, JC polyoma virus; MRI, magnetic resonance imaging; MS, multiple sclerosis; VZV, varicella-zoster virus.

associated with an increased risk of PML. Rare cases of GCN have also been described in patients taking natalizumab. The risk of natalizumab-associated JCV CNS infection can be stratified on the basis of JCV antibody status (commensurate with the strength of the antibody response or index), duration of natalizumab therapy, and prior exposure to immunosuppressant drugs.

Close clinical and radiographic follow-up is important for detecting the onset of symptoms and signs related to JCV infection as opposed to those related to MS. Episodes of inflammatory demyelination are usually acute in onset (hours to days) and self-limited (improve over weeks to months). In contrast, PML presents with subacute onset (weeks to months) of progressive aphasia, hemiparesis, cortical visual deficits, or behavioral and cognitive abnormalities. GCN presents with subacute progressive ataxia, dysarthria, nystagmus, and extraocular movement abnormalities. Progressive MS, which must also be considered in this clinical setting, most commonly presents with insidious (months to years) asymmetric spastic paraparesis, hemiparesis, or quadriparesis. Isolated progressive ataxia without concomitant pyramidal dysfunction is much less common.

MRI in PML classically demonstrates T2-hyperintense and T1-hypointense white matter lesions without enhancement or mass effect. Enhancement and edema can be seen, however, when PML develops in patients with preserved immunity or in those with reconstituting immunity (eg, after natalizumab discontinuation). Progressive cerebellar atrophy is the most common imaging finding in GCN, although white matter changes in the cerebellum and brainstem can occur.

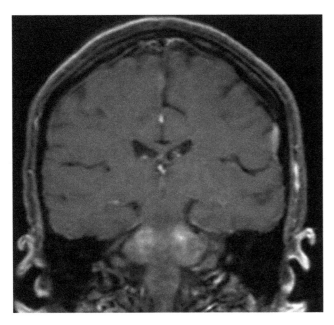

Figure 20.2 T1 Coronal Brain Magnetic Resonance Image, Post Gadolinium.
Enhancement is observed in the bilateral middle cerebellar peduncles, supportive of immune reconstitution inflammatory syndrome.

Table 20.2 | INFECTIONS ASSOCIATED WITH DISEASE-MODIFYING THERAPIES

DISEASE-MODIFYING THERAPY	INFECTIONS OTHER THAN JC POLYOMA VIRUS–ASSOCIATED CNS DISEASE
Alemtuzumab[a]	CMV, HSV, VZV, PML, listeriosis, *Nocardia*, tuberculosis
B-cell depletion therapy,[a] rituximab, ocrelizumab	Enterovirus, CMV, VZV, West Nile virus, Hep B reactivation, PML, *Cryptococcus*, tuberculosis, toxoplasmosis
Dimethyl fumarate	VZV, PML[b]
Fingolimod	VZV, HSV, PML, *Cryptococcus*, listeriosis
Interferons/glatiramer acetate	Low risk of systemic or CNS infection
Natalizumab	VZV, HSV

Abbreviations: CMV, cytomegalovirus; CNS, central nervous system; Hep B, hepatitis B virus; HSV, herpes simplex virus; PML, progressive multifocal leukoencephalopathy; VZV, varicella-zoster virus.

[a] Infection did not necessarily occur in patients receiving this agent as monotherapy or for a primary neurologic indication.

[b] Most cases associated with lymphocyte counts ≤500 cells/μL.

PCR testing of CSF for JCV is highly sensitive and specific but can be falsely negative. If suspicion is high, JCV PCR should be repeated. Biopsy is rarely needed to establish the diagnosis.

There is currently no specific treatment for JCV-associated CNS infection. Natalizumab should be immediately withdrawn if the diagnosis is strongly suspected. Empiric plasma exchange has been used in this setting to hasten elimination of circulating natalizumab, which results in more rapid immune reconstitution. However, evidence is limited to observational retrospective studies, and the benefit of plasma exchange remains unproved. The mainstay of treatment for IRIS is corticosteroids. Although the survival rate is relatively high in natalizumab-associated JCV CNS infection, the vast majority of patients have subsequent moderate to severe disability.

KEY POINTS

- Natalizumab is associated with increased risk of JCV CNS infection.

- Risk is stratified on the basis of antibody index, duration of natalizumab therapy, and prior exposure to other immunosuppressant therapies.

- JCV CNS infection can present as progressive cerebellar atrophy and ataxia in the absence of the white matter lesions most characteristic of PML; this entity is termed *GCN*.

- Discontinuation of natalizumab, with or without plasma exchange, can result in IRIS, which is characterized by paradoxical worsening of symptoms and associated gadolinium enhancement on MRI.

WEAKNESS AND DYSARTHRIA AFTER RADIOSURGERY

Andrew McKeon, MB, BCh, MD

CASE PRESENTATION

HISTORY AND EXAMINATION

A 60-year-old woman with a history of Sjögren syndrome had an episode of painful left eye vision loss. In the course of screening for a cause, brain magnetic resonance imaging (MRI) showed an arteriovenous malformation adjacent to the left ventricular atrium (Figure 21.1A-C). Although this was considered an asymptomatic lesion, the patient underwent stereotactic radiosurgery (Gamma Knife; Elekta AB) to reduce the risk of future growth and hemorrhage. Within days of the surgery, speech disturbance and weakness of the right arm and leg developed. Examination indicated a subcortical language deficit and an upper motor pattern of paresis of right-sided limbs.

TESTING

Considered in the differential diagnosis were new hemorrhage from the arteriovenous malformation, ischemic stroke, radiation-induced necrosis, abscess, and demyelinating disease. MRI of the head with and without gadolinium contrast was used to evaluate for these possibilities. Brain MRI after onset of speech and motor symptoms demonstrated new areas

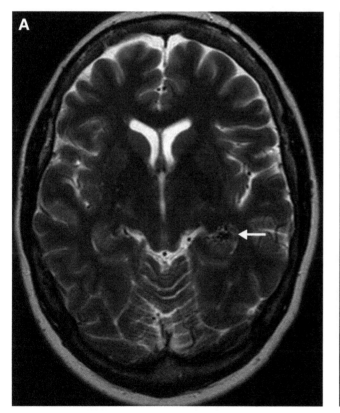

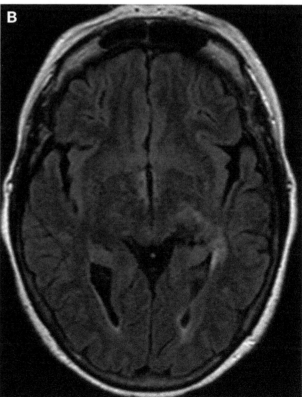

Figure 21.1 Magnetic Resonance Imaging (MRI) Findings for the Case Patient.
Axial brain T2 (A), T2/fluid-attenuated inversion recovery (B, D, and E), and T1 postgadolinium images (C and F). A-C, Before Gamma Knife surgery, a speckled hypointense lesion without mass effect or enhancement was visualized adjacent to the left ventricular atrium (A, arrow). D-F, After Gamma Knife surgery, when new neurologic deficits developed, extensive, new T2 hyperintensities were detected in the brainstem and brachium pontis (D) and deep frontoparietal white matter (E), with accompanying faint enhancement (F).

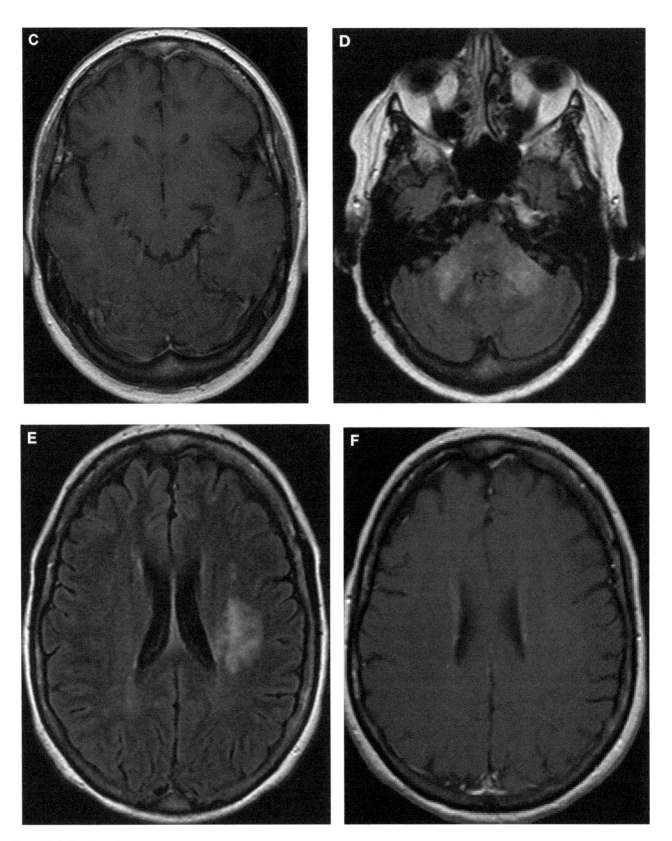

Figure 21.1 **Continued**

of confluent T2 signal abnormality in the brainstem and deep white matter of the left hemisphere, with some accompanying enhancement (Figure 21.1D-F) but without evidence of hemorrhage or acute stroke. Findings of cerebrospinal fluid evaluation were noninflammatory, including negative oligoclonal band testing, but slow conduction was noted in the left optic nerve on visual evoked potentials.

DIAGNOSIS

The patient was diagnosed with optic neuritis, with subsequent evolution to multiple sclerosis (MS) in the setting of radiosurgery.

MANAGEMENT

The patient received corticosteroids (intravenous methylprednisolone 1,000 mg/d for 5 days) with full recovery of language function and partial recovery of the hemiparesis, which improved with rehabilitation such that she could walk without a gait aid. Because the patient had more than 1 episode, she was treated with interferon beta-1a for further prevention of MS relapse.

DISCUSSION

Chronic neurotoxicity leading to subcortical dementia occurs in approximately 25% of patients undergoing whole-brain radiotherapy. Histologically, demyelination, as well as necrosis, can be a prominent feature. Among patients with MS or a clinically isolated syndrome, the risk of demyelinating events appears to increase after brain radiotherapy, within the field of treatment (whole-brain, targeted narrow-field, or stereotactic radiosurgery). Anecdotal reports have noted striking, sometimes fatal, instances of accelerated demyelination in patients with MS receiving external-beam radiotherapy to the brain.

Consistent with the clinical course in the case patient, this form of neurotoxicity generally occurs within 1 year after radiotherapy. In a Mayo Clinic study of 15 patients with MS diagnosed before or after external-beam radiotherapy, no relapses occurred during treatment. However, grade 4 (of 4) neurologic toxicity developed in 5 patients (40%) within a median of 1.0 year (range, 0.2-4.3 years) after irradiation. In all but 1 case, the patients had a preexisting diagnosis of MS or had preexisting symptoms consistent with a diagnosis of demyelinating disease. All occurrences of neurotoxicity were radiologically and/or clinically consistent with demyelinating injury within the volume of brain receiving radiotherapy. No patients appeared to have brain necrosis. Patients who receive bilateral, central brain radiotherapy with opposed fields appeared to be at the highest risk for subsequent neurotoxicity, although neurotoxicity can also occur with peripheral brain irradiation, or even, as illustrated here, with focused Gamma Knife irradiation.

Radiosurgery directed outside the central nervous system, at peripheral trigeminal nerve roots, is an effective therapy for trigeminal neuralgia, including in MS patients. In the largest surgical series reported to date, 80% achieved substantial pain relief for a median of 4 years. The relapse rate for the following year was not reported. Approximately 20% were reported to have facial numbness afterward. However, as this case illustrates, brain-directed radiosurgery may trigger demyelination. This exposure may be avoided by obtaining a careful symptom-based history for possible, prior, undiagnosed demyelinating events and by considering other treatment options (eg, surgical resection).

KEY POINTS

- Brain irradiation, including targeted techniques such as Gamma Knife radiosurgery, can trigger demyelination or exacerbate clinically preexisting disease, even in the absence of a clear MS diagnosis.

- A careful review of prior neurologic history and symptoms should be undertaken before radiotherapy.

SECTION II

AUTOIMMUNE NEUROLOGIC DISORDERS

FATIGUE, BLURRY VISION, AND SWOLLEN OPTIC NERVES

Marie D. Acierno, MD, M. Tariq Bhatti, MD, John J. Chen, MD, PhD,

and Eric R. Eggenberger, DO

CASE PRESENTATION

HISTORY AND EXAMINATION

A 71-year-old woman had development of generalized fatigue over 1 week, along with low-grade fever. The fever resolved, but the fatigue persisted. Subsequently, retro-orbital and head discomfort developed. She had no previous headaches, jaw claudication, scalp tenderness, diplopia, obscurations of vision, or scintillating scotomas. One month later, she had blurred vision. An ophthalmic examination revealed a visual acuity of 20/20 −2 in the right eye and 20/50 −2 in the left eye. She had mild dyschromatopsia, bilateral visual field constriction, bilateral marked optic disc edema (Figure 22.1), and vitreous cells graded as vitreous haze score 2.0. She had no pertinent past illnesses, including no history of prior vascular disease or cancer. Her body mass index was 23.5, and her only medication was amitriptyline. She smoked one-half to 1 pack of cigarettes per day for many years.

TESTING

Magnetic resonance imaging (MRI) of the brain showed confluent abnormal areas of T2 hyperintensity without mass effect or enhancement involving the subcortical and periventricular white matter in the cerebral hemispheres bilaterally, basal ganglia, pons, and left thalamus. MR venography did not show occlusion of the dural venous sinuses. Test results for complete blood cell count, erythrocyte sedimentation rate, vitamin B_{12} level, folate level, anticardiolipin antibodies, coagulation profile, rapid plasma reagin, cholesterol panel, antinuclear antibody, and antineutrophil cytoplasmic antibodies were normal or negative. She had 2 lumbar punctures, which showed normal opening pressures. Cerebrospinal fluid (CSF) analysis showed an increased white blood cell count of 161 cells/µL (reference range, ≤5 cells/µL), which was cytologically consistent with reactive pleocytosis with a predominance of lymphocytes. The CSF protein level was increased, at 77 mg/dL (reference range, ≤35 mg/dL), and cultures were negative for organisms. Immunostain confirmed polyclonal plasma cells and a possible T-cell proliferative disorder. The CSF and serum were positive for collapsin-response mediator protein 5 (CRMP5)-immunoglobulin G (IgG) and microtubule-associated protein 1B (MAP1B)-IgG antibodies at high titers. Computed tomography of the chest, abdomen, and pelvis showed an indeterminate pulmonary nodule in the upper lobe. Bronchoscopy identified thickened mucosa

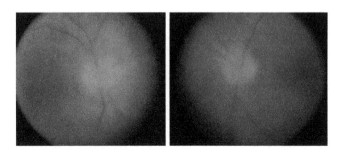

Figure 22.1 Ophthalmic Examination Findings.
Bilateral disc edema and vitritis are seen. The view to the posterior pole is hazy because of the vitritis.

Table 22.1 | **DIFFERENTIAL DIAGNOSIS**

CATEGORY	CONDITIONS
Intracerebral mass lesion	Primary CNS mass lesion
	Secondary (metastatic) CNS lesion
Other causes of increased intracranial pressure	Dural venous sinus thrombosis
	Idiopathic intracranial hypertension
Infectious CNS disease	Fungal
	Syphilis
	Viral encephalitis
CNS vasculitis	Giant cell arteritis
	Neurosarcoidosis
	Granulomatosis with polyangiitis (formerly Wegener granulomatosis)
Neoplastic CNS disease	Lymphoma
	Carcinomatous meningitis
Paraneoplastic disorder	CRMP5 autoimmunity

Abbreviations: CNS, central nervous system; CRMP5, collapsin-response mediator protein 5.

in the right lower lung consistent with small cell carcinoma. Bone scan findings were normal. Positron emission tomography showed abnormal hypermetabolic areas of the ascending colon. Biopsy revealed tubulovillous adenoma of the ascending colon, and the patient underwent a right-sided colon resection and anastomosis. Diagnoses considered for this patient are shown in Table 22.1.

DIAGNOSIS

The patient was diagnosed with paraneoplastic optic neuropathy (PON) (CRMP5-IgG–associated optic neuropathy and vitritis).

MANAGEMENT

Intravenous methylprednisolone at a dosage of 1 g/d was given for 5 days, followed by a prolonged course of oral prednisone, with slight visual improvement. The patient underwent a right-sided thoracotomy with biopsy of the right lower lobe, the results of which were consistent with small cell undifferentiated carcinoma. Mediastinoscopy with biopsy of the pretracheal and azygous lymph nodes indicated no metastatic tumor. Unfavorable results of pulmonary function testing precluded pneumectomy.

DISCUSSION

Paraneoplastic neurologic syndromes are a heterogeneous group of disorders associated with various systemic cancers and with other mechanisms believed to be immune mediated. Paraneoplastic visual syndromes can precede or follow a diagnosis of cancer.

There are 2 paraneoplastic visual disorders with autoantibodies that are primarily related to small cell lung carcinomas: cancer-associated retinopathy and PON. Cancer-associated retinopathy is classically associated with antirecoverin antibody, and PON is most commonly associated with CRMP5-IgG antibodies.

CRMP5 autoimmunity may be accompanied by 1 or more autonomic findings (cerebellar ataxia, chorea, peripheral neuropathy, and myelopathy) and neuro-ophthalmic manifestations, including optic neuropathy, vitritis, retinitis, and diplopia. Patients with CRMP5-IgG–associated optic neuropathy typically have painless bilateral vision loss over weeks to months. At onset, bilateral optic disc edema is typically present without evidence of enhancement of the optic nerve on MRI or increased opening pressure on lumbar puncture. Visual acuity can range from 20/20 to hand motion. Patients typically have coexisting vitritis or retinitis. In addition, patients can have diplopia, typically from cerebellar involvement. Most patients with CRMP5-IgG–associated optic neuropathy will have other neurologic deficits as a result of CRMP5 autoimmunity, such as asymmetric axonal polyradiculoneuropathy. Small cell lung carcinomas and, less commonly, thymoma are the 2 most common neoplasms in patients with CRMP5-IgG autoimmunity.

PON is a diagnostic challenge. PON presents with gradual vision loss, and the underlying cancer may not be initially recognized. In PON, the autoimmune response is directed against an antigen expressed by both tumor and neuronal/glial tissues. Neuro-ophthalmic symptoms of CRMP5 autoimmunity occur before detection of the cancer in about two-thirds of patients. Therefore, adult patients with subacute vision loss, optic disc edema, and vitreous cells should undergo serologic and cerebrospinal evaluations with paraneoplastic autoantibody panels. Autoimmune antibody positivity for markers such as CRMP5 can hasten the search for lung cancer. Similar to our case, patients with CRMP5 autoimmunity are more likely to have had a past smoking history.

In addition to CRMP5 antibody positivity in the serum and CSF, the most frequent laboratory finding for PON and associated neurologic symptoms is CSF lymphocytic pleocytosis and increased protein concentration. Paraneoplastic autoantibodies often coexist with CRMP5-IgG, most commonly antineuronal nuclear antibody type 1 and Purkinje cell cytoplasmic antibody type 2-IgG, which is also known as MAP1B-IgG.

Because of the rarity of the disease, the best treatment for CRMP5-IgG–associated optic neuropathy remains unclear. Vision may recover slightly with therapy directed at the underlying cancer. Improvement in visual acuity may also occur in those receiving systemic corticosteroids in addition to other forms of immunotherapy, including cyclophosphamide, intraocular corticosteroid injections, plasma exchange, and intravenous immunoglobulin.

The combination of papillitis, retinitis, and/or vitritis without optic nerve enhancement on MRI should alert the clinician to initiate serum testing for CRMP5-IgG. Accurate and timely diagnosis may help expedite vision-sparing immunosuppressant therapy and a targeted systemic cancer search.

KEY POINTS

- CRMP5-IgG–associated optic neuropathy is a PON that typically presents with optic disc edema, retinitis, and vitreous inflammatory cells.

- The presenting symptom often is bilateral painless vision loss over weeks to months and is usually accompanied by multifocal neurologic symptoms.

- CRMP5-IgG is a neurologic autoimmunity marker related to lung carcinoma, most commonly small cell carcinoma.

PROGRESSIVE, SYMMETRICAL, PAINLESS VISUAL LOSS

Eric R. Eggenberger, DO, Marie D. Acierno, MD, M. Tariq Bhatti, MD,
and John J. Chen, MD, PhD

CASE PRESENTATION

HISTORY AND EXAMINATION

A 75-year-old woman with a medical history of mixed connective tissue disease (positive for antinuclear antibody and Sjögren syndrome-B antibody) and breast adenocarcinoma (5 years earlier, successfully managed with resection and hormonal therapy) sought care for subacute visual "haze" in both eyes characterized by light sensitivity, particularly with commercial fluorescent lighting, progressing over weeks. Visual acuity was 20/40 in each eye. The pupils were equal in size with no relative afferent pupillary defect but were sluggishly reactive to light. Automated perimetry documented peripheral constriction in both eyes (Figure 23.1). Ocular motility was normal. Ophthalmoscopy showed mild retinal pigment epithelial changes in both maculae with normal optic nerves (Figure 23.2).

Diagnoses considered included causes of symmetric bilateral retinopathies, such as the white dot spectrum disorders (eg, acute zonal occult outer retinopathy and multiple evanescent white dot syndrome), autoimmune or cancer-associated retinopathy (CAR), retinitis pigmentosa variants, idiopathic cone-rod dystrophy, and toxic or metabolic retinopathies such as vitamin A deficiency. Most of these considerations may be distinguished by their retinal findings, historical comorbid conditions, and the pace of visual loss.

TESTING

Optical coherence tomography (OCT) showed macular thinning in both eyes (Figure 23.3). Findings of fundus autofluorescence were normal. Serum testing documented the presence of 3 retinal antibodies, against 30-, 36-, and 46-kDa proteins. A paraneoplastic panel was negative except for low-level ganglionic (alpha 3) acetylcholine receptor autoantibody positivity, at 0.04 nmol/L (reference range, <0.02 nmol/L), which was interpreted as nonspecific autoimmunity. Electroretinography (ERG) indicated severely decreased scotopic and photopic a and b waves. Cranial magnetic resonance imaging and whole-body positron emission

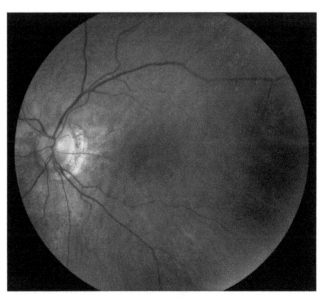

Figure 23.2 Fundus Photography Findings for the Case Patient.
Fundus photograph of the left eye shows retinal pigment epithelial changes, which were symmetrically present in both maculae.

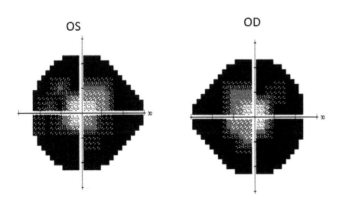

Figure 23.1 Automated Perimetry Findings for the Case Patient.
Gray-scale perimetry documents diffuse constriction in both eyes. OD indicates right eye; OS, left eye.

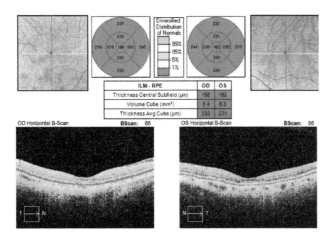

Figure 23.3 Macular Optical Coherence Tomography Findings for the Case Patient.

Thinning is seen in both maculae: average thickness, 233 μm in the right eye and 231 μm in the left eye, with normal average thickness (≈278 μm). T→N indicates temporal to nasal scan direction (OD); N→T indicates nasal to temporal scan direction (OS), through the fovea (the central depression). ILM-RPE indicates retinal thickness, inner limiting layer to retinal pigment epithelium; OD, right eye; OS, left eye.

tomography (PET)/computed tomography (CT) findings were unremarkable.

DIAGNOSIS

A diagnosis of paraneoplastic or nonparaneoplastic autoimmune retinopathy was made, consistent with the clinical presentation, OCT and ERG findings, and the presence of retinal antibodies. Retinal antibodies alone, however, have poor specificity and must be interpreted in the correct clinical context.

MANAGEMENT

There are no established evidence-based guidelines to assist treatment decisions in autoimmune retinopathy, although several lines of therapy have been advocated. In general, no single therapy or combination of therapies has consistently demonstrated significant efficacy.

No specific immunosuppressive therapy was undertaken in this case. However, if her vision had continued to rapidly worsen over time, empiric immunotherapy would have been instituted.

DISCUSSION

Autoimmune retinopathy includes paraneoplastic and nonparaneoplastic forms. The best-characterized autoimmune retinopathy phenotype is CAR, first described in 1976 in 3 patients with small cell lung cancer.

CAR typically presents with subacute, painless, bilateral (although asymmetry has been described) vision loss that is progressive over weeks to months, reflecting both rod and cone dysfunction in most patients. Accordingly, symptoms often include nyctalopia (inability to see in dim light or at night), impaired dark adaptation, photopsia (flashes of light in the field of vision), photosensitivity, dyschromatopsia, and, ultimately, severe visual acuity loss. CAR epidemiology

reflects the most common underlying tumor types, which include small cell lung carcinoma and gynecologic and breast cancers, with an average age at presentation of 65 years and a slight female predilection. Visual symptoms precede recognition of an underlying cancer in approximately 50% of cases.

Perimetry may demonstrate a ring scotoma, generalized constriction, or central defects. Ophthalmoscopy findings are generally unremarkable early and are typically more benign than the level of visual symptoms would suggest, even later in the course when attenuated retinal arteries, retinal pigment epithelial changes, and a mild degree of secondary optic nerve pallor often develop. Less commonly, mild vitreitis and retinal vasculitis have been reported.

Electrophysiologic studies such as ERG, OCT, and laboratory assays for retinal antibodies often make up the initial diagnostic evaluation. The full-field ERG typically documents depressed or extinguished scotopic and photopic a and b waves if there is substantial visual field loss. Multifocal ERG will show diminished central waveforms in patients with predominantly central vision loss. Although the OCT findings may be normal initially, with progressive symptoms, retinal thinning with loss of the photoreceptor layer and inner segment/outer segment junction (ellipsoid zone) usually occurs.

Immunohistochemistry, Western blot, or enzyme-linked immunosorbent assays are used in the detection of retinal antibodies. According to a recent expert consensus panel, a 2-tiered design is recommended, with Western blot to screen for antibodies and follow-up immunohistochemistry for confirmation. The best-studied antigen targeted by autoantibodies is recoverin, a 23-kDa protein that controls phosphorylation of rhodopsin. Although the recoverin autoantibody is the one most specifically associated with cancer, studies suggest that it is found in only 10% of patients with CAR. In addition to recoverin-directed autoimmunity, antibodies to several other targets have been described, including α-enolase (46 kDa), transducin α-subunit (40 kDa), heat shock cognate protein 70 (65 kDa), carbonic anhydrase II (30 kDa), interphotoreceptor retinoid-binding protein (145 kDa), neurofilament proteins, and tubby-like proteins. These antibodies have much lower specificity for autoimmune retinopathy than antirecoverin. Although the presence of antirecoverin tends to indicate an underlying cancer, all of these other antibodies may be detected in healthy persons (40% prevalence) without cancer or autoimmune retinopathy.

Other primary retinopathies and comorbid conditions have a higher incidence of nonspecific retinal antibodies, which further hinders the diagnostic usefulness of laboratory testing; these include inflammatory bowel disease, Behçet syndrome, systemic lupus erythematosus, multiple sclerosis, age-related macular degeneration, and uveitis such as Vogt-Koyanagi-Harada syndrome and sympathetic ophthalmia. Often, multiple retinal antibodies are expressed in the same patient, which suggests a possible synergism leading to CAR or autoimmune retinopathy. How these antibodies cross the blood-retinal barrier and the exact pathophysiologic mechanisms of these diseases remain under investigation. In addition, other than antirecoverin, retinal antibodies have poor specificity and therefore must be interpreted in the correct clinical context.

In some patients with autoimmune retinopathy, fundus autofluorescence shows a ring of hyperautofluorescence in the parafoveal region, corresponding to thinning in the outer nuclear layer segment on OCT and loss of the photoreceptor inner-outer segment junction. Fluorescein angiography is generally not useful but may document vasculitis in rare cases and helps narrow the differential diagnosis in other cases.

Imaging in autoimmune retinopathies is essential for excluding an underlying malignant process. Although CT of the chest-abdomen and pelvis is a common screening procedure for this purpose, the addition of PET/CT increases the detection of underlying cancer in high-risk patients. In addition, selected sex- and age-specific tests such as mammography and ultrasonography may also be indicated in certain cases.

Treatment of autoimmune retinopathy is heterogeneous and lacks evidence-based support. In general, treatment of the underlying cancer does not appear to affect the course of CAR-related visual loss; this may reflect delayed diagnosis, permanent retinal cell loss preceding therapeutic interventions, ineffective therapies, or a combination of these factors. In patients with small cell lung cancer, those with recoverin autoantibodies have longer recurrence-free survival than those without such antibodies; it is possible that the anti-recoverin immune response produces a robust anticancer response, at the expense of retinal degeneration. Treatment of autoimmune retinopathy often includes systemic corticosteroids, cytotoxic agents, or immunomodulatory agents such as intravenous immunoglobulin or plasma exchange and has produced mixed results. Immunomodulatory therapies may be effective in preventing further vision loss in some patients but cannot reverse retinal cell loss. Therefore, if a patient has continued progressive vision loss from autoimmune retinopathy, empiric immunotherapy is typically instituted in hopes of preventing further vision loss.

Other less-common paraneoplastic retinopathies include melanoma-associated retinopathy, paraneoplastic vitelliform maculopathy, and bilateral diffuse uveal melanocytic proliferation. Melanoma-associated retinopathy most often occurs in patients with a preceding melanoma diagnosis, with an average latency from the diagnosis of cutaneous melanoma to visual symptoms of several years.

In contrast to CAR, nonparaneoplastic autoimmune retinopathies are heterogeneous diseases that lack well-defined or specific antibody associations. The diagnosis is made via clinical suspicion in patients with decreased visual acuity, varied field defects, and symptoms dependent on rod (vs cone) dysfunction and findings on electrophysiologic testing. These syndromes may mimic a CAR-like presentation but have no underlying malignant process. The currently available retinal antibody tests lack specificity and are not recommended for routine clinical use. Specific biomarkers in the investigation of nonparaneoplastic autoimmune retinopathy remain an unmet need.

KEY POINTS

- Autoimmune retinopathies are a varied, incompletely understood, and heterogeneous group of disorders.

- CAR with antibodies against the 23-kDa retinal antigen recoverin is the best understood among this group and typically presents with subacute, painless, symmetric vision loss.

- Initial retinal examination findings in these disorders are generally benign; however, with time, retinal artery attenuation and a degree of secondary optic atrophy typically develop.

- Although retinal antibodies are an often-emphasized feature of these diseases, the specificity and sensitivity of non-23-kDa (CAR) antibodies remain poor. OCT and ERG are useful diagnostic tests.

- Treatment remains suboptimal in these diseases because diagnosis is often delayed until permanent retinal cell loss has occurred.

PERSONALITY CHANGES, COGNITIVE DECLINE, AND JERKING MOVEMENTS[a]

A. Sebastian Lopez Chiriboga, MD

CASE PRESENTATION

HISTORY AND EXAMINATION

A 64-year-old man had development of abnormal movements characterized by grimacing of the left hemiface and posturing of the ipsilateral arm, occurring up to 40 times per day. Four weeks later, he started to experience visual and auditory hallucinations, prominent anxiety, and personality changes. He was diagnosed with tics and late-onset psychosis and was admitted to a psychiatric ward; he was discharged on olanzapine therapy. He continued to experience additional symptoms, and 2 weeks later he had a generalized tonic-clonic seizure, followed by cognitive decline requiring assistance for most activities of daily living. He was readmitted to the hospital for neurologic evaluation.

His heart rate was 120 beats/min, he was afebrile, and other vital signs and general physical examination findings were normal. On neurologic examination, he had a Mini-Mental State Examination (MMSE) score of 16/30 (points were missed for orientation, attention, calculation, registration, and recall). The patient was oriented to person only, and he had multiple, frequent, left hemibody jerks during the neurologic examination, but findings were otherwise normal. Diagnoses considered at the time are shown in Table 24.1.

TESTING

Laboratory investigations for reversible causes of encephalopathy, including complete blood cell count, chest radiography, blood culture, urine culture, ammonia levels, liver and kidney function, HIV, rapid plasma reagin (syphilis), and serum levels of thyrotropin, vitamins, and micronutrients, were unrevealing. Cerebrospinal fluid (CSF) analysis indicated increased protein concentration but otherwise normal findings. Results of extensive testing for infectious agents,

including polymerase chain reaction and cultures, were negative; real-time quaking-induced conversion analysis was negative for Creutzfeldt-Jakob disease, and neural autoantibodies were not detected.

Laboratory abnormalities included a serum sodium concentration of 126 mmol/L (reference range, 135-145 mmol/L), and cell-based assay identified antibodies to leucine-rich, glioma-inactivated protein 1 (LGI1). Electroencephalography revealed diffuse slowing and bilateral temporal lobe epileptiform discharges. Extensive oncologic investigations, including ^{18}F-fludeoxyglucose–positron emission tomography (FDG-PET) and testicular ultrasonography, were negative. Magnetic resonance imaging of the brain showed T2/fluid-attenuated inversion recovery hyperintensities in the bilateral hippocampi and amygdalae (Figure 24.1A) and gadolinium enhancement in the same regions (Figure 24.1B). Brain FDG-PET demonstrated hypermetabolism in the mesiotemporal lobes bilaterally (Figure 24.1C). There was no diffusion restriction or cortical ribboning.

DIAGNOSIS

A diagnosis of limbic encephalitis associated with LGI1-immunoglobulin G (IgG) antibodies was confirmed on the basis of the clinical presentation, imaging findings, and seropositivity for LGI1-IgG. The unilateral facial and arm movements were consistent with faciobrachial dystonic seizures (FBDS) and are pathognomonic of the disorder.

MANAGEMENT

The patient's seizure frequency did not improve with antiepileptic drug therapy, including the combination of levetiracetam and lamotrigine. The patient was then treated with intravenous methylprednisolone 1 g/d for 5 days, followed by plasmapheresis. This resulted in substantial improvement of

[a] Portions previously published in Lopez Chiriboga AS, Siegel JL, Tatum WO, Shih JJ, Flanagan EP. Striking basal ganglia imaging abnormalities in LGI1 AB faciobrachial dystonic seizures. Neurol Neuroimmunol Neuroinflamm. 2017;4:e336; used with permission of Mayo Foundation for Medical Education and Research.

Table 24.1 | POSSIBLE CAUSES OF SYMPTOMS IN CASE PATIENT

CATEGORY	CAUSES
Viral agents	Human herpesviruses (HHVs): HHV-1, HHV-2, HHV-3/VZV, HHV-4/EBV, HHV-5/CMV, HHV-6, HHV-7
	Enteroviruses
	Arboviruses
	HIV
Bacterial infections	Neurosyphilis
	Whipple disease
	Listeriosis
	Tuberculosis
	Lyme disease
Fungal agents	*Aspergillus*
	Cryptococcus
Other infectious causes	Toxoplasmosis
Immune-mediated causes	Behçet disease
	Nonlimbic antibody-associated encephalitis, paraneoplastic or idiopathic (eg, NMDA receptor encephalitis)
	Sjögren syndrome
	Kikuchi-Fujimoto disease
	X-linked lymphoproliferative disease
	Posterior reversible leukoencephalopathy syndrome
	Susac syndrome
	Neurosarcoidosis
	Encephalitis post immune checkpoint inhibitors
Other causes	Glioma: gliomatosis cerebri-CNS metastasis
	Leptomeningeal metastases
	Primary or secondary CNS lymphoma
	Neurodegenerative disorders (FTD, LBD, CJD)
	Psychiatric disorders (schizophrenia, bipolar disorder)
	Nutritional deficiencies (vitamins B_1, B_{12})
	Mitochondrial disorders
	Toxins/drugs/withdrawal
	Paroxysmal dyskinesias

Abbreviations: CJD, Creutzfeldt-Jakob disease; CMV, cytomegalovirus; CNS, central nervous system; EBV, Epstein-Barr virus; FTD, frontotemporal dementia; LBD, Lewy body dementia; NMDA, *N*-methyl-ᴅ-aspartate; VZV, varicella-zoster virus.

his cognitive dysfunction (MMSE score, 27/30) and decrease in the FBDS frequency (1-5 per day). Therapy was transitioned to oral prednisone (1 mg/kg), and the patient was discharged from the hospital. When prednisone was decreased from 20 to 10 mg daily, clinical relapse occurred, characterized by increased frequency of FBDS (up to 10 episodes daily), which required reinstitution of high-dose oral prednisone and initiation of mycophenolate mofetil and a slow oral prednisone taper. The FBDS frequency decreased after 1 week and continued to improve over time. The patient remained cognitively stable and was able to return to work. He was seizure free at last follow-up 48 months after onset.

DISCUSSION

This patient had classic features of LGI1 antibody encephalitis: FBDS, personality changes, subacute cognitive decline, hyponatremia, and improvement with immunotherapy.

Limbic encephalitis is an inflammatory process that affects the limbic cortex, hippocampus, amygdala, hypothalamus, and cingulate gyrus. It presents with cognitive dysfunction, behavioral changes, prominent amnesia, and seizures. Limbic encephalitis can be secondary to infectious or autoimmune processes.

Infections affecting predominantly the limbic system can be associated with several microorganisms, but viral causes are the most common (Table 24.1). Temporal lobe abnormalities are encountered in approximately 60% to 80% of patients, whereas CSF oligoclonal bands and increased white blood cell counts are rare.

Autoimmune limbic encephalitis can be divided into paraneoplastic and nonparaneoplastic; it has also been reported in patients treated with immune checkpoint inhibitors. Although encephalitis can be a manifestation of multiple neural autoantibodies, classic limbic encephalitis is more commonly seen in patients who are seropositive for antineuronal nuclear antibody type 1 (ANNA-1/anti-Hu) and antibodies to Ma2, CV2/collapsin-response mediator protein 5, γ-aminobutyric acid$_B$ receptor, α-amino-3-hydroxy-5-methyl-4-isoxazolepropionic acid (AMPA) receptor, metabotropic glutamate receptor 5, LGI1, contactin-associated protein 2 (CASPR2), and neurexin.

After excluding other toxic, metabolic, neoplastic, and infectious causes of encephalopathy, a trial of immunotherapy

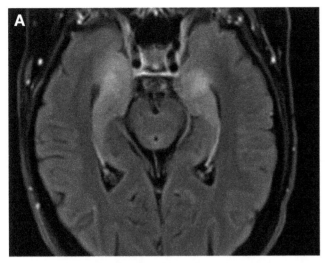

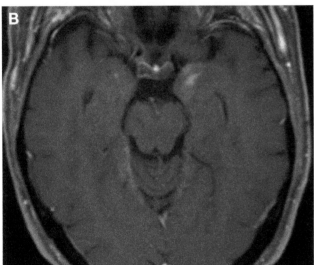

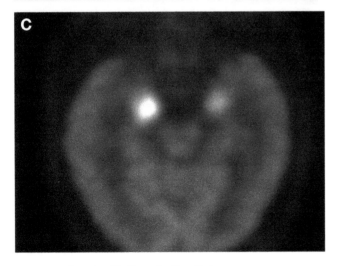

Figure 24.1 Imaging Findings for Case Patient.
A and B, Magnetic resonance imaging of the brain demonstrates T2/fluid-attenuated inversion recovery hyperintensities in the bilateral hippocampus and amygdalae (A) and gadolinium enhancement in the same regions (B). C, ¹⁸F-Fludeoxyglucose–positron emission tomography of the brain shows hypermetabolism in the mesial temporal lobes bilaterally.

can be initiated while waiting for the results of neural antibody testing.

Given that limbic encephalitis is considered a classic paraneoplastic syndrome, an oncologic evaluation should be undertaken. Antibody testing helps with cancer screening and has prognostic implications. Typically, paraneoplastic limbic encephalitis associated with antibodies targeting onconeural antigens that are intracellular proteins (eg, ANNA-1 or Ma2) has a strong cancer association. Although symptoms can improve or stabilize, cognitive outcomes are typically poor. This is in contrast to autoimmune limbic encephalitis associated with antibodies against neuronal surface antigens, particularly the voltage-gated potassium channel complex proteins LGI1 and CASPR2, and AMPA receptor, in which most patients have substantial improvement with immunotherapy.

There is no US Food and Drug Administration–approved medication for limbic encephalitis. Similar to other autoimmune neurologic disorders, first-line immunotherapy comprises intravenous high-dose corticosteroids, plasma exchange, or intravenous immunoglobulin, sometimes used in combination. Seizures in the setting of limbic encephalitis are typically resistant to antiepileptic drug therapy, but immunotherapy can be effective. Most patients respond within weeks of first-line therapy, but recovery can be slow. Patients who have no response to first-line therapy are usually treated with rituximab or cyclophosphamide; other agents such as bortezomib and natalizumab have also been used successfully.

KEY POINTS

- Limbic encephalitis is characterized by seizures, cognitive dysfunction, behavioral changes, and short-term memory loss.

- The differential diagnosis includes primarily infectious encephalitis.

- Serum and CSF should be tested for neural autoantibodies.

- Normal imaging findings and noninflammatory CSF are unusual, but they do not exclude the diagnosis.

- Early administration of immunotherapy can prevent long-term cognitive dysfunction.

RAPIDLY PROGRESSIVE MEMORY LOSS, MOOD CHANGE, MUTISM, AND ABNORMAL MOVEMENTS

Shailee S. Shah, MD, and Marie F. Grill, MD

CASE PRESENTATION

HISTORY AND EXAMINATION

A 24-year-old woman with a medical history pertinent only for migraine sought care for 2 weeks of disorientation and short-term memory difficulties, as well as diffuse tremor of all extremities. A flulike illness was initially suspected given the presence of low-grade fever and tachycardia. One week later, she returned with further decline in memory and new severe headaches. Her family reported that she had intermittent agitation and emotional outbursts of crying or laughing, as well as insomnia over the preceding 4 days. Spells had also developed consisting of disorganized speech and episodes of intermittent right gaze deviation with facial twitching and lip smacking. Within several days she was nearly mute. Her appetite had decreased substantially and she had not had a bowel movement in several days. She was noted to have significant tachycardia to 170 beats/min and was intermittently febrile. Within several days of her subsequent admission to the hospital, she became unresponsive to all external stimuli, with nonpurposeful eye movements and frequent dyskinesias observed, and ultimately required ventilator support.

Diagnoses considered at the time included herpes simplex virus or other infectious encephalitis, autoimmune encephalitis, toxic-metabolic encephalopathy, central nervous system inflammatory disease, vasculitis, and psychosis secondary to an underlying primary psychiatric disorder (Table 25.1).

TESTING

Findings on contrast-enhanced brain magnetic resonance imaging (MRI) were normal. Results of extensive serum testing for toxic-metabolic derangements, including toxicology and thyroid studies, were negative. Testing of the cerebrospinal fluid (CSF) showed 236 white blood cells/µL (reference range, 0-5 cells/µL; lymphocyte predominant), mildly increased protein concentration of 50 mg/dL (reference range, 15-45 mg/dL), and normal glucose values. Extensive CSF studies for herpes simplex virus and other viral, bacterial, and fungal organisms were negative. Electroencephalography (EEG) initially demonstrated generalized slowing and generalized periodic epileptiform discharges, with progression to right temporal subclinical seizures and clinical and electrographic status epilepticus. EEG was also notable for an extreme delta brush pattern (Figure 25.1). There was no EEG correlate with the patient's emotional outbursts or dyskinesias.

Bilateral ovarian masses were identified on pelvic ultrasonography, and subsequent computed tomography (CT) of the abdomen and pelvis showed bilateral teratomas. Whole-body positron emission tomography–CT findings were negative. An autoimmune encephalitis autoantibody panel was positive for antibodies targeting the *N*-methyl-D-aspartate (NMDA) receptor in the serum and CSF, by both cell-based and immunofluorescence assays (titer, 1:128 [reference range, <1:2]).

DIAGNOSIS

The patient was diagnosed with anti-NMDA receptor encephalitis.

MANAGEMENT

The patient initially received a 5-day course of intravenous (IV) methylprednisolone 1 g/d, followed by IV immunoglobulin (2 g/kg divided over 5 days). Benzodiazepines and propranolol were used to manage agitation and dysautonomia. Antiepileptic drugs were initiated for seizures, with frequent escalation required for status epilepticus. She required mechanical ventilation and parenteral nutrition given her persistent profound encephalopathic state. Ten days into her hospitalization, she underwent left ovarian cystectomy and right salpingo-oophorectomy. Despite teratoma resection, minimal improvements were noted at hospital week 3, and she was treated with several rounds of high-dose rituximab and repeated courses of methylprednisolone. Given only minimal improvement 6 to 8 weeks into her hospitalization, cyclophosphamide was also administered, and within several weeks, more substantial improvements were noted, with resolution of catatonia and improvement in dyskinesias.

Table 25.1 DIFFERENTIAL DIAGNOSIS FOR CASE PATIENT

DIAGNOSIS	PERTINENT DISTINGUISHING FEATURES
Infectious encephalitis: viral (eg, herpes simplex virus, SSPE), bacterial, fungal	Negative CSF infectious studies
Alternate autoimmune encephalitis (LGI1, AMPA receptor, GABA$_B$ receptor antibodies)	Prominent early neuropsychiatric manifestations, dysautonomia, mutism and speech abnormalities, demographic features (young woman)
Metabolic or nutritional derangements (hyperthyroid, vitamin B$_{12}$ or thiamine deficiency)	Absence of acute, severe symptoms; seizures, dysautonomia, inflammatory CSF
Neuroleptic malignant syndrome or drug toxicity	No identified drug exposure, no prominent early rigidity or high-grade fevers
Psychosis due to underlying psychiatric disorder such as schizophrenia or bipolar disorder	Seizures, inflammatory CSF
CNS demyelinating disease (multiple sclerosis, neurosarcoidosis)	Lack of abnormalities on brain MRI
Postinfectious encephalitis, acute disseminated encephalomyelitis	Lack of abnormalities on brain MRI
Primary or secondary CNS vasculitis	Lack of abnormalities on brain MRI
Rapidly progressive neurodegenerative disorders, prion disease	Viral-like prodrome, rapid progression over days to weeks rather than weeks to months, CSF pleocytosis
Malignant process (metastasis, lymphoma)	Lack of abnormalities on brain MRI
Inherited disorders (mitochondrial cytopathies)	Inflammatory CSF, subacute onset, lack of abnormalities on brain MRI

Abbreviations: AMPA, α-amino-3-hydroxy-5-methyl-4-isoxazolepropionic acid; CNS, central nervous system; CSF, cerebrospinal fluid; GABA$_B$, γ-aminobutyric acid$_B$; LGI1, leucine-rich, glioma-inactivated protein 1; MRI, magnetic resonance imaging; SSPE, subacute sclerosing panencephalitis.

After a 3-month hospitalization, she was discharged with tracheostomy and gastrostomy tube to intensive multidisciplinary rehabilitation. She was treated with a prolonged course of oral prednisone 60 mg daily followed by a gradual taper over 1 year. Neurologic improvement continued over 24 months post hospitalization, with good seizure control and improved performance on neuropsychometric testing. She required management of spasticity and dystonia with botulinum toxin injections and pharmacotherapy. She regained ambulatory function within 6 months, and her tracheostomy

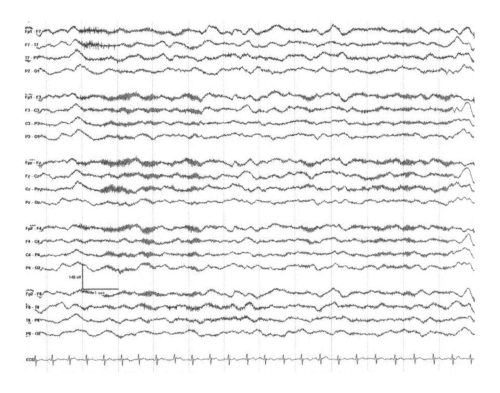

Figure 25.1 Electroencephalography (EEG) Findings for the Case Patient.
EEGs demonstrate rhythmic, generalized delta activity at 1-3 Hz with superimposed bursts of rhythmic 20-30–Hz beta activity compatible with an extreme delta brush pattern, a pattern described in adults with anti-*N*-methyl-D-aspartate receptor encephalitis.

and gastrostomy tubes were removed after 12 and 18 months, respectively. Chronic sleep disturbances, mood disorder, and headaches persisted, but she recovered to the point of independence in activities of daily living. Outpatient management in the Autoimmune Neurology Clinic focused on careful tapering of antiseizure medications and immunosuppressants (with intermittent clinical and EEG surveillance), as well as management of sleep, mood, and headaches. She returned to employment within 36 months of symptom onset.

DISCUSSION

This patient's history highlights the progressive clinical features characteristic of anti-NMDA receptor encephalitis and the long but often complete or near-complete recovery. A viral-like prodrome often manifests first, at which time neurologic symptoms are minimal, if present, and underrecognized. Neuropsychiatric symptoms including mood disturbance, psychosis, agitation, insomnia, mutism, memory impairment, and speech abnormalities typify the early illness. Additionally, patients may have visual or auditory hallucinations. As cognition further declines, mutism, coma, prominent dyskinesias (≈75% of adult patients), and seizures (57%-82% of patients) are frequently observed. Other possible causes of these symptoms, such as toxic and metabolic derangements, infections, and other inflammatory processes, should be diligently excluded. Initial CSF studies are abnormal in up to 80% of patients early in the disease course when lymphocytic-predominant pleocytosis is typically seen. In later stages, abnormalities such as increased CSF protein concentration and oligoclonal bands may be detected and are compatible with an evolving inflammatory process. Brain MRI abnormalities may be observed in up to 50% of patients, with fluid-attenuated inversion recovery abnormalities most commonly seen in the hippocampi, cerebral cortex, insula, basal ganglia, brainstem, and cerebellum; rarely, signal changes may be identified in the spinal cord. MRI abnormalities are more common among patients with coexisting autoimmunity targeting glial fibrillary acidic protein, aquaporin-4, and myelin oligodendrocyte glycoprotein.

EEG abnormalities are common and range from generalized or focal slowing to rhythmic delta activity to electrographic seizures. The presence of an extreme delta brush pattern on EEG (Figure 25.1) is supportive of (although not entirely specific for) severe anti-NMDA receptor encephalitis.

The diagnosis is confirmed by the presence of antibodies against the GluN1 subunit of the NMDA receptor in the CSF because false-negatives or false-positives (2%-14%) occur in serum testing, particularly when there has been a delay in diagnosis or if immunotherapies have already been initiated.

Admission to the intensive care unit for respiratory compromise, coma, and dysautonomia is common, and aggressive supportive care is necessary to prevent severe complications such as cardiac arrest and bradyarrhythmias. Care must be taken in the management of agitation because adverse reactions to antipsychotics, including neuroleptic malignant syndrome, appear to be higher in this population.

Treatment should not be delayed while confirmatory antibody testing results are pending if clinical suspicion is high, because earlier treatment predicts better outcomes. Tumors have been noted in 26% to 59% of patients, most commonly ovarian teratoma, and are more common in women (particularly Black women). If a tumor is detected, surgical resection is recommended. Treatment also includes a 2-fold immunotherapy approach, which is based on expert opinion (rather than controlled trial data). First-line therapy is considered to include corticosteroids, plus IV immunoglobulin or plasma exchange. Second-line immunosuppressive therapy is considered to include rituximab, cyclophosphamide, or sometimes both, administered consecutively. In reality, many patients are treated early with second-line immunosuppressants without waiting to gauge the outcomes of first-line therapy, because most patients do not have brisk responses to immunotherapy by which an outcome can be judged. This is in contrast to anti–leucine-rich, glioma-inactivated 1 encephalitis, whereby a robust early response to first-line immunotherapies is typical.

In patients who receive prompt immunotherapy and undergo tumor removal, up to 81% have favorable outcomes at 2 years. Seizures are well controlled in most patients, although psychiatric issues, memory or executive dysfunction, sleep disturbances (frequently hypersomnia), and mobility restrictions can persist for months to years, as seen in this patient. A multidisciplinary approach to optimize symptom management and minimize disability should be adopted.

KEY POINTS

- Anti-NMDA receptor encephalitis should be considered in patients with new-onset neuropsychiatric symptoms, including memory impairment, language difficulties, sleep disturbances, and behavioral changes, often preceded by a viral-like prodrome, with progression to catatonia or coma with prominent dyskinesias, seizures or status epilepticus, and dysautonomia frequently seen.

- Thorough diagnostic evaluation should be pursued to evaluate for presence of an underlying neoplasm, most often ovarian teratoma in young women.

- Treatment consists of tumor resection, if applicable, and immunotherapy (IV corticosteroids, IV immunoglobulin, and/or plasmapheresis as first-line therapy, followed by rituximab and/or cyclophosphamide as second-line immunosuppression) and should not be delayed while awaiting CSF NMDA receptor antibody confirmation.

BEHAVIORAL AND COGNITIVE CHANGES FOLLOWED BY COMA

Anastasia Zekeridou, MD, PhD

CASE PRESENTATION

HISTORY AND EXAMINATION

A 60-year-old woman who was a current smoker (20 pack-years) with no other past medical history sought care for behavioral and cognitive changes over 1 week. She became irritable, could not run her daycare facility, and had short-term memory loss and confusion (she could not recognize her grandchildren and was asking repetitive questions). She was admitted to the hospital, where decreased consciousness developed over 2 to 3 days. She became comatose and needed to be intubated because of an aspiration event. She had no fever and had a history of a tick bite 6 months prior with negative Lyme disease serologic tests and without any skin changes at that time.

Her clinical examination at admission showed short-term memory and attention deficits and generalized hyperreflexia without any meningeal signs or myoclonic jerks. She also had evidence of left axillary and retroclavicular lymphadenopathy.

Diagnoses considered at the time included an infectious or inflammatory encephalitis/meningoencephalitis, prion disease, status epilepticus with partial and partial-complex seizures due to brain lesions (abscesses, primary or metastatic cancer, infection), central nervous system vasculitis, or an autoimmune or paraneoplastic encephalopathy.

TESTING

Magnetic resonance imaging (MRI) of the brain showed T2 and fluid-attenuated inversion recovery (FLAIR) bilateral hyperintensities in the caudate nuclei and putamina, without any diffusion abnormalities (Figure 26.1A and B). Cerebrospinal fluid (CSF) analysis showed lymphocytic pleocytosis (37 white blood cells/μL [reference range, <5 cells/μL; 75% lymphocytes]), increased protein concentration (63 mg/dL [reference range, 0-35 mg/dL]), and CSF-restricted oligoclonal bands. Testing for bacterial, fungal, and viral infections was negative, including herpes simplex virus polymerase chain reaction, as was real-time quaking-induced conversion testing

for prion disease. Electroencephalography showed diffuse slowing with no epileptiform activity. Neural autoantibody testing was positive for immunoglobulin G (IgG) antibodies to α-amino-3-hydroxy-5-methyl-4-isoxazolepropionic acid (AMPA) receptor in the serum and CSF by indirect tissue immunofluorescence and antigen-specific cell-based assays. Because of suspicion for paraneoplastic neurologic disease, positron emission tomography of the body was performed and showed hypermetabolic axillary, retropectoral, and retroclavicular lymph nodes (Figure 26.1C-E). Lymph node biopsy showed metastatic melanoma of unknown primary.

DIAGNOSIS

A diagnosis of paraneoplastic anti-AMPA receptor encephalitis was made.

MANAGEMENT

The patient received treatment for melanoma (vemurafenib and cobimetinib) and encephalitis (intravenous methylprednisolone, 1 g/d for 5 days, followed by weekly infusions) and plasma exchange (7 exchanges, 1 every other day for 14 days), followed by rituximab (1 g, 2 doses, 2 weeks apart). She continued to have a Glasgow Coma Scale score of 3 for 6 weeks and remained intubated and unresponsive but subsequently recovered substantially. By 3 months the patient had minimal short-term memory loss; at 2-year follow-up her function had returned to baseline and her cancer was in remission.

DISCUSSION

Anti-AMPA receptor encephalitis can be severe, necessitating a protracted immunotherapy course and cancer treatment, if necessary. In more than half of patients with AMPA receptor–IgG, a cancer is detected. The more common tumors described are thymoma and small-cell lung carcinoma, followed by breast and ovarian adenocarcinomas. Even though anti-AMPA receptor encephalitis is often paraneoplastic, patients can respond favorably to immunotherapy

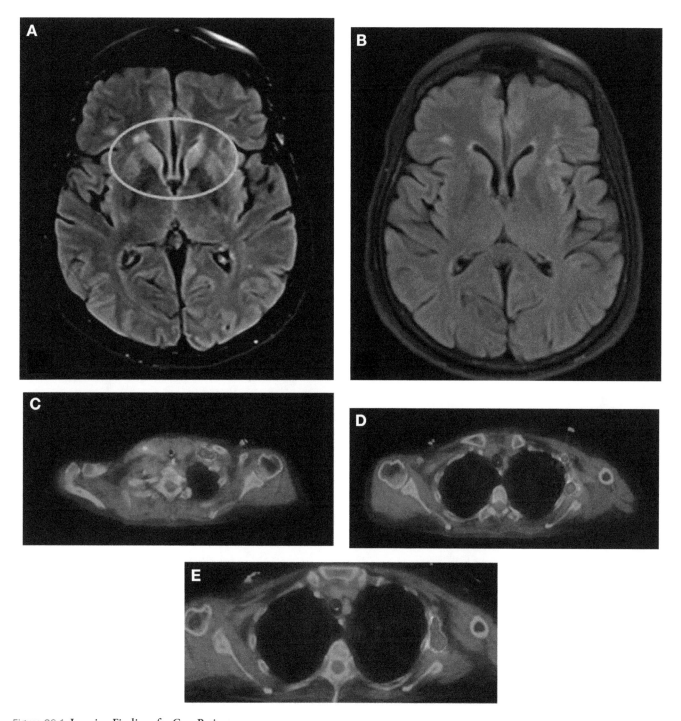

Figure 26.1 **Imaging Findings for Case Patient.**
A and B, Axial fluid-attenuated inversion recovery magnetic resonance images of the brain show bilateral basal ganglia hyperintensities (circled, A) that resolved after immunotherapy (B). C-E, Positron emission tomography of the body shows hypermetabolic retroclavicular, retropectoral, and axillary lymph nodes.

and appropriate cancer treatment. As demonstrated by this patient, even in presentations with severe encephalopathy necessitating an intensive care unit stay, there is potential for full recovery, especially if the cancer is treatable. If AMPA receptor–IgG is accompanied by antibodies to intracellular neural antigens, the prognosis is worse.

The incidence of encephalitis of autoimmune origin is comparable to that for infectious origins. The presence of cancer or central nervous system or systemic infections has been implicated as a possible trigger of paraneoplastic, autoimmune, and postinfectious encephalitides. If a neural autoantibody is present, the cellular location of its antigenic target defines the effectors of the specific autoimmune response: In cases with autoantibodies targeting membrane proteins in neuronal or glial synapses, the antibodies are potentially pathogenic; if the respective antigen is located intracellularly, the neural autoantibodies are just a biomarker of the effector cytotoxic T cells of the same specificity.

An autoimmune or paraneoplastic encephalitis should be suspected in patients with subacute onset of cognitive and behavioral difficulties associated with treatment-refractory epilepsy, movement disorders, or autonomic dysfunction and in patients with a personal history of autoimmunity or cancer or with systemic manifestations at presentation (eg, weight loss, night sweats). Neural autoantibody biomarkers aid in timely diagnosis of both autoimmunity and cancer and guide appropriate treatment. Clinical clues suggesting a specific neural autoantibody are summarized in Table 26.1. Brain MRI can show mesial temporal lobe T2/FLAIR hyperintensities, with or without gadolinium enhancement (limbic encephalitis) or extratemporal lesions. Cortical and subcortical multifocal, nonenhancing, T2/FLAIR hyperintensities should raise suspicion for anti-γ-aminobutyric acid$_A$ receptor encephalitis. Basal ganglia T2/FLAIR hyperintensities can be seen in patients with collapsin-response mediator protein 5-IgG– or phosphodiesterase 10A-IgG–related autoimmunity, whereas periventricular, linear, radial, perivascular enhancement can be seen in patients with autoimmune glial fibrillary acidic protein astrocytopathy. CSF can be inflammatory with increased white blood cell count, IgG index, and/or CSF-restricted oligoclonal bands. Increased protein concentration alone is not a specific marker of autoimmune encephalitis.

Cancer screening is essential in these cases, especially if a cancer-predictive autoantibody is detected. ^{18}F-Fludeoxyglucose-positron emission tomography–computed tomography of the body increases the yield of cancer detection, but computed tomography of the chest or dedicated MRI might be more helpful in the detection of thymoma. In women, a gynecologic examination with ultrasonography and mammography is suggested; in men, testicular ultrasonography for seminoma is recommended. Depending on the risk factors and presentations, dermatologic examination and gastrointestinal tract endoscopic examination can be useful.

If an underlying cancer is found, treating it is crucial. Similar to the current case, if the identified cancer is commonly treated with immune checkpoint inhibitors, these medications should be avoided if possible—by enhancing immune responses they can aggravate the paraneoplastic neurologic syndrome. In addition, early immunotherapy is warranted; first-line intravenous methylprednisolone or plasma exchange is often used, with or without intravenous immunoglobulin. In cases of synaptic autoimmunity, rituximab, which targets B cells, is efficient and is often used as first-line treatment. Depending on the presentation and autoantibody profile, cyclophosphamide might be necessary (2 mg/kg orally or monthly infusions at 1 g/m², usually for 6 months), along with treatment of the underlying cancer, if found. Some patients with encephalitis

Table 26.1 **CLINICAL CLUES SUGGESTING A SPECIFIC DIAGNOSIS IN PATIENTS WITH AUTOIMMUNE ENCEPHALITIS**

CLINICAL PHENOTYPE	ASSOCIATED NEURAL AUTOANTIBODY SPECIFICITIES
Faciobrachial dystonic seizures	LGI1
Dizzy spells	LGI1
Status epilepticus, seizure-predominant presentation	GABA$_A$R, GABA$_B$R, GAD65 (multiple others)
Myoclonus	DPPX, glycine receptor, neurexin 3a
Opsoclonus-myoclonus	ANNA2 (Ri), rare; ANNA1 in children with neuroblastoma
Psychosis	NMDAR (multiple others)
Coexisting ataxia	GAD65, ANNA1 (Hu), CASPR2 (episodic)
Progressive encephalopathy with rigidity and myoclonus; exaggerated startle	Glycine receptor, DPPX
Stiff-person syndrome	Amphiphysin, GAD65, glycine receptor
Peripheral nerve hyperexcitability	CASPR2, LGI1
Coexisting gastrointestinal tract dysmotility	ANNA1 (Hu)
Coexisting gastrointestinal tract hypermotility	DPPX
Morvan syndrome (central, peripheral, and autonomic nervous system hyperexcitability)	CASPR2
Coexisting sensory neuronopathy	ANNA1 (Hu)
Prominent meningeal involvement	GFAP
Coexisting myelopathy	GFAP, amphiphysin, ANNA1, CRMP5, MOG
Encephalitis in children	Aquaporin-4, MOG, NMDAR, GABA$_A$R

Abbreviations: ANNA1, antineuronal nuclear antibody type 1; ANNA2, antineuronal nuclear antibody type 2; CASPR2, contactin-associated protein 2; CRMP5, collapsin-response mediator protein 5; DPPX, dipeptidyl peptidase-like protein 6; GABA$_A$R, γ-aminobutyric acid$_A$ receptor; GABA$_B$R, γ-aminobutyric acid$_B$ receptor; GAD65, glutamic acid decarboxylase 65-kDa isoform; GFAP, glial fibrillary acidic protein; LGI1, leucine-rich, glioma-inactivated protein 1; MOG, myelin oligodendrocyte glycoprotein; NMDAR, N-methyl-D-aspartate receptor.

have a monophasic course, whereas others have a relapsing course requiring long-term immunosuppression with medications such as rituximab or mycophenolate mofetil.

KEY POINTS

- Anti-AMPA receptor encephalitis can be severe but is potentially treatable. The disease course can be protracted, with long recovery periods.

- Autoimmune encephalitis should be suspected in patients with subacute onset of cognitive decline, especially when associated with treatment-refractory epilepsy, movement disorders, or autonomic dysfunction and in patients with a history of autoimmunity or cancer.

- Early recognition and appropriate immunotherapy and cancer treatment may lead to favorable outcomes.

EPISODIC HEMIPARESIS, COGNITIVE DECLINE, AND SEIZURES IN A WOMAN WITH PERNICIOUS ANEMIA

Cristina Valencia-Sanchez, MD, PhD, and Andrew McKeon, MB, BCh, MD

CASE PRESENTATION

HISTORY AND EXAMINATION

A 46-year-old woman with a history of pernicious anemia, treated with intramuscular vitamin B$_{12}$ injections (1 per month for 3 months), sought care for intermittent episodes of weakness in her right upper extremity and speech difficulties lasting for minutes to hours over the course of 2 months. Each episode was followed by a headache. It was initially thought that she had migraine headaches. Blood tests showed increased thyrotropin and low free thyroxine levels, and she was diagnosed with Hashimoto thyroiditis. She initiated treatment with levothyroxine. One month later, the patient had a confusional episode during which she was talking about her mother as if she was still alive, though she had been deceased for several years.

She was seen at a local emergency department and was given a 6-day course of oral methylprednisolone. She experienced complete recovery of her symptoms for 6 weeks. Recurrent episodes of right-sided weakness, fluctuating confusion, and abnormal behavior then developed. On one occasion, she drove to a mall, parked her car, and walked in her bare feet through the parking lot. She also left the kitchen stove on, not having made any food. Over the course of the following 2 months, the cognitive difficulties progressed. She became less interactive and more confused. She again was brought to the emergency department after a generalized tonic-clonic seizure. On examination, she was profoundly encephalopathic. Formal bedside cognitive testing could not be obtained. She had no focal deficits on neurologic examination. Diagnoses considered at the time are shown in Table 27.1.

TESTING

Findings of magnetic resonance imaging (MRI) of the brain were normal. Electroencephalography (EEG) revealed diffuse slowing. Cerebrospinal fluid (CSF) analysis showed increased protein concentration of 81 mg/dL (reference range, ≤35 mg/dL) and lymphocytic pleocytosis (white blood cell count, 25/μL; reference range, ≤5/μL). Thyroid peroxidase (TPO) antibody value was markedly increased (>13,000

Table 27.1 | **DIFFERENTIAL DIAGNOSIS FOR THE CASE PATIENT**

POSSIBLE DIAGNOSES	PERTINENT NEGATIVES
Infectious encephalitis	No febrile illness
Virus: herpesviruses (HSV1/2, VZV, EBV, HHV-6, CMV), arbovirus, HIV	No history of immunosuppression
Bacterial: Lyme disease, TB, listeria, syphilis	Negative serum and CSF studies
Immunocompromised: JC polyoma virus, fungal/parasitic	Negative serum and CSF studies
Autoimmune encephalitis as defined by a neural antibody, such as anti-NMDA receptor encephalitis	Negative antibodies in serum and CSF
Inflammatory encephalitis, such as sarcoidosis, ADEM	MRI unremarkable
Metabolic/endocrine encephalopathy: uremic, hepatic, hyponatremia, hypo/hyperthyroid, hypoglycemia, vitamin B$_{12}$ deficiency	Laboratory studies unremarkable
Toxic encephalopathy: alcohol, chemotherapy, carbon monoxide	No history of exposure
Neoplastic: CNS lymphoma, primary CNS cancer, brain metastases	No history of cancer
Creutzfeldt-Jakob disease	No other associated signs (ataxia, myoclonus)
	MRI and EEG not typical

Abbreviations: ADEM, acute disseminated encephalomyelitis; CMV, cytomegalovirus; CNS, central nervous system; CSF, cerebrospinal fluid; EBV, Epstein-Barr virus; EEG, electroencephalography; HHV, human herpesvirus; HSV, herpes simplex virus; MRI, magnetic resonance imaging; NMDA, *N*-methyl-D-aspartate; TB, tuberculosis; VZV, varicella-zoster virus.

IU/mL; reference range, <9.0 IU/mL). Thyroglobulin antibody value was also increased at 284 IU/mL (reference range, <4.0 IU/mL). Findings of complete metabolic panel, thyroid function tests, and vitamin B_{12} levels were normal. Consistent with her history of pernicious anemia, she was positive for gastric parietal cell antibodies. Other nonneural autoantibodies were negative. Testing for neural autoantibodies was negative in serum and CSF. Infectious studies of the serum and CSF were also negative.

DIAGNOSIS

The clinical presentation—with fluctuating cognitive decline, strokelike episodes, and seizures, encephalopathic EEG findings, inflammatory CSF and markedly increased thyroid autoantibodies, and complete (although short-lived) response to initial empiric treatment with corticosteroids—was compatible with steroid-responsive encephalopathy associated with autoimmune thyroiditis (SREAT), also known as Hashimoto encephalopathy.

MANAGEMENT

The patient started levetiracetam therapy and had no further seizures. She received intravenous methylprednisolone 1,000 mg/d for 5 days. At the completion of treatment, her confusion rapidly and substantially improved. She was discharged home 1 week after admission on oral prednisone 80 mg/d, with planned gradual taper by 10 mg per month. She also started pantoprazole, calcium, and vitamin D supplementation and *Pneumocystis jirovecii* prophylaxis (trimethoprim-sulfamethoxazole, double strength, 1 tablet 3 times per week). For long-term immunotherapy, she initiated methotrexate 10 mg weekly.

Three months later, the patient and her family reported 90% improvement in her cognitive functioning and resolution of the episodes of hemiparesis. On the Kokmen Short Test of Mental Status (which is similar to the Mini-Mental Status Examination), the patient missed 1 point for calculation and 1 point for immediate recall (36/38). Otherwise her examination was unremarkable.

The patient continued tapering prednisone by 10 mg per month, until she was taking 10 mg/d, and then tapered by 1 mg per month thereafter until discontinuation. It was recommended that she continue methotrexate for 5 years before discontinuing.

DISCUSSION

SREAT, also known as Hashimoto encephalopathy, was initially described by Brain et al in 1966 in a 48-year-old man with strokelike episodes and subacute encephalopathy months after the onset of autoimmune (Hashimoto) thyroiditis.

It remains a controversial entity, but focusing on several key points can assist in the diagnosis. First, patients with one autoimmune disease are at risk for development of another. Second, autoimmune thyroid disease is common, and in some patients with that disorder, other autoimmune diseases, sometimes neurologic, can develop. Third, the disorder is defined by the presence of a subacute-onset brain syndrome (encephalopathy), with thyroid antibodies detected and objective neurologic improvement after immunotherapy (usually with corticosteroids), with no detection of other neural autoantibody biomarkers. Fourth, detection of thyroid antibodies reflects a predisposition to an autoimmune neurologic disorder but does not imply a neurological pathogenic role for those antibodies. Finally, thyroid autoantibodies are common in the general population and of themselves are not diagnostic of any disease, although in the right clinical context they may assist in making an autoimmune encephalopathy diagnosis.

The clinical manifestations are variable, with subacute cognitive impairment and behavioral changes, typically fluctuating, associated with other features such as tremor, myoclonus, transient aphasia, lateralized motor or sensory deficits (strokelike episodes), sleep abnormalities, seizures, and gait difficulties. It is 4 to 5 times more likely to affect women than men.

MRI findings may be normal or demonstrate nonspecific T2-signal abnormalities. CSF frequently shows abnormal features, although often with nonspecific findings such as increased protein level. EEG abnormalities are nonspecific—commonly diffuse background slowing consistent with encephalopathy. TPO antibodies are increased, and antibody levels do not correspond to the severity of the clinical deficits. Thyroglobulin antibodies are increased in up to 70% of cases.

TPO and thyroglobulin autoantibodies are serologic markers of autoimmune thyroiditis. The prevalence of TPO antibodies in the general population is high, 2% to 10% in younger adults and 5% to 20% in healthy older adults. It is also detected in coexistence with other systemic autoantibodies and in patients with autoimmune neurologic disorders with neural antibodies (such as anti–*N*-methyl-D-aspartate receptor encephalitis). Advances in autoimmune neurology have revealed new neuron-specific autoantibodies as the cause of or biomarkers of reversible cognitive decline in some patients previously diagnosed with SREAT.

A diagnosis of SREAT should only be considered after exclusion of other infectious and autoimmune causes of encephalitis (Table 27.1) and should not be made without objective evidence of encephalopathy. An abnormality on cognitive testing, brain imaging (MRI or positron emission tomography–computed tomography), or EEG may assist in that regard and may also serve as a baseline for future posttreatment comparison.

Initial treatment is with high-dose intravenous corticosteroids. Most patients have a favorable outcome, and lack of response should prompt review of the diagnosis. This is usually followed by slow oral corticosteroid tapering. In patients who regain normal cognition after immunotherapy, observation without immunosuppression is reasonable. Long-term immunotherapy should be considered in patients who have relapse. Maintenance immunotherapy includes steroid-sparing agents such as azathioprine, mycophenolate mofetil, or methotrexate. Cyclophosphamide and rituximab are generally reserved for patients with refractory disease.

KEY POINTS

- A diagnosis of SREAT should be considered only in patients with clinical and paraclinical neurologic findings to support encephalopathy in whom other metabolic, toxic, infectious, and autoimmune causes of encephalopathy have been excluded.

- Required features include:
  - Subacute and fluctuating encephalopathy, with 1 or more of strokelike episodes, seizures, myoclonus, and tremor

- Detection of thyroid autoantibodies; these reflect a predisposition to an autoimmune neurologic disorder but do not imply a pathogenic role for those antibodies
- An objective neurologic response to immunotherapy
- Encephalopathic-appearing EEG findings and inflammatory CSF support the diagnosis.

- Thyroid antibody levels do not correspond to the severity of the clinical deficits, and changes in those values do not serve as a surrogate of treatment response or outcome.

RAPIDLY PROGRESSIVE DEMENTIA AND THYROID ANTIBODIES

Amy C. Kunchok, MBBS, and Eoin P. Flanagan, MB, BCh

CASE PRESENTATION

HISTORY AND EXAMINATION

A 70-year-old right-handed woman sought care for subacute cognitive decline. Before these symptoms began, she was cognitively normal, including driving her car and managing her own finances without difficulty. She initially began to get lost in familiar places. She was then amnestic for a vacation she had taken, would repeat questions, and had become more withdrawn. She also reported multiple episodes of hot flashes accompanied by an unusual abdominal sensation that lasted 90 seconds each, which were suspicious for sensory seizures. After symptom onset, her cognition rapidly deteriorated over the subsequent 6 weeks such that she had difficulty with activities of daily living.

Initial investigations at her local hospital included normal brain magnetic resonance imaging (MRI) findings, vitamin B_{12} level, and thyroid function. She was initially diagnosed with dementia due to Alzheimer disease and prescribed donepezil, without improvement in her symptoms. Her cognition continued to worsen and additional testing was undertaken. Cerebrospinal fluid (CSF) analysis showed a normal white blood cell count and protein concentration and was negative for oligoclonal bands. CSF polymerase chain reaction testing for herpes simplex virus type 1 and 2 was negative. Serologic testing for syphilis and HIV was negative. However, her thyroid peroxidase antibodies were increased (469 IU/mL; reference range, <9 IU/mL) and she had hyponatremia (sodium, 126 mmol/L; reference range, 135-145 mmol/L). She was then diagnosed with Hashimoto encephalitis. She was treated with oral prednisone 40 mg/d, which resulted in complete resolution of cognitive symptoms, but her memory problems began to return with tapering of corticosteroids. She was referred to the Autoimmune Neurology Clinic at Mayo Clinic for further evaluation.

Her medical history included herpes zoster ophthalmicus, essential hypertension, ischemic heart disease, and bilateral cataracts. She had a 20-pack-year smoking history and had quit 30 years earlier. Her family history included breast cancer in 2 sisters and her mother. Her medications included amlodipine, aspirin, hydrochlorothiazide, metoprolol, and simvastatin.

Her neurologic examination at our institution (during her oral corticosteroid taper) was normal except for a Kokmen Short Test of Mental Status score of 30/38, in which she lost 3 points for delayed recall, 2 points for calculation, 1 for abstraction, 1 for construction, and 1 for information. Neuropsychological testing indicated problems with delayed recall, but other cognitive domains were preserved. The Beck Depression Inventory score was normal. Diagnoses considered at the time are shown in Table 28.1.

TESTING

On neural autoantibody testing, serum and CSF were positive for α-amino-3-hydroxy-5-methyl-4-isoxazolepropionic acid (AMPA) receptor immunoglobulin G (IgG) autoantibody by tissue-based indirect immunofluorescence assay (Figures 28.1A and B), which was molecularly confirmed by AMPA receptor–specific cell-based assay. Because of the paraneoplastic significance of AMPA receptor–IgG, a comprehensive search for cancer followed. Findings of mammography were normal, as were electroencephalography findings, although it was performed 12 weeks after symptom onset and after initiating oral corticosteroids.

[18]F-Fludeoxyglucose (FDG) positron emission tomography (PET)-computed tomography (CT) of the body demonstrated increased FDG uptake (hypermetabolism) in the right hilum and numerous mediastinal lymph nodes, suggestive of malignancy (Figures 28.2A and B). Dedicated PET-CT brain imaging demonstrated generalized atrophy, without abnormal uptake. Bronchoscopy with lymph node biopsy was undertaken. Small cell carcinoma of the lung (SCLC) was found on histopathologic analysis.

Table 28.1 | DIFFERENTIAL DIAGNOSIS FOR THE CASE PATIENT

DIAGNOSIS	INDICATIONS FOR	INDICATIONS AGAINST
Alzheimer dementia	Short-term memory loss, disorientation and visuospatial difficulties, noninflammatory CSF, no response to donepezil	Subacute onset, rapid deterioration, response to corticosteroids
Lewy body dementia	Fluctuations, normal brain MRI, noninflammatory CSF	No parkinsonism, visual hallucinations, or REM sleep behavior disorder
Creutzfeldt-Jakob disease	Rapidly progressive dementia, noninflammatory CSF	Normal brain MRI, response to corticosteroids
Vascular (vascular dementia, subdural hematoma, PRES)	Vascular risk factors, age, noninflammatory CSF	Normal brain MRI
Pseudodementia	Loss of interest in activities, withdrawn, metoprolol use	No prior depression history, response to corticosteroids, depression rating scales normal
Other infections (HIV, Whipple disease, syphilis)	Rapidly progressive dementia	No infectious symptoms or risk factors, noninflammatory CSF, normal brain MRI, negative serologic findings for infections
Toxic-metabolic (alcohol, medications, electrolyte disturbance, infection)	Fluctuating cognitive state, hyponatremia	No recent changes in medication, response to corticosteroids
Neoplastic	Rapidly progressive dementia, noninflammatory CSF	Normal brain MRI
Autoimmune/paraneoplastic	Rapidly progressive dementia, history of smoking, corticosteroid responsiveness, thyroid antibodies	Noninflammatory CSF, normal brain MRI

Abbreviations: CSF, cerebrospinal fluid; MRI, magnetic resonance imaging; PRES, posterior reversible encephalopathy syndrome; REM, rapid eye movement.

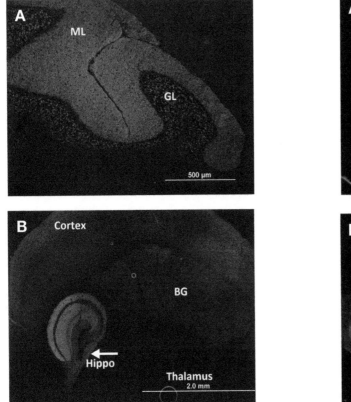

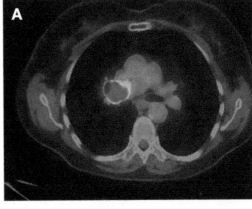

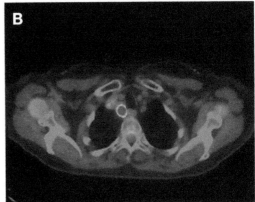

Figure 28.1 Tissue-Based Indirect Immunofluorescence Assay.
Immunofluorescent staining for immunoglobulin G antibodies to α-amino-3-hydroxy-5-methyl-4-isoxazolepropionic acid (AMPA) receptor shows typical intense staining in (A) the cerebellar molecular layer (ML) and granular layer (GL) and (B) the hippocampus (Hippo), cortex, and basal ganglia (BG), but not in the thalamus.

Figure 28.2 ^{18}F-Fludeoxyglucose-Positron Emission Tomography–Computed Tomography Findings for the Case Patient.
Imaging of the body shows avid glucose uptake (red) in the right hilum (A) and right paratracheal regions (B) supportive of a malignant process.

DIAGNOSIS

The patient was diagnosed with paraneoplastic autoimmune dementia in the setting of AMPA receptor autoantibodies and stage IIIB SCLC.

MANAGEMENT

The metastatic SCLC was treated with chemotherapy (carboplatin and etoposide) and radiation, with disease resolution. For her cognitive symptoms, she was given intravenous methylprednisolone 1 g per week for 12 weeks, with resolution of symptoms. Unfortunately, the patient was logistically unable to complete the planned follow-up neuropsychological testing to objectively quantify this improvement.

DISCUSSION

An insidious onset of cognitive decline in older persons is suggestive of a neurodegenerative dementia. However, a rapidly progressive dementia or a subacute or fluctuating course should raise suspicion for an autoimmune/paraneoplastic cause, which is critical to identify given the potential for reversibility. In the case patient, in addition to the rapidly progressive dementia, the history of smoking and family history of breast cancer were clues to a paraneoplastic autoimmune encephalitis. Objective testing of cognition with bedside cognitive testing or neuropsychological testing is useful in autoimmune dementia to serve as a baseline from which response to immunotherapy treatment can be judged. Assessing for MRI abnormalities suggestive of autoimmunity (eg, unilateral or bilateral mesial temporal T2 hyperintensity on MRI) or CSF inflammation (eg, increased white blood cell count, markedly increased protein concentration [>100 mg/dL], or positive oligoclonal bands) can help support a diagnosis of autoimmune dementia; these features were not present in this case and are absent in up to 23% of older persons with autoimmune encephalitis/dementia. The detection of thyroid peroxidase antibodies was a clue to a general predisposition to autoimmunity, but these antibodies lack specificity and can be present in up to 20% of healthy controls. Testing serum and CSF for neural autoantibodies is crucial in cases of suspected autoimmune dementia because it can help confirm the diagnosis and be a clue to an underlying cancer. The detection of AMPA receptor–IgG in this case helped indicate a likely diagnosis of SCLC, which PET-CT and subsequent biopsy helped confirm.

AMPA receptor–IgG is a neuronal antibody biomarker associated with autoimmune paraneoplastic syndromes. The most common associated cancers include SCLC, thymoma, breast cancer, and ovarian teratoma. It is more often found in older patients (median age, 62 years). Although limbic encephalitis typically presents with severe short-term memory loss, confusion, seizures, and psychiatric symptoms, the spectrum can include more subtle presentations of confusion and cognitive impairment that can mimic neurodegenerative diseases.

In this case, the patient had resolution of symptoms with corticosteroids and oncologic treatment and did not require additional acute immunotherapy (such as intravenous immunoglobulin or plasma exchange) or longer-term steroid-sparing immunosuppression (such as rituximab, mycophenolate mofetil, or azathioprine) that may be considered in cases of autoimmune dementia.

KEY POINTS

- Autoimmune and paraneoplastic causes should be considered in the differential diagnosis of a rapidly progressive dementia, and evaluation for neural autoantibodies is crucial in confirming the diagnosis.

- Detection of inflammation on brain MRI or in CSF is a potential clue to an autoimmune dementia but is not universally present.

GOOSE BUMPS AND MEMORY LOSS

Jeffrey W. Britton, MD, Bhavya Narapureddy, MBBS, and Divyanshu Dubey, MBBS

CASE PRESENTATION

HISTORY AND EXAMINATION

A 46-year-old man had an episode of loss of awareness while driving home. He was found in a cul de sac by his neighbor and was acting confused. He was brought to the emergency department; while there, he started having recurrent episodes of goose bumps (goose flesh) involving half of his body (5-10 episodes per hour) associated with a "wavelike" sensation that would typically begin in the lower extremities and spread upward. Each episode lasted for 20 to 60 seconds. Some episodes involved the right side of his body and others, the left side. During some of the longer goose bump episodes, he also had some speech difficulty. However, he never had loss of awareness, convulsive activity, tongue biting, or bowel or bladder incontinence. Physical and neurologic examinations were unremarkable, except for mild cognitive deficits.

Findings on initial laboratory workup, including complete blood cell count with differential, electrolyte values, thyroid function tests, erythrocyte sedimentation rate, C-reactive protein level, antinuclear antibodies, extractable nuclear antigen antibodies, toxicology screen, and computed tomography of the head, were unremarkable. Diagnoses considered at the time are shown in Table 29.1.

TESTING

Video electroencephalographic (EEG) monitoring showed frequent independent left and right temporal ictal and interictal discharges. Magnetic resonance imaging of the brain showed fluid-attenuated inversion recovery (FLAIR) hyperintensity in the bilateral hippocampi (Figure 29.1). Cerebrospinal fluid (CSF) analysis showed a mildly increased total protein concentration of 65 mg/dL (reference range, ≤35 mg/dL) but no supernumerary oligoclonal bands and normal nucleated cell count and immunoglobulin G (IgG) index. CSF analysis for infection was negative, including fungal complement fixation, blastomyces and cryptococcal antibodies, Gram stain and cultures, and polymerase chain reaction testing for herpes simplex virus (type 1 and type 2), *Toxoplasma*, human herpesvirus 6, varicella-zoster virus, and *Tropheryma whipplei*. Computed tomography of the chest, abdomen, and pelvis detected no underlying malignancy.

Serum autoimmune epilepsy evaluation was remarkable for leucine-rich, glioma-inactivated protein 1 (LGI1)-IgG seropositivity.

DIAGNOSIS

The patient was diagnosed with LGI1-IgG antibody–associated autoimmune seizures presenting with pilomotor seizures.

MANAGEMENT

Before autoimmune workup, the patient had been treated with a gradual escalation of the following antiseizure medications twice daily: levetiracetam 1,500 mg, followed by sodium valproate 750 mg, and then oxcarbazepine 150 mg.

Table 29.1 | **DIFFERENTIAL DIAGNOSIS FOR THE CASE PATIENT**

POSSIBLE DIAGNOSES	PERTINENT NEGATIVES
Focal seizures without impaired awareness, nonmotor, autonomic	
Autonomic dysreflexia	No additional sympathetic or parasympathetic dysautonomic signs/symptoms
Arrhythmias	Stereotypical spells, no arrhythmias reported on cardiac telemetry
Transient ischemic attack	Recurrent episodes (>50 per day) without any lasting deficits
Substance abuse/withdrawal	No prior history of substance abuse, normal toxicology screen
Panic attacks	Brief events, multiple per day
Psychogenic nonepileptic spells	Stereotypical spells, brief

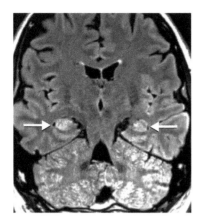

Figure 29.1 Magnetic Resonance Imaging (MRI) Findings for Case Patient.
MRI of the brain demonstrates fluid-attenuated inversion recovery hyperintensity involving the bilateral hippocampi (arrows).

The seizures continued. He was subsequently started on intravenous methylprednisolone (IVMP) 1,000 mg daily for 5 days. He was seizure free by day 3 of the 5-day course of IVMP and was transitioned to an oral prednisone taper starting at 60 mg/d. His pilomotor seizures recurred, however, a month after his initial evaluation. He was again treated with a 3-day course of high-dose IVMP, but the seizures remained refractory. He was subsequently started on a 6-week regimen of intravenous immunoglobulin (IVIG), with a starting dosage of 0.4 g/kg daily for 3 days, followed by 0.4 g/kg every week for 5 weeks. He again achieved seizure freedom while on IVIG. He was also started on mycophenolate mofetil at 1,000 mg twice daily.

On follow-up clinic visits, the patient had no recurrence of seizures and disclosed no cognitive dysfunction except for mild inattention. Three years after the patient's initial episode, the antiseizure medications and mycophenolate mofetil were gradually tapered, without recurrence.

DISCUSSION

LGI1-IgG–associated autoimmunity is typically seen among older patients (>50 years), more commonly men. Symptoms commonly include seizures and cognitive dysfunction, presenting as memory loss and disorientation.

Pilomotor seizures presenting as multiple brief episodes of unilateral piloerection have been described in association with LGI1 antibodies. Other characteristic seizure semiology associated with LGI1-IgG is faciobrachial dystonic seizures (FBDS), manifesting as stereotypic contraction of the face, arm, and leg. Semiologies other than FBDS also may be present. For example, paroxysmal dizzy spells (recurrent brief episodes of dizziness) were recently described. These episodes preceded the development of autoimmune encephalitis by weeks to months. Also, sensory and "thermal" seizure semiology has been described. Seizures associated with LGI1-IgG encephalitis are noted to be significantly shorter in duration

and to occur at a significantly higher frequency than limbic seizures of other causes.

A considerable proportion of patients with LGI1 autoimmune epilepsy have normal findings on EEG. However, in some cases ictal or interictal temporal and/or frontal discharges on EEG can be detected. Brain magnetic resonance imaging may be normal or may demonstrate temporal lobe T2/FLAIR hyperintensities (unilateral or bilateral). Hippocampal atrophy may also occur with disease progression, especially if immunotherapy is not initiated early in the disease course. Serum is more sensitive than CSF for detection of LGI1 antibodies. HLA-DRB1*07:01 has been demonstrated to have strong association with LGI1 autoimmunity. Paraneoplastic association with thymoma has been reported in a minority of cases (10%).

Treatment of LGI1-IgG–associated autoimmune seizures is primarily focused on early initiation of immunotherapy. Acute-phase treatment includes high-dose IVMP 1 g daily for 5 treatments, followed by plasma exchange (5-7 exchanges over 10-14 days) or IVIG (0.4 g/kg daily for 5 days). The use of IVIG is supported by a randomized clinical trial, although corticosteroids seem particularly effective from clinical experience. Continuation of immunotherapy for at least 6 to 9 months is needed. This can be accomplished by the use of high-dose oral prednisone with a slow taper, gradually widening intervals of IVMP or IVIG infusions (weekly, alternate week, every third week, monthly, then discontinue), or early use of rituximab. Even though seizures in autoimmune epilepsy are characteristically resistant to antiseizure medications alone, such medications can help prevent transition of focal to bilateral convulsive seizures. Some recent studies have found sodium channel–blocking agents such as carbamazepine, phenytoin, oxcarbazepine, and lacosamide to be relatively more efficacious than other antiseizure medications, but these are only effective in 15% of patients. Oxcarbazepine was ineffective in this case patient. Relapses occur in 10% to 30% of patients. To prevent relapses or for management of refractory cases, second-line immunotherapies such as mycophenolate mofetil, rituximab, or azathioprine are also used.

KEY POINTS

- Most cases of LGI1-IgG antibody encephalitis include seizure semiology other than FBDS.

- Characteristic features of non-FBDS seizures in LGI1-IgG antibody encephalitis include sensory, "thermal," and autonomic symptoms. Seizure frequency tends to be very high (daily to multiple per day), with seizure duration shorter than focal limbic seizures of other causes.

- Early initiation of first-line immunotherapy (IVMP, IVIG, or plasma exchange), followed by slow tapering over 6 to 9 months, is critical for favorable clinical outcomes.

- Chronic immunotherapy in the form of mycophenolate mofetil, rituximab, or azathioprine can help prevent relapses.

A PATIENT WITH HEADACHE AND PROGRESSIVE TREMOR

Anastasia Zekeridou, MD

CASE PRESENTATION

HISTORY AND EXAMINATION

A 50-year-old man with no prior medical history sought care for new-onset daily headaches persisting for 3 months that did not improve after taking over-the-counter analgesics. In addition, he described asymmetric upper extremity action tremor and clumsiness affecting predominantly the right side, particularly his handwriting. In the past month, the patient's wife also noted personality changes, anxiety, and depression. The review of systems was pertinent for a flulike syndrome in the weeks before his symptoms started.

Neurologic examination showed reduced digit span, pyramidal signs with asymmetric hyperreflexia (right greater than left), and bilateral subtle lower extremity spasticity. He also had cerebellar ataxia and postural and action tremor of the upper extremities (right predominant). Ophthalmologic examination indicated mild bilateral optic disc edema with normal visual acuity.

The timing of the patient's symptoms suggested a probable infectious, postinfectious, autoimmune, inflammatory, neoplastic, or paraneoplastic etiology. Viral and mycobacterial infections could be considered, but bacterial would be less likely because of the 3-month evolution. Given the flulike prodrome and the subacute onset, postinfectious and autoimmune causes (either neurologic autoimmunity or systemic autoimmunity with neurologic manifestations) including paraneoplastic disease could occur. The myelopathy and the optic disc edema suggest possible myelin oligodendrocyte glycoprotein and aquaporin-4 autoimmunity, but these would be less likely because of the mild myelopathic symptoms and no symptoms of optic neuritis. There was no evidence of systemic autoimmunity in the history or the examination. A primary central nervous system malignant process, including lymphoma, or metastatic disease, including leptomeningeal carcinomatosis, are part of the differential diagnosis in this otherwise healthy 50-year-old man. Metabolic and genetic causes seem less likely given the subacute onset of the disease;

the neurologic examination abnormalities make primary headache disorders unlikely.

TESTING

Brain magnetic resonance imaging (MRI) showed linear radial perivascular enhancement in both cerebral hemispheres without associated T2 hyperintensities (Figure 30.1A). MRI of the spine showed some hazy T2 hyperintensity in the thoracic cord with subtle gadolinium enhancement (Figure 30.1B and C).

Cerebrospinal fluid (CSF) examination showed an opening pressure of 21 cm H_2O, 63 white blood cells/μL with lymphocytic predominance, increased protein concentration of 130 mg/dL, and no oligoclonal bands. CSF cytologic analysis showed no malignancy, and flow cytometric assays were negative for lymphoma. Gram stain and bacterial, mycobacterial, viral, and fungal cultures were negative, as was polymerase chain reaction testing for selected viruses and *Tropheryma whipplei*. Serologic tests for syphilis, Lyme disease, and HIV were negative. Levels of vitamin B_{12}, copper, zinc, vitamin E, hemoglobin A_{1c}, and connective tissue biomarkers, celiac disease serologic testing, and protein electrophoresis with immunofixation were all negative or normal.

Positron emission tomography-computed tomography of the body showed no cancer (lymphoma) or signs of inflammation, including sarcoidosis. Computed tomography of the chest and ultrasonography of the testes were normal.

The patient's CSF was positive for immunoglobulin G (IgG) antibodies specific for glial fibrillary acidic protein (GFAP); no other neural autoantibodies were found in the serum or CSF.

DIAGNOSIS

The patient was diagnosed with autoimmune GFAP astrocytopathy.

MANAGEMENT

The patient was treated with high-dose intravenous corticosteroids (1 g methylprednisolone for 5 days) followed

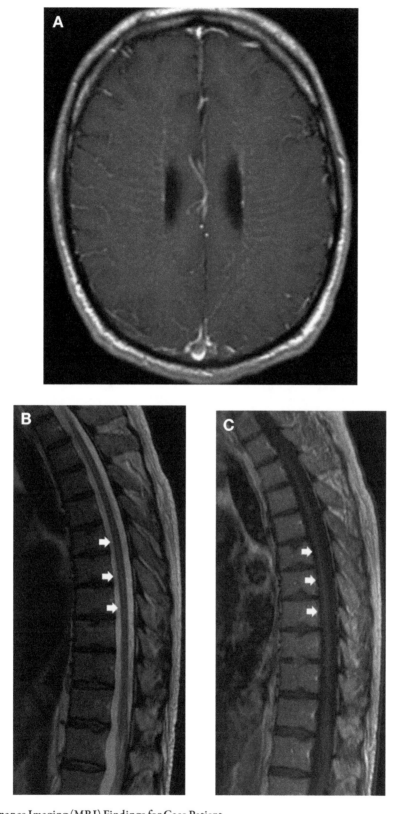

Figure 30.1 **Magnetic Resonance Imaging (MRI) Findings for Case Patient.**

A, Postgadolinium axial T1 MRI of the brain shows linear radial perivascular enhancement in both cerebral hemispheres without associated T2 hyperintensities (not shown). B and C, MRI of the spine shows some hazy T2 hyperintensity (arrows) more prominent in the thoracic cord (B) with subtle gadolinium enhancement (arrows) (C).

by oral prednisone 1 mg/kg per day, which was tapered over 1 month. The patient improved after the first 2 weeks of treatment, the headaches disappeared, and he had only mild persistent tremor. After the corticosteroids were discontinued, he had an early relapse with increased headaches, confusion, and ataxia. At that time, CSF reevaluation again showed lymphocytic pleocytosis, and the patient was treated with oral prednisone 1 mg/kg per day for 3 months. The patient recovered completely and the corticosteroids were tapered over 6 months. Repeated imaging showed resolution of the abnormalities. At 3-year follow-up, the patient was relapse free.

DISCUSSION

Autoimmune GFAP astrocytopathy, first described in 2016, is defined by the presence of GFAP-IgG in the CSF. The highest sensitivity and specificity for diagnosis is achieved by testing CSF for a pattern of astrocytic staining of rodent brain tissue by patient IgG and then confirming positivity by a GFAPα isoform-specific cell-based assay. Serum testing is neither sensitive nor specific.

This disorder manifests as meningoencephalomyelitis or limited forms thereof. Headaches, encephalopathy with confusion, psychiatric symptoms, seizures, ataxia, and tremor are some of the common manifestations. Patients also can have blurry vision or asymptomatic optic disc edema, most often with normal visual acuity. If signs of myelopathy are present, they are often mild. Preceding flulike symptoms are common.

Approximately one-fourth of cases have a paraneoplastic cause, and an associated cancer is detected. In women, the most common neoplasm encountered is ovarian teratoma, but multiple other cancers have been described. It affects men and women equally and is also common in children, who have similar clinical manifestations but lack associated cancers. Coexisting neural autoantibodies are more commonly found in patients with ovarian teratoma and

include N-methyl-D-aspartate receptor and aquaporin-4 autoantibodies.

MRI findings are abnormal in most patients. Postgadolinium T1 images reveal linear, radial, perivascular enhancement throughout the cerebral white matter in half the patients. Leptomeningeal and ependymal enhancement are also encountered. Extensive T2 fluid-attenuated inversion recovery hyperintensities are rare but have been described in severe, untreated cases. Spinal cord MRI shows hazy T2 hyperintensities and subtle gadolinium enhancement. The CSF is almost always markedly inflammatory with lymphocytic pleocytosis (average of 80/μL), increased protein concentration, and oligoclonal bands.

Prolonged use of corticosteroids is the cornerstone of treatment. As demonstrated by the case patient, the patients may have disease relapse if corticosteroids are tapered prematurely. Treatment with high-dose corticosteroids (prednisone 60 mg or 1 mg/kg daily) for 3 months before tapering is suggested. Even in these cases, some patients will have relapses and will need a steroid-sparing agent; options include azathioprine, mycophenolate mofetil, or others.

KEY POINTS

- Autoimmune GFAP astrocytopathy manifests as a potentially relapsing, corticosteroid-responsive meningoencephalomyelitis, or limited forms thereof.

- Patients have lymphocytic pleocytosis and characteristic findings on MRI of the brain and/or spinal cord.

- One-fourth of patients have an accompanying neoplasm; ovarian teratoma is most common in women.

- GFAP-IgG is detected in the CSF by indirect tissue-based immunofluorescence and confirmed by a cell-based GFAP-IgG–specific assay. Serum positivity alone is neither as sensitive nor as specific.

A MAN WITH FLULIKE SYMPTOMS AND HEMORRHAGIC BRAIN LESIONS

Michel Toledano, MD

CASE PRESENTATION

HISTORY AND EXAMINATION

A 52-year-old man is admitted to a neurosciences intensive care unit during winter for management of seizures requiring mechanical ventilation. Two days earlier he reported cough and myalgia. On the day of admission, he was found by his brother seated on the couch with altered mental state and was minimally responsive.

Upon arrival to the emergency department he was febrile at 38.8 °C and tachycardic. Complete blood cell count showed leukocytosis (11.1×10⁹ cells/L, neutrophilic predominance). Chest radiography and urinalysis were normal. Inflammatory markers were within normal limits. Computed tomography (CT) of the head showed an area of hypodensity in the left temporal lobe. During CT, the patient had generalized convulsions requiring lorazepam, fosphenytoin, and levetiracetam, followed by initiation of a continuous midazolam infusion before seizures were controlled.

He was started on broad-spectrum antimicrobials, including acyclovir, and a lumbar puncture was performed. Cerebrospinal fluid (CSF) protein concentration was 196 mg/dL, and he had 10 white blood cells/μL (reference range, ≤5 cells/μL) with lymphocyte predominance. There was no hypoglycorrhachia.

After 24 hours, the patient was weaned from the midazolam infusion and maintained on levetiracetam monotherapy. He was extubated but remained encephalopathic. Magnetic resonance imaging performed the day after admission demonstrated numerous T2 hyperintense lesions throughout both cerebral hemispheres including both mesial temporal lobes and right thalamus. Some of these lesions had associated marginal restricted diffusion and gadolinium enhancement in association with subacute blood products (Figure 31.1).

The patient was up to date on cancer screening and had never smoked. His family was not aware of any recent history of weight loss, other constitutional symptoms, headache, or confusion. HIV and syphilis screening were negative. He took no regular medications, and there was no known history of substance abuse.

Because of the patient's seizures in the setting of flulike symptoms and hemorrhagic lesions on magnetic resonance imaging, infectious and autoimmune parainfectious (or postinfectious) causes were suspected, although neoplastic or other inflammatory causes were also considered (Table 31.1).

TESTING

Transesophageal echocardiography was negative for endocarditis. Magnetic resonance angiography was not suggestive of underlying vasculopathy. CT of the chest, abdomen, and pelvis, as well as testicular ultrasonography, were negative for cancer.

There were no CSF oligoclonal bands, and the immunoglobulin G index was normal. Gram stain and cultures were negative. Polymerase chain reaction (PCR) testing for herpes simplex virus (HSV), varicella-zoster virus, cytomegalovirus, and enterovirus were negative, as was cryptococcal antigen. Neural autoantibody profiles of serum and CSF, including Ma antibodies, were negative. Nasopharyngeal PCR was positive for influenza virus A, which was later typed further and identified as pandemic 2009 H1N1 virus (H1N1 pdm09).

DIAGNOSIS

A diagnosis of influenza-associated encephalopathy/encephalitis (IAE) was made.

MANAGEMENT

The patient was treated with oseltamivir, as well as a 5-day course of high-dose intravenous methylprednisolone (1,000 mg each infusion). His encephalopathy gradually improved. Repeated imaging at 3-month follow-up showed resolution of the previously seen abnormalities. His neurologic examination was normal.

DISCUSSION

Postinfectious or parainfectious autoimmunity syndromes refer to neurologic signs and symptoms that develop during or after an infection but are not thought to be caused by direct infection of the nervous system. The vast majority of these, including acute disseminated encephalomyelitis, Guillain-Barré syndrome and variants, and postinfectious cerebellitis, are thought to be mediated by an aberrant immune response triggered by a microorganism, but the exact pathophysiologic mechanism remains unknown. More recently, a link has been established between herpesvirus infections, HSV-1 encephalitis in particular, and the development of anti–N-methyl-D-aspartate receptor encephalitis in some patients (see also Case 25).

A broad spectrum of central and peripheral neurologic complications have been documented in association with seasonal influenza type A (H1N1 and H3N2), as well as influenza type B. IAE ranges from mild encephalopathy to acute necrotizing encephalopathy (ANE), which is associated with a poor prognosis. Although IAE is more common in children, it is increasingly recognized in adults. The underlying

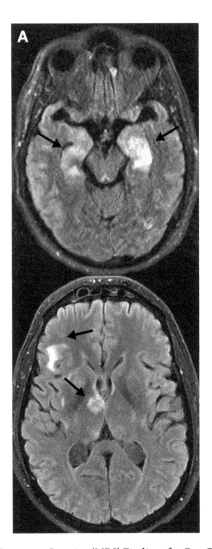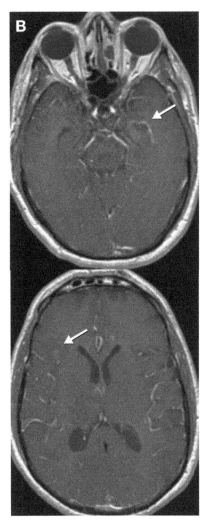

Figure 31.1 Magnetic Resonance Imaging (MRI) Findings for Case Patient.
A, MRI of the brain at 2 levels (top and bottom) demonstrates T2 fluid-attenuated inversion recovery signal change and swelling in the left greater than right mesiotemporal structures, right thalamus, and right frontal operculum (arrows). B-D, There is associated linear and blush enhancement on T1 postgadolinium sequences (arrows, B), as well as restricted diffusion on diffusion-weighted imaging (arrows, C), and blooming artifact on susceptibility-weighted imaging suggestive of subacute blood products (arrows, D).

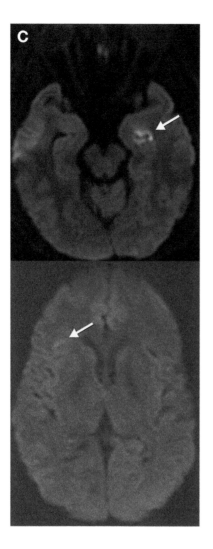 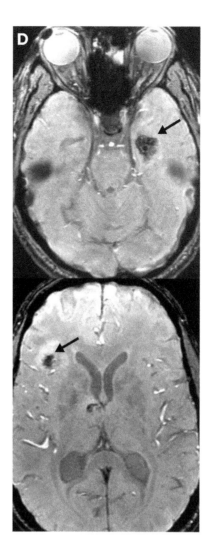

Figure 31.1 **Continued**

pathophysiologic mechanism remains unclear, but neither direct viral infection nor an unequivocal inflammatory process appears to cause the condition. Results of CSF studies are often normal, although a mildly increased white blood cell count may be seen. Similarly, direct evidence for viral invasion on CSF and histopathologic analysis is rare. Given the varying manifestations of IAE, more than 1 mechanism of injury may be possible.

Reported imaging abnormalities range from scattered white matter or cortical abnormalities to diffuse cerebral edema. A more distinct imaging pattern is reversible focal swelling and restricted diffusion in the corpus callosum. This pattern, termed *mild encephalitis/encephalopathy with reversible splenial lesion*, has been described with other infectious or metabolic derangements and is associated with a good prognosis. Another radiographic pattern associated with IAE is that of symmetric necrotizing lesions in the bilateral thalami

or brainstem. This pattern is associated with ANE, which has a more severe course and is associated with poor outcomes. Familial and recurrent ANE has been associated with mutations in RAN binding protein 2.

There is no demonstrated treatment for IAE. The neuraminidase inhibitor oseltamivir can be considered if patients are seen within 48 hours of onset of flulike symptoms. A short course of high-dose corticosteroid or intravenous immunoglobulin can be considered, but efficacy has not been demonstrated.

Although the World Health Organization declared the end of the 2009 H1N1 influenza pandemic in 2010, H1N1 pdm09 continues to circulate as a seasonal flu virus and appears to be associated with a higher number of neurologic complications. Our patient had never been vaccinated, but annual vaccination is associated with a decreased rate of infection, as well as decreased morbidity and mortality rates.

Table 31.1 **DIFFERENTIAL DIAGNOSIS FOR THE CASE PATIENT**

POSSIBLE DIAGNOSIS	MITIGATING FACTORS
Immune-mediated	
Acute disseminated encephalomyelitis/acute hemorrhagic leukoencephalopathy	Rare in this age group
	No history of vaccination
	Short latency between viral prodromal stage and onset of neurologic symptoms
	Dearth of white matter lesions on MRI
PACNS	Main radiographic finding tends to be ischemic strokes of different ages, which are absent in this case
	Acute onset—PACNS usually characterized by subacute prodromal period (weeks to months)
Systemic vasculitis with CNS involvement	No prior history of systemic symptoms
	Absent leptomeningeal and pachymeningeal involvement
Neurosarcoidosis	Hemorrhagic lesions rare
	Absent perivascular or meningeal enhancement
Paraneoplastic autoimmune encephalitis	Acute onset
	Hemorrhagic lesions not characteristic
Infectious	
Viral	
Varicella-zoster virus	Not immunocompromised
	Absent zoster rash
	Ischemic stroke more common than hemorrhagic stroke
Influenza-associated ANE	Usually affects children
	CSF pleocytosis—ANE usually associated with normal CSF cell count
	ANE characterized by bilateral symmetric hemorrhagic thalamic lesions
Arthropod-borne encephalitis	Wrong season
Fungal	
Aspergillus or other angioinvasive fungal infections (*Fusarium*, *Mucor*)	Patient not immunocompromised
	No history of diabetes
	No history of sinusitis
	Negative chest radiography
Bacterial	
Endocarditis	Lesions not respecting vascular territories
	Signal change in limbic system argues against purely embolic phenomena
	Short latency between flulike symptoms and neurologic decline
Meningovascular syphilis	Ischemic stroke of different ages usually present on imaging
	Hemorrhagic stroke less common
	No history of rash
	Short latency between flulike symptoms and neurologic decline
Neoplasm	
Hemorrhagic metastasis (melanoma, renal cell carcinoma, choriocarcinoma, thyroid carcinoma, breast and lung adenocarcinoma)	No history of weight loss
	No history of smoking
	Mixture of discrete lesions with more diffuse limbic involvement is atypical
	Fever, cough at onset
Multifocal glioblastoma	Imaging atypical

Abbreviations: ANE, acute necrotizing encephalopathy; CNS, central nervous system; CSF, cerebrospinal fluid; MRI, magnetic resonance imaging; PACNS, primary angiitis of the central nervous system.

KEY POINTS

- Parainfectious or postinfectious neurologic syndromes refer to signs and symptoms that develop during or after an infection, on an autoimmune basis, but are not thought to result from direct infection itself.

- Acute demyelinating encephalomyelitis, Guillain-Barré syndrome, and post-HSV anti–*N*-methyl-D-aspartate receptor encephalitis, are immune-mediated neurologic syndromes that can be triggered by infection.

- IAE occurs more commonly in children but is increasingly recognized in adults.

- Although it remains unclear whether an immune-mediated mechanism is responsible for the neurologic injury observed in IAE, a course of high-dose corticosteroids or intravenous immunoglobulin can be considered.

HEARING LOSS, IMBALANCE, AND DIPLOPIA IN A 44-YEAR-OLD MAN

Michelle F. Devine, MD, Divyanshu Dubey, MBBS, and Sean J. Pittock, MD

CASE PRESENTATION

HISTORY AND EXAMINATION

A 44-year-old man sought care for new right-sided tinnitus and sensorineural hearing loss. Brain magnetic resonance imaging (MRI) did not indicate a cause, so he was treated with 7 days of high-dose oral prednisone and acyclovir for a presumed viral cause. This provided only partial improvement of his auditory symptoms and audiography findings. A few weeks later, mild, intermittent dizziness developed (without frank vertigo or oscillopsia), which progressed to constant, moderate dizziness. This dizziness was exacerbated by sudden head movements but not by complex visual stimuli. He participated in vestibular rehabilitation with only mild improvement. Within 5 months of tinnitus onset, horizontal binocular diplopia also developed.

Examination showed spontaneous left-beating torsional nystagmus in primary gaze, down-beating nystagmus with leftward gaze, and right-beating torsional nystagmus in rightward gaze. Head impulse testing to the right produced a catch-up saccade. Dix-Hallpike maneuver in both positions did not elicit vertigo symptoms but led to leftward torsional nystagmus followed by down-beating nystagmus. He had full range of eye motion without ocular misalignment, head tilt, lid lag, or ptosis. There was evidence of asymmetric hearing loss on the right and moderate gait unsteadiness; he was able to complete only a few steps in tandem. Neurologic examination findings were otherwise normal, including for the remaining cranial nerves, strength, and reflexes. Possible diagnoses considered for the patient are shown in Table 32.1.

TESTING

Oculomotor testing demonstrated abnormalities supportive of a central nervous system disorder. These included excessive square-wave jerks, impaired smooth pursuit, and direction-changing nystagmus.

Repeated MRI of the brain and auditory canals showed normal findings. Results of cerebrospinal fluid (CSF) studies included a normal opening pressure, pleocytosis with 17 white blood cells/μL (90% lymphocytes), 4 erythrocytes/μL, and increased protein concentration of 64 mg/dL (reference range, 0-35 mg/d). There were no oligoclonal bands, and immunoglobulin G (IgG) index was normal. Testing for Ma1, Ma2, and GQ1b antibodies and Lyme disease serologic testing were negative. Serum and CSF paraneoplastic evaluations showed a unique immunofluorescence staining pattern on rodent brain tissue by patient IgG, which was later confirmed to be IgG antibodies to KLHL11 (kelch like family member 11). Findings of scrotal ultrasonography were negative. Whole-body positron emission tomography (PET) showed a single anterior mediastinal mass (Figure 32.1), which was then resected. Pathologic analysis of the resected tissue indicated seminoma and normal thymic tissue.

Table 32.1 DIFFERENTIAL DIAGNOSIS FOR THE CASE PATIENT

POSSIBLE DIAGNOSIS	PERTINENT NEGATIVES
Miller Fisher syndrome or Bickerstaff brainstem encephalitis	Normal reflexes Subacute to chronic progression
Acoustic nerve tumor	No mass or lesions on brain MRI
Neurosarcoidosis	Normal MRI
Lyme disease	No systemic manifestations of Lyme disease
Whipple disease	Subacute to chronic progression Hearing loss is atypical
Cogan syndrome	No fevers, weight loss, or eye pain
Anti-Ma1/Ma2 encephalitis	Hearing loss is atypical
Chronic basilar meningitis	No fevers, headaches, or meningism Normal MRI

Abbreviation: MRI, magnetic resonance imaging.

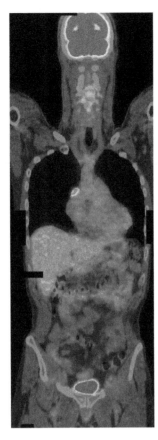

Figure 32.1 Positron Emission Tomography Findings for Case Patient.
A hypermetabolic mediastinal mass is detected.

DIAGNOSIS

The patient was diagnosed with a paraneoplastic anti-KLHL11 rhombencephalitis with an extratesticular seminoma.

MANAGEMENT

After removal of the mediastinal mass, intravenous (IV) methylprednisolone was started at 1,000 mg daily for 3 consecutive days, followed by weekly doses for a total of 6 weeks. The patient had symptom stabilization but no clinical improvement. A second-line agent, cyclophosphamide (50 mg twice daily orally [100 mg/d], later increased to 75 mg twice daily [150 mg/d]) was added to the weekly pulse-dose IV corticosteroids. After 8 weeks on this regimen, he had mild improvement in vertigo and gait imbalance. For symptomatic management of the vertigo, he received baclofen, citalopram, and vestibular rehabilitation. He continued to have slow improvement.

After approximately 1 year of cyclophosphamide treatment, his gait normalized and nystagmus diminished, although he had persistent neurologic deficits including spontaneous down-beating nystagmus and a few intermittent square-wave jerks. Given the patient's prolonged stability, the IV methylprednisolone infusions were tapered, with continued examination stability. He was able to resume work full time. After stable symptoms and examination

findings for several additional months, cyclophosphamide was discontinued.

The patient remained neurologically stable for 3 years without immunosuppression. However, 3½ years after discontinuation of cyclophosphamide, new central sensorineural hearing loss developed suddenly in his left ear. This improved with additional IV methylprednisolone treatment. Mycophenolate mofetil was also started, and corticosteroids were tapered. Repeated PET of the body showed no recurrence of seminoma. Symptoms and audiography findings were stable after 10 months, so the patient elected to discontinue immunosuppression again and has remained stable.

DISCUSSION

KLHL11 autoimmunity is a distinct paraneoplastic syndrome associated with encephalitis and testicular germ cell tumors (including seminoma). The clinical phenotypes include rhombencephalitis (brainstem and/or cerebellar features), limbic encephalitis, or a combination. The most common symptoms are gait instability and diplopia; however, vertigo, tinnitus, and hearing loss can occur weeks to months before incoordination or oculomotor manifestations. Slurred speech, seizures, and encephalopathy can also occur. Findings of CSF studies are often inflammatory, with increases in protein concentration, white blood cell count, and oligoclonal bands. MRI of the brain can be normal or can demonstrate T2 hyperintensities involving the temporal lobe, cerebellum, and brainstem; intracranial mass effect can occur. Testicular germ cell tumors are found in the majority of patients on cancer screening; some of these are extratesticular, which supports the need for full-body PET-computed tomography if testicular ultrasonography findings are normal.

The differential diagnosis for paraneoplastic brainstem encephalitis includes Ma1/Ma2 autoimmunity (associated with germ cell tumors of testes in men or diverse cancer types in women) and antineuronal nuclear antibody type 2 (anti-Ri) autoimmunity (associated with breast cancer in women or, occasionally, small cell carcinoma in either sex).

In the current case, detection and treatment of a seminoma along with aggressive immunotherapy were associated with a favorable outcome. However, even with optimal tumor treatment, anti-KLHL11 encephalitis is a severe paraneoplastic condition. Symptoms can be refractory, requiring multiple immunosuppressive agents to achieve stability. The goal of treatment is to halt progression, although some patients achieve improvement. Residual symptoms and relapses can occur. In some cases, death has occurred within 10 years of symptom onset.

KEY POINTS

- Paraneoplastic neurologic disorders should be considered in patients with subacute brainstem features including ataxia, sensorineural hearing loss, vertigo, diplopia, and nystagmus.

- The strong association between KLHL11 autoimmunity and testicular germ cell tumors should direct a thorough cancer screen, including scrotal ultrasonography and possibly whole-body PET.

- In most cases, the goal of immunotherapy is symptom stabilization; however, some patients may improve.

- A trial of discontinuing immunosuppression can be considered with prolonged stability of symptoms and examination findings, but relapses can occur in some cases.

CHOREA, ATAXIA, AND DISTURBED SLEEP

John C. Feemster, and Erik K. St. Louis, MD, MS

CASE PRESENTATION

HISTORY AND EXAMINATION

A 72-year-old White man with a medical history pertinent for type 2 diabetes, spinal stenosis, and obstructive sleep apnea sought care for predominant choreiform movements, mild gait ataxia, urinary dysfunction, and abnormal nocturnal behaviors for the past 2 years. Choreiform movements were nearly constant while awake, vanished during sleep, and predominantly involved his lower extremities and trunk. He also had significant urinary dysfunction, with severe urinary hesitancy and frequency during both day and night. Sleep-related behaviors included sleep talking, sleep singing, sudden single-limb jerking movements, and complex hand movements that emulated typing on a keyboard. The patient had only rare dream recall that paralleled these behaviors. He also had daytime sleepiness, with an Epworth Sleepiness Scale score of 16 (abnormal, >10).

On neurologic examination, his mental status was normal, as were cranial nerves, motor and sensory surveys, muscle stretch reflexes, and coordination. Abnormal findings included postural instability at baseline with eyes open and a slightly wide-based tentative gait and inability to execute tandem walking. Rest tremor, bradykinesia, and rigidity were absent. He had intermittent choreiform movements of the legs and the left shoulder. He also had occasional repetitive, periodic, voluntary-appearing, triple flexion–type movements of both legs, which he reported as being unassociated with any sense of an urge to move the legs. Diagnoses considered at the time are shown in Table 33.1.

TESTING

Overnight polysomnography (PSG) was ordered to evaluate nocturnal movements and behaviors and for assurance of obstructive sleep apnea management. PSG confirmed effective positive airway pressure titration at 12 cm H_2O pressure level, consistent with the patient's chronic home prescription pressure, and also revealed rapid periodic leg movements of sleep and rapid eye movement (REM) sleep without atonia (RSWA) (Figure 33.1). Sleep architecture was mildly deranged, with electroencephalographic alpha intrusion throughout non-REM sleep, as well as absent N3 (slow-wave sleep). However, N2 architecture was normally formed, with K complexes and spindles clearly present. Ferritin level was suboptimal at 41 μg/L (reference range, 24-336 μg/L). Evaluation of serum for autoimmune encephalitis demonstrated IgLON family member 5 (IgLON5) antibody positivity by tissue immunofluorescence assay, confirmed by cell-based assay.

Table 33.1 | DIFFERENTIAL DIAGNOSIS

POSSIBLE DIAGNOSES	PERTINENT NEGATIVES
Huntington disease	Older age at symptom onset, absence of cognitive impairment or behavioral changes
Wilson disease	Older age at symptom onset, absence of parkinsonism or hepatic disease
Dentatorubral pallidoluysian atrophy	Not of Asian ethnicity, absence of cognitive decline or myoclonic seizures
Spinocerebellar ataxia	Absence of limb ataxia, pyramidal or extrapyramidal signs, sensory loss, or cognitive impairment
Neuroferritinopathy	Absence of parkinsonism, dystonia, or cognitive impairment
Neuroacanthocytosis (chorea-acanthocytosis)	Absence of dystonia, tics, parkinsonism, behavioral changes, seizures, or cognitive impairment

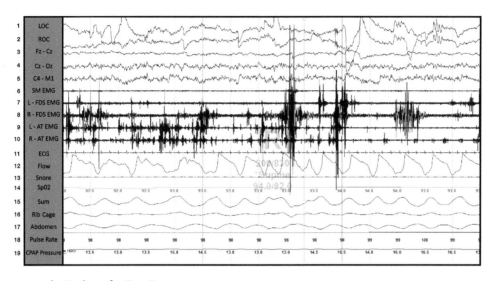

Figure 33.1 Polysomnography Findings for Case Patient.
A 30-second polysomnogram epoch shows frequent bursts of abnormally excessive phasic muscle activity during rapid eye movement (REM) sleep, most evident in the limbs (channels 7-10), whereas relatively normal levels of REM sleep atonia are seen in the chin (channel 6). Channels 1 and 2, left outer canthus (LOC) and right outer canthus (ROC) electrooculogram; channels 3-5, frontocentral (FZ-CZ), centrooccipital (CZ-OZ), and right central (C4-M1) electroencephalogram; channels 6-10, submental (SM), left (L) and right (R) flexor digitorum superficialis (FDS) (arm) and anterior tibialis (AT) (leg) electromyogram (EMG); channel 11, electrocardiogram (ECG); channel 12, airflow (Flow) through positive airway pressure mask; channel 13, sonogram (snoring detection [Snore]); channel 14, oxyhemoglobin saturation (Spo$_2$); channels 15-17, Sum/chest (Rib Cage)/abdominal (Abdomen) respiratory effort; channel 18, Pulse Rate; channel 19, continuous positive airway pressure (CPAP) pressure level.

DIAGNOSIS

The patient was diagnosed with IgLON5 autoimmune encephalitis and symptomatic REM sleep behavior disorder (RBD).

MANAGEMENT

The patient was instructed to maintain a safe sleep environment at home and to begin taking melatonin 3 mg at bedtime, which was eventually increased to 6 mg to control dream enactment behaviors. Positive airway pressure was maintained. A therapeutic trial of intravenous methylprednisolone 1 g weekly for 3 months, together with mycophenolate mofetil 1 g twice daily (2 g/d), was followed by improvement in memory, confusion, and hallucinations, waking involuntary movements, bladder dysfunction, and sleep quality. At last neurologic follow-up 2 years later, choreiform movements had greatly improved, dream enactment had resolved, and gait ataxia was markedly improved.

DISCUSSION

RBD is a parasomnia characterized by RSWA, the loss or dysregulation of normal REM sleep atonia, which is its pathophysiologic signature, and which is permissive for dream enactment behaviors during REM sleep. PSG is required for confirmatory diagnosis of RBD, which requires the presence of RSWA. Early detection of RBD is of high clinical importance because patients are vulnerable to sleep-related injuries, either to themselves from falls from bed, or to their bedpartner through inadvertent punching or kicking movements that frequently accompany the often-violent nightmares patients experience with this disorder.

The diagnosis is also of key importance given that in most older adults with this parasomnia, a defined neurodegenerative disease may later develop, specifically α-synucleinopathies including Parkinson disease, dementia with Lewy bodies, or multiple system atrophy. Early detection, therefore, provides an opportunity to proactively track the progression of common clinical manifestations of these diseases. This also allows for early symptomatic treatment with pharmacotherapy for motor or cognitive consequences. RBD has also been associated with medications, especially antidepressant use, and psychiatric conditions such as depression, anxiety disorders, and posttraumatic stress disorder. Other sleep disorders such as narcolepsy type 1 (narcolepsy with cataplexy), or brain lesions of specific pontine REM sleep atonia control regions and, rarely, autoimmune encephalitis, may be alternative causes of RBD, as in this case patient.

IgLON5 is an immunoglobulinlike cell adhesion molecule that is widely expressed in the central nervous system (CNS). Despite its widespread distribution, the exact function of the molecule is currently unknown. Autoimmune targeting of this molecule has been associated with heterogeneous waking and sleep neurologic disorders, including gait instability, movement disorders, abnormal eye movements, bulbar symptoms and signs, neuropsychiatric symptoms, dysautonomia, peripheral nervous system disorders, and abnormal oneiric behaviors during sleep with symptomatic RBD, sleep apnea, and, in some cases, sleep-related stridor. Unfortunately, many cases have progressed to premature death, often involving sudden death during sleep, which is thought to be facilitated by respiratory failure. Additionally, rapid periodic limb movements during sleep have been reported to recur, such as those seen in our patient.

IgLON5 was first identified as the antigen associated with other waking neurologic and sleep disorders by Sabater and colleagues in 2014. Unlike many autoimmune CNS disorders, autoimmunity targeting IgLON5 may be associated with either subacute onset and rapid symptom progression or a more indolent and chronically progressive course. The course of IgLON5 autoimmunity syndrome is often that of a progressive CNS disorder, similar to previously reported tauopathies such as progressive supranuclear palsy or corticobasal degeneration, with which it may be confused. Previous research has found tauopathies and IgLON5 autoimmunity to be frequently comorbid. Neuropathologic findings in patients with IgLON5 autoimmunity include a lack of inflammatory infiltrates, neuronal loss, gliosis, and neuronal accumulation of hyperphosphorylated tau protein (3R + 4R isoforms) found in the hypothalamus and tegmental brainstem nuclei.

Evidence regarding treatment for IgLON5 autoimmunity syndrome is currently limited. Symptomatic treatment of RBD related to IgLON5 autoimmunity has largely been the same as that recommended for idiopathic RBD. Melatonin and clonazepam are the pharmacotherapies of choice, with melatonin showing less frequent and severe adverse effects in general, although no studies have systematically evaluated its efficacy for control of dream enactment behaviors in RBD associated with IgLON5 autoimmunity syndrome. The reported success of disease-specific or -modifying therapy with immunosuppressive/modulatory agents has been mixed. Earlier reports of a relatively homogeneous phenotype of IgLON5 autoimmunity syndrome were universally discouraging and suggested a fatally progressive course. However, a more heterogeneous set of clinical phenotypes and more favorable responses to immunotherapy were reported by Honorat and colleagues.

Other autoimmune serologic-clinical encephalomyelitides classically accompanied by sleep disorders include those associated with contactin-associated protein 2 (CASPR2) antibody, antineuronal nuclear antibody type 2 (ANNA-2; anti-Ri), Ma2 antibody, and dipeptidyl-peptidase-like protein-6 (DPPX) antibody. Sleep disorders, including insomnia, RBD, and sleep apnea, are commonly encountered during or after autoimmune encephalitis, including in seronegative cases.

KEY POINTS

- RBD is characterized by vocal and complex motor behaviors during REM sleep, accompanied by RSWA during PSG.

- Melatonin or clonazepam may be helpful in the symptomatic treatment of violent dream enactment behaviors.

- IgLON5 autoimmunity syndrome is characterized by a heterogeneous autoimmune encephalitis phenotype, usually involving prominent bulbar symptoms, hypokinetic or hyperkinetic movement disorders, gait impairment, RBD, highly disturbed sleep architecture, sleep apnea, and, in some cases, sleep stridor.

- The reported response to immunotherapy in IgLON5 autoimmunity syndrome has been variable, but it was helpful in a substantial proportion of patients in a recently reported case series.

RAPIDLY PROGRESSIVE GAIT AND COORDINATION DIFFICULTIES

Andrew McKeon, MB, BCh, MD

CASE PRESENTATION

HISTORY AND EXAMINATION

A 59-year-old woman noted sudden onset of slurred speech. Within a few days, she noted double vision, gait unsteadiness, and incoordination of her limbs. All of these symptoms progressed over 1 week, and she sought care at her local emergency department. Computed tomography and magnetic resonance imaging (MRI) of the head were negative for stroke, and she was discharged from the emergency department. Her symptoms persisted. Upon evaluation at Mayo Clinic 7 months later, neurologic examination indicated a moderate pancerebellar ataxia, without additional abnormalities. Her pursuit eye movements were saccadic. She had binocular diplopia with horizontal, gaze-evoked nystagmus. She had ataxic dysarthria and dysmetria of all limbs. Her steps and walking were irregular and she could not accomplish tandem gait, although she did not require a walking aid (❍ Video 34.1).

Because she is a woman and had subacute-onset ataxia, a classic paraneoplastic disorder characterized by the detection of Purkinje cell cytoplasmic antibody type 1 (PCA-1, also known as Yo antibody) was suspected. A broad evaluation for paraneoplastic antibodies in serum and cerebrospinal fluid (CSF) was ordered, as well as mammography and ultrasonography of the pelvis. Infectious disease testing was also performed because of the subacute onset of symptoms, her residence in a Lyme disease–endemic region, and a history of tick bites. The cancer imaging tests were negative. CSF basic parameters were normal (including protein concentration, blood cell count, immunoglobulin G [IgG] index and synthesis rate, and oligoclonal band numbers), as were Lyme disease test results. In addition, the standard evaluations of serum and CSF were negative for paraneoplastic antibodies, including PCA-1.

Subacute infarction, demyelinating disease, and space-occupying lesions had all been excluded by head MRI. Metabolic causes, including vitamin B_{12} deficiency and folate deficiency, had also been excluded. There were no additional

clinical or radiologic findings to support prion disease. No features of synucleinopathy (anosmia, dysautonomia, myelopathy, parkinsonism, or rapid eye movement sleep behavior disorder) were present to suggest multiple system atrophy. The patient did not have celiac disease.

TESTING

Additional neural antibody testing was undertaken, beyond the classic paraneoplastic antibodies (Table 34.1). Metabotropic glutamate receptor 1 (mGluR1)-IgG was detected in the serum and CSF.

DIAGNOSIS

The patient was diagnosed with autoimmune cerebellar ataxia.

MANAGEMENT

Because of the reported association of mGluR1-IgG with Hodgkin disease and non-Hodgkin lymphoma, positron emission tomography–computed tomography of the trunk (orbits to thighs) was performed, which was negative. After 6 weeks of intravenous methylprednisolone therapy (1,000 mg intravenously daily for 3 days, followed by 1 infusion weekly for 5 weeks), the patient returned for evaluation. She had a mild ataxic dysarthria and minimal dysmetria of her left upper extremity only. She could tandem walk almost without error, and her gait appeared normal (no longer broad-based). At that point, immunotherapy was discontinued. At last follow-up, 1 year after completing treatment, her neurologic examination findings remained stable.

DISCUSSION

The subacute onset and rapid progression of ataxic symptoms in this adult patient led to suspicion for an autoimmune cause. CSF may indicate general inflammatory clues, but these also may be lacking, as was the case in this patient. Radiologic evidence of cerebellar atrophy might become apparent in patients

Table 34.1 | AUTOANTIBODIES ASSOCIATED WITH AUTOIMMUNE CEREBELLAR ATAXIA

NEURONAL NUCLEAR, CYTOPLASMIC IgGs	CANCER ASSOCIATION	ION CHANNEL OR RECEPTOR IgGs	CANCER ASSOCIATION
ANNA-1 (anti-Hu)	Small cell carcinoma[a]	P/Q- and N-type calcium channel antibodies	Various[b]
ANNA-2 (anti-Ri)	Small cell carcinoma, breast adenocarcinoma[a]		
AGNA (SOX1-IgG)	Small cell carcinoma	mGluR1	Hodgkin disease, non-Hodgkin lymphoma, prostate adenocarcinoma[b]
PCA-1 (anti-Yo)	Breast and gynecologic adenocarcinomas[a]		
MAP1B (PCA-2)	Small cell carcinoma	DNER	Hodgkin or non-Hodgkin lymphoma[a]
Ma2	Testicular germinomas[a]		
CRMP5-IgG	Small cell carcinoma, thymoma[a]	DPPX	B-cell neoplasms[b]
GAD65-IgG	Occasional cases of thymoma and carcinomas	IgLON5	None recognized
		GABA$_B$R	Small cell carcinoma[a]
Amphiphysin-IgG	Small cell carcinoma, breast adenocarcinoma[a]		
ITPR1-IgG	None recognized		
GRAF-IgG	None recognized		
Septin-5-IgG	None recognized		
AP3B2-IgG	None recognized		

Abbreviations: AGNA, antiglial/neuronal nuclear antibody; ANNA, antineuronal nuclear antibody; AP3B2, adaptor protein 3B2; CRMP5, collapsin-response mediator protein 5; DNER, delta/notch like EGF repeat; DPPX, dipeptidyl-peptidase-like protein-6; GABA$_B$R, γ-aminobutyric acid receptor, type B; GAD65, glutamic acid decarboxylase 65-kDa isoform; GRAF, GTPase regulator associated with focal adhesion kinase; IgG, immunoglobulin G; IgLON5, IgLON family member 5; ITPR1, inositol 1,4,5-trisphosphate receptor type 1; MAP1B, microtubule-associated protein 1B; mGluR1, metabotropic glutamate receptor 1; PCA, Purkinje cell cytoplasmic antibody.

[a] Majority have neoplasm detected.

[b] Minority have neoplasm detected.

with advanced paraneoplastic cerebellar degeneration, but this is generally not evident early on. Thus, in the absence of other diagnostic clues, autoantibody testing of serum and CSF becomes pertinent in these cases. Furthermore, the IgG profile is informative regarding cancer diagnosis and sometimes prognosis. In children, autoimmune ataxia is generally a postinfectious cerebellitis without IgG biomarkers.

In the case patient, given her sex and the neurologic presentation, the prototypic example of paraneoplastic ataxia (PCA-1 neurologic autoimmunity) was suspected. These patients, almost always female, typically have accompanying breast or müllerian adenocarcinoma (uterine, ovarian, fallopian tubal, or primary pelvic peritoneal), little to no response to immunotherapies, and a very poor neurologic prognosis. In contrast, the case patient had no cancer detected and responded well to immunotherapy, both of which were predicted by the detection of mGluR1-IgG. The number of neural IgG biomarkers of autoimmune ataxia has increased substantially in the past 3 decades. The most common antibodies are glutamic acid decarboxylase 65-kDa isoform (GAD65)-IgG and PCA-1-IgG. Patients with GAD65 autoimmunity may have overlap of ataxia and stiff-person syndrome. Although patients with celiac disease might have development of gait ataxia, this is usually sensory ataxia secondary to dorsal column disease or sensory neuronopathy secondary to malabsorption of 1 or more of vitamin B_{12}, vitamin E, folate, or copper.

Overall, even with treatment, just 25% of patients with autoimmune ataxia remain ambulatory without a walking aid, and almost 50% become wheelchair dependent. In general,

patients with antibodies to neural ion channels or receptors (Table 34.1, right) less frequently have cancer and have better neurologic prognoses than do patients with neuronal nuclear or cytoplasmic IgGs (Table 34.1, left). Nonetheless, trials of immunotherapy are generally undertaken in all patients, and improvement may also accrue from treatment of any underlying neoplasm. Immunotherapies generally include several-week courses of intravenous methylprednisolone, intravenous immunoglobulin, or plasma exchange. Patients with neuronal nuclear or cytoplasmic IgGs are generally postulated to have a cytotoxic T-cell–mediated disorder, which sometimes prompts the use of cyclophosphamide in severely affected patients. Patients with plasma membrane protein–directed IgGs are generally postulated to have an IgG-mediated disorder, which sometimes prompts the use of anti–B-cell therapy (ie, rituximab).

KEY POINTS

- Autoimmune ataxia should be suspected in patients with subacute onset of ataxia and rapid progression of symptoms.

- Head MRI findings and general inflammatory markers in CSF help exclude other causes of ataxia but are generally not informative for the diagnosis.

- Testing for a broad profile of neural IgGs in serum and CSF may be informative for neurologic and cancer diagnoses, likely treatment response, and prognosis.

DANCELIKE MOVEMENTS IN A PATIENT WITH A HISTORY OF RASH

Andrew McKeon, MB, BCh, MD

CASE PRESENTATION

HISTORY AND EXAMINATION

A 67-year-old man visited the neurology clinic for new-onset, generalized, uncontrollable movements. Six months earlier, his wife noticed onset of some unusual facial expressions and facial movements. This then evolved over the course of 2 months to him having some writhing movements of the left upper and left lower extremity. His speech and swallowing also became affected. He noted a tendency to bite his tongue, which was moving uncontrollably. Shortly before his neurology clinic visit, the same writhing movements of right-sided limbs developed. No cognitive or behavioral changes were reported.

He had been diagnosed with cutaneous lupus erythematosus 5 years previously after a malar rash of his face developed after sun exposure. His rash resolved after a course of topical corticosteroids and did not relapse after he started hydroxychloroquine therapy. He also had white hair from the age of 25 years. The patient had a strong family history of autoimmunity, with 3 sisters having systemic lupus erythematosus (SLE). The patient was a nonsmoker. There was no family history of hyperkinetic movement disorders. On physical examination, he had marked chorea, hyperkinetic movements that were unpredictable, primarily affecting his facial expression, head, neck, and jaw. Hyperkinetic movements were also noted of the limbs, of lower amplitude and frequency. No cerebellar ataxia or upper motor neuron signs were present. He had some mild reduction in temperature and vibration sensation in his feet, but ankle reflexes were preserved, and plantar reflexes were flexor. When he walked in the hallway, he had a narrow-based gait. Some mild upper extremity hyperkinetic movements could be seen as he walked, along with persistence of the marked facial grimacing and other movements. Diagnoses considered at the time are shown in Table 35.1.

TESTING

Findings on magnetic resonance imaging of the head were unremarkable. Genetic testing for Huntington disease was negative. Because of the time course and the personal and family history of autoimmunity, autoimmune chorea was suspected. Neuronal autoantibody testing was negative in serum and cerebrospinal fluid. His cerebrospinal fluid demonstrated normal protein concentration, blood cell count, immunoglobulin G (IgG) index and synthesis rate, and oligoclonal bands. Neural IgG testing was negative. Indirect immunofluorescence assays using HEp-2 substrate (although not bead-based multiplex enzyme-linked immunosorbent assay) were positive for antinuclear antibody and Sjögren syndrome-A antibody (anti-Ro). Antiphospholipid antibodies, anti–double-stranded DNA antibodies, and other rheumatologic-pertinent autoantibodies were negative.

DIAGNOSIS

Autoimmune chorea was diagnosed in the context of a known history of a limited form of SLE.

MANAGEMENT

The patient received intravenous methylprednisolone infusions, 1,000 mg daily for 3 days, followed by 1,000 mg weekly for 6 weeks. Trimethoprim-sulfamethoxazole, double strength, 1 tablet by mouth 3 days per week was given for *Pneumocystis jirovecii* prophylaxis. A rash developed, and the patient was determined to be sulfa allergic. Instead, he received atovaquone 1,500 mg by mouth daily as prophylaxis. Calcium (1,500 mg/d) and vitamin D (1,000 U/d) were used as osteopenia prophylaxis while the patient was taking corticosteroids. During the 6 weeks of corticosteroid treatment, his chorea resolved, except for some occasional adventitious tongue and face movements. Oral azathioprine was initiated after thiopurine methyltransferase activity testing demonstrated normal values. Azathioprine dosing was 2.5 mg/kg per day in 2 divided doses. Oral hydroxychloroquine was continued. Monthly monitoring of complete blood cell count and liver function tests showed leukopenia and thrombocytopenia, which resolved after halving the azathioprine dose. Over the following 6 months, the corticosteroids were slowly tapered by gradually reducing

Table 35.1 DIFFERENTIAL DIAGNOSIS FOR THE CASE PATIENT

POSSIBLE DIAGNOSES	PERTINENT NEGATIVES
Autoimmune	NA
Neural IgG biomarkers	
CRMP5-IgG	
ANNA-1 (anti-Hu)	
ANNA-2 (anti-Ri)	
Amphiphysin-IgG	
GAD65-IgG	
LGI1-IgG	
CASPR2-IgG	
Idiopathic	
Systemic lupus erythematosus	
Antiphospholipid syndrome	
Poststreptococcal	
Sydenham chorea (in children)	
Degenerative causes	
Parkinson disease with treatment producing generalized dyskinesias	No levodopa therapy
Huntington disease	No family history of Huntington disease, neuropsychiatric symptoms, or caudate atrophy on MRI
C9ORF72 repeat expansions (rarely presents with chorea)	No Huntington disease phenocopy
Huntington disease–like syndromes 1-4 (very rare genetic disorders)	No Huntington disease phenocopy
Benign hereditary chorea	Presents in infancy

Abbreviations: ANNA-1, antineuronal nuclear antibody type 1; ANNA-2, antineuronal nuclear antibody type 2; CASPR2, contactin-associated protein 2; CRMP5, collapsin-response mediator protein 5; GAD65, glutamic acid decarboxylase 65-kDa isoform; IgG, immunoglobulin G; LGI1, leucine-rich, glioma-inactivated protein 1; MRI, magnetic resonance imaging; NA, not applicable.

dosing frequency from weekly, to alternate week, to every third week, then monthly, and then stopping. The patient remained stable for 2 years, at which time more prominent choreiform tongue movements then developed, inhibiting his ability to eat, along with bilateral choreiform lower extremity movements. Again, the patient had near-complete response to corticosteroids. Because of prior leukopenia and thrombocytopenia at therapeutic doses of azathioprine, it was discontinued in favor of mycophenolate mofetil 1,000 mg twice daily, which was well tolerated. Three years later, the patient remained in remission from his chorea except for mild occasional hyperkinetic movements of his tongue.

DISCUSSION

In adults, autoimmune chorea is the most common form of chorea after levodopa-induced dyskinesias and Huntington disease. Patients have a subacute onset of symptoms and rapid progression. Patients may have accompanying neuropsychiatric symptoms. Autoimmune chorea can be categorized into 2 broad forms. Paraneoplastic chorea is more common among older men with coexisting peripheral neuropathy and weight loss. Some other patients have an idiopathic autoimmune form, sometimes with neural antibody positivity (⬤ Video 35.1). Patients with SLE or antiphospholipid syndrome–associated chorea respond well to corticosteroids. The idiopathic form is typically robustly corticosteroid responsive, in contrast to the paraneoplastic

form. The most common accompanying cancer in paraneoplastic chorea is small cell lung carcinoma. Other reported cancer types include adenocarcinomas of the breast, lung, colon, prostate, and pancreas and chronic myeloid leukemia.

Other hyperkinetic movement disorders recognized in an autoimmune context include dyskinetic and stereotyped movements observed in anti-N-methyl-D-aspartate receptor encephalitis, faciobrachial dystonic seizures in leucine-rich, glioma-inactivated protein 1 (LGI1)-IgG encephalitis (⬤ Video 35.2), and myoclonus (with or without opsoclonus) (⬤ Video 35.3).

Autoantibody testing should be broad and include biomarkers of SLE (antinuclear antibody, anti–double-stranded DNA antibody), antiphospholipid syndrome (antiphospholipid antibodies and lupus anticoagulant), and neural IgGs. Recognized serologic associations in autoimmune chorea include IgGs specific for small cell carcinoma–related paraneoplastic disorders (such as collapsin-response mediator protein 5–IgG and antineuronal nuclear antibody type 1) and IgGs with some occasional association with thymoma (LGI1 and contactin-associated protein 2 antibodies). Antinuclear antibody is most sensitively detected by indirect immunofluorescence assay and then with reflex to anti–double-stranded DNA antibody. Magnetic resonance imaging of the head may occasionally demonstrate inflammatory-appearing basal ganglial abnormalities.

As is typical for most corticosteroid-responsive autoimmune encephalitides, a short duration of treatment (days) is insufficient, and longer treatment (weeks to months) is required, with taper usually over several months. For patients with relapsing symptoms, a steroid-sparing agent may be introduced as the corticosteroids are being tapered, with an aim of maintaining remission over years and avoiding long-term corticosteroid adverse effects. Examples of steroid-sparing agents include azathioprine, mycophenolate mofetil, and methotrexate (all by mouth) and rituximab (intravenous). Patients with paraneoplastic disorders may respond to cancer treatment or immunotherapies (corticosteroids, plasma exchange, or intravenous immunoglobulin), although the overall prognosis is poor. Prophylaxis against pneumocystis infection should include oral trimethoprim-sulfamethoxazole. Oral atovaquone, dapsone, or aerosolized pentamidine are alternatives for sulfa-allergic patients.

Prophylaxis against osteopenia should include calcium and vitamin D. If bone density demonstrates osteopenia or osteoporosis, a bisphosphonate such as alendronate 70 mg/wk by mouth should be started.

KEY POINTS

- Autoimmunity should be considered as a cause of chorea in patients with subacute onset and rapidly progressive symptoms and no family history of Huntington disease.

- Workup should include testing for neural IgGs, lupus, and phospholipid IgG biomarkers.

- Trials of immunotherapy should be undertaken but are more likely to be successful in those with SLE.

BODY SPASMS IN A WOMAN WITH THYROID DISEASE

Andrew McKeon, MB, BCh, MD

CASE PRESENTATION

HISTORY AND EXAMINATION

A 46-year-old woman with a history of autoimmune Hashimoto thyroiditis sought care for a 6-month history of spasms affecting her back and bilateral proximal lower extremities. Initially, these spasms occurred episodically and seemed to be triggered by loud noises only. Later on, these episodes would occur when one of her children would touch her or if she was feeling anxious, and they became superimposed on a persistent feeling of stiffness in her back and thighs. In the previous month, on 2 occasions, the spasms generalized and resulted in falls. On both occasions, she fell forward to the ground, injuring her face.

On examination, the patient appeared anxious, and her whole body seemed to stiffen when the examiner entered the room. Her cognitive, cranial nerve, and upper extremity examinations were normal, except for brisk deep tendon reflexes. Examination of the patient's spine indicated hyperlordosis of the lumbar region, which was not eliminated by lying supine (● Video 36.1). There was visible hypertrophy of the lumbar paraspinal muscles. When asked to walk, the patient took short, tentative steps, despite having normal strength in her lower extremities. Her lower extremity tone demonstrated diffuse rigidity. Her deep tendon reflexes were brisk. Babinski signs were absent, and sensory and cerebellar

examinations were normal. Diagnoses considered at the time are shown in Table 36.1.

TESTING

Magnetic resonance imaging of the brain and whole spine showed normal findings. Cerebrospinal fluid (CSF) evaluation showed isolated increased protein concentration (62 mg/dL; reference range, ≤36 mg/dL). Autoantibody testing of the serum and CSF showed markedly increased levels of glutamic acid decarboxylase 65-kDa isoform (GAD65)–immunoglobulin G (IgG) antibody: 550 nmol/L in serum and 5.10 nmol/L in CSF (reference range, ≤0.02 nmol/L). Testing for antibodies to glycine receptor α1 subunit (GlyRα1) and amphiphysin was negative. Neurophysiologic studies in a movement disorders laboratory indicated a nonhabituating, exaggerated, acoustic startle response.

DIAGNOSIS

Stiff-person syndrome (SPS) was diagnosed.

MANAGEMENT

The patient received diazepam 5 mg 3 times daily for symptomatic relief, with a gradual, careful increase to 10 mg 3 times daily over the following 3 weeks. At her follow-up visit,

Table 36.1 | **DIFFERENTIAL DIAGNOSIS**

POSSIBLE DIAGNOSES	PERTINENT NEGATIVES
Myelopathy	No other myelopathic features (sensory, bowel, bladder), abnormal spinal cord imaging
Amphiphysin "stiff-person"–like syndrome	No coexisting lower motor neuron symptoms and signs; no back involvement
Amyotrophic lateral sclerosis	No fasciculations, atrophy; no fasciculations or fibrillations on electromyography
Peripheral nerve hyperexcitability (eg, Isaac syndrome)	No neuropathic (burning) pain or paresthesias, fasciculations
Mechanical low back pain	No predominance of localized pain and tenderness
Fibromyalgia	No predominance of diffuse pain and tenderness

the patient reported reduction in frequency and severity of spasms but persistent stiffness throughout the lower back and lower extremities. Intravenous immunoglobulin (IVIG) was prescribed at a dosage of 2 g/kg of ideal body weight in 4 divided doses each month, in addition to the diazepam. After 3 months, the patient reported a 50% further improvement in stiffness and spasms but still required a walking aid. The patient expressed fear of injurious falls. After 8 weekly physical therapy sessions focused on gait and safety, the patient was able to resume ambulation with a cane, without further falls. Thiopurine methyltransferase activity was normal, and thus azathioprine was started at a full dosage of 2.5 mg/kg per day in 2 divided doses. Complete blood cell count with differential white blood cell count and liver function tests were performed on a deescalating schedule, from weekly initially, to once every 3 months eventually, to monitor for azathioprine toxicity. After 3 months of IVIG, the dosing frequency was gradually reduced over 9 months until discontinued, without evidence of further relapse.

DISCUSSION

SPS was described by Moersch and Woltman at Mayo Clinic in 1956. It most commonly arises in women of middle age but can affect men, women, and children. It is an autoimmune disorder of brainstem and spinal cord inhibitory interneuronal pathways, leading to what is termed *central hyperexcitability*. Disorders on the SPS spectrum most commonly arise in patients with GAD65-IgG autoimmunity (80%), with about one-fourth of the remaining 20% having GlyRα1-IgG positivity. Phenotypes include classic SPS (as in this case patient), stiff-limb syndrome, and a more widespread and often fatal form known as *progressive encephalomyelitis with rigidity and myoclonus* (PERM). Although either GAD65 or GlyRα1 autoimmunity (or both) may be encountered with any SPS spectrum phenotype, PERM predominates among patients who are GlyRα1-IgG positive. Occasionally there is a paraneoplastic cause, but not one specific cancer type. Amphiphysin autoimmunity is comparatively rare and phenotypically has features of a myeloneuropathy accompanying limb stiffness and spasms. Breast adenocarcinoma and small cell carcinoma

should be excluded in those cases. GAD65-IgG antibody titers should be interpreted with caution. GAD65-IgG antibody at low titers is encountered in 5% to 8% of the healthy general population (<2.00 nmol/L; reference range, ≤0.02 nmol/L) and in those with type 1 diabetes, autoimmune thyroid disease, or pernicious anemia. GAD65-IgG antibody values in SPS are typically in the hundreds of nmol/L. Similarly, GlyRα1-IgG may be encountered in some healthy persons and non-SPS neurologic phenotypes, but the clinical significance is unclear.

Neurophysiologic testing may be a useful adjunct to other testing, particularly in uncertain cases, but the results may be falsely negative in patients already taking benzodiazepines to manage symptoms.

Overall, approximately 50% of patients with SPS have substantial improvement with immunotherapies. IVIG (2 g/kg ideal body weight per month) was demonstrated to improve stiffness and spasms in a randomized clinical trial, although off-label treatments including corticosteroids, rituximab, and cyclophosphamide often provide benefit. Oral mycophenolate mofetil (1 g twice daily) and azathioprine can serve as infusion-sparing maintenance immunotherapies. Symptomatic therapies including high doses of diazepam (5-20 mg 3 or 4 times daily by mouth) and baclofen (10-20 mg 3 times daily by mouth) are used instead of or in conjunction with immunotherapies. For patients with refractory lower extremity spasms, intrathecal baclofen may be used.

KEY POINTS

- SPS disorders affect central inhibition, leading to stiffness and spasms of trunk and limbs.

- Positive clinical signs on examination or electrophysiologic testing are critical to the diagnosis.

- Serologic testing for antibodies (high-titer antibodies to GAD65, GlyRα1, and amphiphysin) aid confirmation of the diagnosis.

- One or more of immunotherapies or symptomatic therapies can lead to substantial improvement.

STIFFNESS, SPASMS, AND FREQUENT FALLS IN A 41-YEAR-OLD MAN

Michelle F. Devine, MD, and A. Sebastian Lopez Chiriboga, MD

CASE PRESENTATION

HISTORY AND EXAMINATION

A 41-year-old man sought care for 3 years of right-sided muscle stiffness. He also had 5- to 10-minute episodes of severe muscle spasms. One year after the onset of the muscle stiffness, he noted development of daily episodes of sudden, severe stiffness, often triggered by unexpected stimuli (eg, a touch or loud sound). These lasted 1 to 2 seconds and were often associated with anxiety. Occasionally, these led to falls and injuries, including a subdural hematoma requiring evacuation. There was no accompanying impaired consciousness, aura, presyncopal prodrome, or postictal phenomenon. He started using a walker and stopped driving. He stopped working as a bank manager because of increasing difficulty with mobility and cognition.

At his first evaluation at Mayo Clinic, his medications included baclofen, 20 mg 4 times a day; gabapentin, 900 mg at bedtime; escitalopram, 20 mg daily; and diazepam, 5 mg 3 times a day. These medications had partially reduced his stiffness, pain, and falls.

Review of systems at his first clinic visit was notable for 1 year of diplopia and 3 years of new anxiety. He had no prior mood symptoms.

His medical history was pertinent for rapid eye movement sleep behavior disorder (onset concurrent with stiffness symptoms) and obstructive sleep apnea controlled with continuous positive airway pressure (diagnosed 2 years before our evaluation).

On neurologic examination, he had a Kokmen Short Test of Mental Status score of 28/38, with points lost for orientation, attention, calculation, and recall. Cranial nerve examination showed bilateral ptosis and hypometric saccadic eye movements. He had normal strength but diffuse rigidity with increased tone, most severe in the right lower extremity. He had mildly brisk deep tendon reflexes in the right arm and bilateral legs. He had extensor plantar responses bilaterally. Mild difficulty with rapid alternating movements in bilateral legs was also noted, and his gait was spastic and unsteady, which necessitated walking assistance for short distances. Diagnoses considered at the time are shown in Table 37.1.

TESTING

Magnetic resonance imaging of the brain indicated right parietal postoperative changes (post hematoma evacuation). Electromyography–nerve conduction studies showed no evidence of neurogenic, myopathic, or neuromuscular junction pathologic processes. Electroencephalography showed dysrhythmia grade 1 over the right frontotemporal region (above the prior hematoma). Cerebrospinal fluid (CSF) was inflammatory, with mildly increased protein concentration of 54 mg/dL (reference range, 0-35 mg/dL) and 6 supernumerary oligoclonal bands. Other CSF findings were benign (1 white blood cell/μL, 2 erythrocytes/μL, negative immunoglobulin G [IgG] index, and negative synthesis rate). CSF was also negative for 14-3-3 protein and real-time quaking-induced conversion.

Movement laboratory evaluation demonstrated an exaggerated startle and abnormal exteroceptive response consistent with central nervous system (CNS) hyperexcitability.

Neural-specific autoantibody testing was positive for glycine receptor α1 subunit (GlyRα1)-IgG in both serum and CSF. Other autoantibodies were negative, including glutamic acid decarboxylase 65-kDa isoform (GAD65), amphiphysin, and dipeptidyl-peptidase-like protein-6 (DPPX).

No malignancy was found on cancer screening, including positron emission tomography–computed tomography and testicular ultrasonography.

DIAGNOSIS

He was diagnosed with progressive encephalomyelitis with rigidity and myoclonus (PERM) with positive GlyRα1-IgG.

Table 37.1 | DIFFERENTIAL DIAGNOSIS FOR THE CASE PATIENT

POSSIBLE DIAGNOSES	PERTINENT POSITIVES/NEGATIVES
Psychogenic nonepileptic spells	Multiple injuries suggesting impaired control during episodes
Corticobasal syndrome	Rigidity without other signs of parkinsonism
	No dystonia
Creutzfeldt-Jakob disease	Relatively slow progression over past 3 years
	Presence of brainstem dysfunction
Cramp-fasciculation syndrome	No fasciculations on examination or neurodiagnostic studies
Fibromyalgia	Positive antibody correlating with clinical phenotype
	Positive brainstem signs
Hereditary spastic paraparesis	Lack of family history
	Presence of brainstem dysfunction
Myasthenia gravis	Myasthenia gravis is not associated with rigidity
	Normal electromyography and nerve conduction studies

MANAGEMENT

Given the immune-mediated cause of PERM, he was started on a 12-week trial of intravenous methylprednisolone and concurrent rituximab. With this immunosuppression trial, the patient markedly improved. He no longer had leg spasms but continued 25 mg diazepam per day for residual stiffness. He no longer needed a walker and was able to drive again. His anxiety was still severe, however, and required increased escitalopram and cognitive behavioral therapy to control.

Over several months, he was tapered off intravenous methylprednisolone. He was maintained on rituximab (2 doses of 1 g rituximab every 6 months, each dose separated by 2 weeks). On this regimen, his symptoms eventually resolved. He remained stable at 2-year follow-up after initiating immunosuppression.

DISCUSSION

PERM is considered a variant of stiff-person syndrome (SPS) (discussed in Chapter 36). There is clinical overlap between PERM and classic SPS, which are both characterized by CNS hyperexcitability with exaggerated startle, muscle rigidity, and painful spasms.

Compared with classic SPS, PERM is typically more severe and more rapidly progressive. PERM also often has encephalopathy and brainstem features. In addition to the progressive rigidity, patients may have ophthalmalgia, ptosis, dysphagia, dysarthria, autonomic dysfunction, and respiratory events. Neuropsychiatric symptoms (particularly anxiety) and falls are common in both SPS and PERM. PERM can be fatal, particularly if untreated.

GlyRα1-IgG is detected in 20% of patients with PERM. GlyRα1-IgG can also be associated with classic SPS and other neurologic phenotypes (eg, demyelinating disease, epilepsy). Development of GlyRα1-IgG antibodies is usually idiopathic, but paraneoplastic cases have been described. DPPX-IgG has also been described in a few PERM cases and can be associated with B-cell lymphoma and leukemia. GAD65-IgG can be found in PERM cases as well as classic SPS. GlyRα1-IgG and GAD65-IgG may also coexist.

PERM management includes symptomatic control, immunosuppression, and tumor treatment (if present). PERM seems to have a more favorable response to immunosuppression than classic SPS. The presence of GlyRα1-IgG is associated with a higher rate of response to immunosuppression compared with SPS spectrum disorders associated with GAD65-IgG alone.

Symptomatic control includes the use of γ-aminobutyric acid-ergic medications (including baclofen and benzodiazepines) and physical therapy. Optimization of anxiety control should involve a psychiatrist/psychologist and may require inpatient psychiatric treatment if anxiety is severe.

KEY POINTS

- PERM has clinical overlap with classic SPS, including CNS hyperexcitability with exaggerated startle, muscle rigidity, and painful spasms.

- Compared with the classic SPS phenotype, PERM has additional features, including encephalopathy and brainstem dysfunction.

- GlyRα1-IgG is detected in 20% of PERM cases. DPPX-IgG and GAD65-IgG antibodies can also accompany the PERM phenotype.

- The presence of GlyRα1-IgG is associated with a favorable response to immunosuppression.

RAPID-ONSET WEAKNESS AND NUMBNESS IN A PATIENT WITH SYSTEMIC LUPUS ERYTHEMATOSUS

Floranne C. Ernste, MD

CASE PRESENTATION

HISTORY AND EXAMINATION

A 33-year-old woman with systemic lupus erythematosus (SLE), diagnosed 2 years prior and treated with hydroxychloroquine, sought care for a 4-week history of pain and paresthesias in her low back and lower extremities. She described a bandlike sensation of numbness starting in her midback which descended to both legs. Her symptoms progressed to constipation and inability to urinate adequately. She reported difficulty with ambulation. She reported no fevers, headaches, or neck stiffness. She did not have cognitive dysfunction or confusion. Over the course of 1 week of hospitalization, urinary and fecal incontinence developed.

On examination, she was alert and appropriately oriented. She had a malar rash and swelling of the metacarpophalangeal joints consistent with bilateral hand synovitis. Neurologic examination indicated hyperreflexia with brisk patellar and Achilles tendon reflexes bilaterally; the biceps, triceps, and brachioradialis reflexes were normal in the upper extremities. She had trace motor weakness of the hip flexors, quadriceps, and hamstrings. She had loss of pinprick and temperature sensation in the lower extremities, extending beyond the saddle area to the T12 dermatome. Vibration perception and proprioception were preserved. She had a positive Babinski sign in the left foot. Her cerebellar examination showed slowing of rapid alternating movements in the left hand. Diagnoses considered at the time are shown in Table 38.1.

TESTING

Magnetic resonance imaging of the brain and thoracic spine showed normal findings. Magnetic resonance imaging of the lumbosacral spine indicated subtle T2 signal change of the intramedullary conus and enhancement of the cauda equina nerve roots (Figure 38.1). Cerebrospinal fluid (CSF) analysis showed an increased protein concentration (60 mg/dL; reference range, ≤35 mg/dL). Two white blood cells/μL were found in the CSF. The CSF glucose level was normal. Oligoclonal bands were not detected. Viral, bacterial, and fungal cultures were negative, as was cytologic examination. Serum paraneoplastic antibodies were negative. The serum antinuclear antibody was strongly positive, and the anti–double-stranded DNA antibody level was greater than 1,000 IU/mL (reference range, <30 IU/mL). The serum complement levels were low: C3, 60 mg/dL (reference range, 75-175 mg/L) and C4, less than 3 mg/dL (reference range, 14-40 mg/dL). The serum was negative for antiribosomal P antibody, aquaporin-4–immunoglobulin G (IgG), and myelin oligodendrocyte glycoprotein–IgG. Lupus anticoagulant, beta-2 glycoprotein antibodies (IgG and IgM), and antiphospholipid antibodies (IgG and IgM) were increased, at greater than twice the upper limits of normal. Electromyography indicated multiple sacral radiculopathies.

DIAGNOSIS

The patient was diagnosed with autoimmune myeloradiculitis as a neuropsychiatric manifestation of SLE (*neuropsychiatric SLE* [NPSLE]).

Table 38.1 **DIFFERENTIAL DIAGNOSIS FOR THE CASE PATIENT**

POSSIBLE DIAGNOSES	PERTINENT NEGATIVES
Aseptic meningitis	Fever, headache, neck stiffness, cranial nerve involvement
Acute inflammatory demyelinating polyneuropathy	Ascending flaccid paralysis
Stroke	Abrupt unilateral neurologic dysfunction
Posterior reversible encephalopathy syndrome	Headaches, seizures
Mononeuritis multiplex	Asymmetric upper/lower extremity weakness

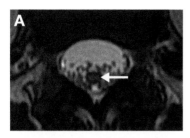
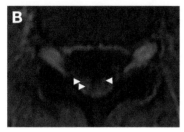

Figure 38.1 **Magnetic Resonance Imaging Findings for Case Patient.**

Axial images of conus medullaris and nerve roots show T2 signal change of the intramedullary conus (A, arrow) and faint enhancement of the cauda equina nerve roots (B, arrowheads).

MANAGEMENT

The patient received 1 g of methylprednisolone on 3 consecutive days, followed by 1 mg/kg of prednisone per day, with a gradual taper. Her hospital course was complicated by the development of deep venous thromboses in the bilateral lower extremities. She was started on heparin and transitioned to warfarin therapy. She started mycophenolate mofetil at a dosage of 500 mg twice daily; it was titrated to a dosage of 1,000 mg twice daily within 1 month. Hydroxychloroquine was continued. She reported a mild relapse of the paresthesia in her legs at a return visit; therefore, the prednisone taper was slowed. After 9 months, full neurologic remission had been achieved. Glucocorticoids were discontinued within 12 months of her initial evaluation. At a 24-month follow-up visit, the patient remained in neurologic remission while continuing mycophenolate mofetil at 1,000 mg twice daily, hydroxychloroquine, and anticoagulation.

DISCUSSION

NPSLE events consist of a heterogeneous array of neurologic and psychiatric disorders including intractable headaches, cognitive dysfunction, psychosis, seizure disorders, transverse myelitis, aseptic meningitis, cranial neuropathies, and acute inflammatory demyelinating polyneuropathy. By the 1999 American College of Rheumatology criteria, the prevalence of NPSLE is 21% to 95% with 19 case definitions, but attributing causality of neurologic events to SLE often remains challenging. Secondary factors can contribute to neurologic events in patients with SLE, such as metabolic abnormalities, drug adverse effects, and infections. Clinical judgment remains paramount in identifying NPSLE for the prompt initiation of immunosuppressive therapy.

Transverse myelitis is a rare and serious complication of SLE and is reported in 1% to 2% of patients. The clinical

manifestations involve abrupt onset of pain, paresthesia, weakness, sensory loss at the level of cord involvement, and sphincter dysfunction. Much of the longitudinally extensive transverse myelitis that occurs in SLE is now accounted for by aquaporin-4 autoimmunity (neuromyelitis optica [NMO] spectrum disorders). Patients with aquaporin-4 autoimmunity typically have a relapsing course and may have other manifestations such as optic neuritis or, rarely, encephalitis. Myelitis accompanying SLE, beyond NMO, has traditionally been described in 2 groups. Patients with gray matter myelitis may have fever, flaccid paralysis, and hyporeflexia within hours and often have active SLE, increased anti–double-stranded DNA antibodies, and urinary retention. In contrast, patients with white matter myelitis have spasticity and hyperreflexia; this subtype may be associated with thrombotic events and the presence of antiphospholipid antibodies and anti-Ro antibodies. Many other patients, such as the case patient, have disorders beyond the classic NMO phenotypes or straightforward transverse myelitis and often have poorly understood pathogeneses.

The pathogenesis of NPSLE, in general, is incompletely understood. Common findings on autopsy are microthromboses, microinfarctions, intimal proliferation of small vessel walls, and thrombotic occlusion of major blood vessels. The presence of overt cerebral vasculitis is uncommon. Several other autoantibodies may be detected in NPSLE. For example, antiphospholipid antibodies are associated with transverse myelitis, chorea, and ischemic strokes; N-methyl-D-aspartate receptor antibodies are encountered in the CSF of some patients with coexisting autoimmune encephalitis; antiribosomal P antibodies may be detected in patients with depression and psychosis. Some autoantibodies may be pathogenic.

The diagnostic workup is complex. Testing often includes serologic autoantibody testing, CSF analysis, electroencephalography, electromyography with nerve conduction studies, and magnetic resonance imaging of the brain and spinal cord, with and without intravenous contrast. Treatment should be targeted to controlling the inflammation and reducing the thrombotic burden. A delay in treatment may lead to substantial neurologic dysfunction and irreversible damage, resulting in decreased 5- and 10-year survival rates. High-dose glucocorticoids are indicated, followed by a prolonged corticosteroid taper. A regimen of pulse cyclophosphamide at 0.6 to 1.0 g/m² administered monthly for 6 months is often used. For patients with rapid deterioration, several courses of plasma exchange may be used. Additional immunosuppressive therapies include intravenous immunoglobulin, mycophenolate mofetil, azathioprine, or methotrexate.

KEY POINTS

- Neuropsychiatric events have varied presentations and may be difficult to attribute to SLE.

- Extensive testing is required for exclusion of confounders.

- Prompt initiation of high-intensity immunosuppression can result in improved neurologic outcomes.

PROGRESSIVE QUADRIPARESIS AND CANCER

Elia Sechi, MD, and Eoin P. Flanagan, MB, BCh

CASE PRESENTATION

HISTORY AND EXAMINATION

A previously healthy 67-year-old White man with a history of cigarette smoking (27 pack-years) sought care at the emergency department for nonspecific dizziness and fatigue. During evaluation, chest radiography showed a right upper lobe mass, and he subsequently underwent right upper lobectomy. Histologic analysis of resected tissue showed the mass to be small cell lung carcinoma. In the first few weeks after surgery, progressive myelopathy developed. Adjuvant chemotherapy with carboplatin and etoposide was begun after neurologic symptom onset. His neurologic symptoms continued to worsen, with development of slowly progressive quadriparesis with gait imbalance, along with numbness and dysesthesias of the 4 limbs and trunk, with a sensory level at C3-C4. He also reported severe bowel and bladder dysfunction. At his neurologic nadir, he had severe quadriparesis and was wheelchair dependent.

TESTING

Initial magnetic resonance imaging (MRI) of the head and cervical and thoracic spine was unremarkable (Figure 39.1A). Cerebrospinal fluid (CSF) analysis showed lymphocytic pleocytosis of 9 white blood cells/μL (reference range, 0-5/μL), erythrocyte count of 2/μL, and normal protein and glucose values. CSF cytologic findings were negative. Serum neural autoantibody screening revealed the presence of collapsin-response mediator protein 5 (CRMP5)–immunoglobulin G (IgG) antibodies on both tissue-based indirect immunofluorescence assay and Western blot. CSF neural antibody testing was not performed.

DIAGNOSIS

The patient was diagnosed with paraneoplastic myelopathy.

MANAGEMENT

The patient was initially treated acutely with a combination of high-dose oral prednisone and plasmapheresis, without improvement. Subsequently, a combination of intravenous immunoglobulin (IVIG) and rituximab resulted in partial improvement, allowing the patient to ambulate with the aid of a cane or a walker. Approximately 2 years after symptom onset, immunotherapy was stopped. Soon after treatment discontinuation, his symptoms returned with worsening weakness, numbness, and neuropathic pain. Monthly IVIG and rituximab were reinitiated, with improvement again noted. Oral corticosteroids, methadone, and high-dose gabapentin (3,300 mg/d) were also administered, with mild

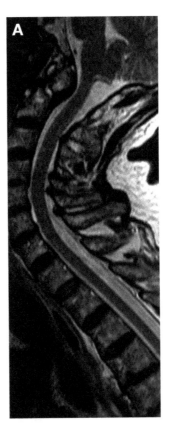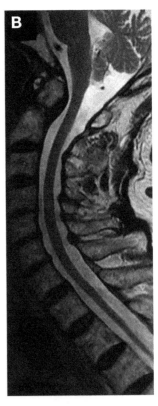

Figure 39.1 **Magnetic Resonance Imaging Findings for Case Patient.**
Sagittal T2-weighted spine images at symptom onset (A) and after 3 years (B) show the development of spinal cord atrophy in the absence of signal abnormalities.

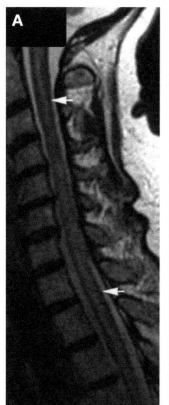

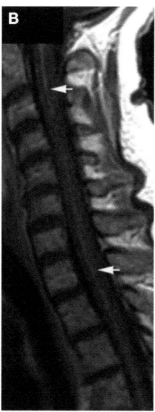

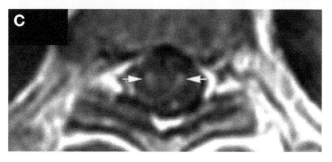

Figure 39.2 Examples of Typical Magnetic Resonance Imaging Abnormalities in Paraneoplastic Myelopathy.

A and B, Sagittal spine images show longitudinally extensive T2-hyperintense lesions along the spinal cord (A, arrows), which enhance after gadolinium administration (B, arrows). C, Axial images show tract-specific involvement of the lateral columns (arrows).

(From Flanagan EP, McKeon A, Lennon VA, Kearns J, Weinshenker BG, Krecke KN, et al. Paraneoplastic isolated myelopathy: clinical course and neuroimaging clues. Neurology 2011 Jun 14;76:2089-95; used with permission.)

benefit for neuropathic pain. Follow-up spine MRI 3 years after symptom onset showed evidence of spinal cord atrophy (Figure 39.1B). At 5-year follow-up after symptom onset, he remained in remission from small cell lung cancer but was wheelchair dependent.

DISCUSSION

Paraneoplastic myelopathy is a rare and underrecognized neurologic disorder that most often manifests before cancer detection, although it may occur concomitantly with cancer diagnosis (as in this case patient) or after a cancer has been treated (in which case it can be a clue to recurrence).

Paraneoplastic myelopathy may occur in isolation or be accompanied by various other peripheral or central nervous system manifestations. Paraneoplastic myelopathies typically affect patients between age 60 and 70 years with a current or past history of cigarette smoking or a known history of cancer. Clinical presentation is generally subacute or slowly progressive over months, but acute onset is possible. CSF typically shows lymphocytic pleocytosis, as in this case patient.

Spinal cord MRI findings are normal in one-third of cases, but a longitudinally extensive, tract-specific, T2 hyperintensity along dorsal or lateral columns with accompanying tract-specific gadolinium enhancement is suggestive of a paraneoplastic cause (Figure 39.2). Similar tract-specific signal changes can occur with nutritional deficiency (eg, vitamin B_{12} or copper deficiency), toxicity (eg, methotrexate), or hereditary conditions (eg, Friedreich ataxia). The CSF pleocytosis and enhancement with gadolinium may help distinguish paraneoplastic myelopathy from other noninflammatory processes in which such findings would be atypical. Paraneoplastic myelopathy may mimic primary progressive multiple sclerosis. The most frequently detected neural antibodies are CRMP5-IgG and amphiphysin-IgG, and there are some seronegative cases. The most frequently detected cancers are small cell lung and breast adenocarcinomas. Occasionally, aquaporin-4–IgG and glial fibrillary acidic protein–IgG can occur in a paraneoplastic context with teratoma or other cancers.

Prognosis is generally poor in patients with paraneoplastic myelopathies. Neurologic responses to cancer treatment and immunotherapy are often limited. However, there may be an augmented antitumor immune response in patients with paraneoplastic disorders which contributes to longer-than-typical survival (as in this case patient). Approximately 90% of patients require a cane, walker, or wheelchair after a median of 17 months from symptom onset. In patients with paraneoplastic neurologic disorders, the benefits and risks of immunotherapy must be carefully considered because immunotherapy could, in theory, hamper the antitumor immune response. However, neurologic manifestations are often severe and life-threatening, and immunotherapy may be necessary in addition to cancer treatment.

In this patient with severe quadriparesis, concomitant immunotherapy with a B-cell–depleting agent (ie, rituximab) and IVIG were used in conjunction with carboplatin and etoposide chemotherapy. He had partial neurologic improvements without cancer recurrence at last follow-up. Evidence from pathologic and in vitro laboratory studies supports CD8+ T cells as prominent effectors in classic paraneoplastic neurologic disorders, if the antigen (such as CRMP5) is intracellular. Rituximab depletes B cells, both antigen presenters (to T cells) or precursors of neural plasma membrane IgG effector-producing plasma cells.

KEY POINTS

- Neurologic manifestations of paraneoplastic myelopathy usually begin before the cancer is detected, and the presence of risk factors for cancer (eg, long history of smoking) may be a clue.

- Symmetric, longitudinally extensive, tract-specific (dorsal or lateral columns), T2 hyperintensities with gadolinium enhancement are a clue to a paraneoplastic myelopathy, although spine MRI findings are normal in one-third of patients.

- The most common neural autoantibodies associated with paraneoplastic myelopathy are CRMP5- and amphiphysin-IgG, and the most common neoplasms are small cell lung and breast carcinomas.

- Rapid detection and treatment of cancer with additional immunotherapy is recommended, but prognosis is poor and most patients become wheelchair dependent.

PROGRESSIVE NUMBNESS, BURNING PAIN, IMBALANCE, AND DRYNESS

Shahar Shelly, MD, and Divyanshu Dubey, MBBS

CASE PRESENTATION

HISTORY AND EXAMINATION

A 65-year-old woman was evaluated for progressive numbness and tingling involving different body parts. Onset was approximately 2 years earlier, starting with her right foot. Within a few weeks, the numbness and paresthesia progressed to her left hand and then left foot. Six months later, numbness and tingling of her right hand also developed. She described severe burning pain in the left palm and both lower limbs, along with joint pain and morning stiffness. Progressive gait instability also developed, leading to frequent falls. She started using a cane to walk. She also reported severe dry eyes and mouth and noticed an inability to sweat in hot weather, leading to recurrent "heat strokes" in summers. She disclosed no history of orthostatic intolerance or bowel or bladder incontinence.

Her neurologic examination showed pseudoathetosis with eye closure and sensory gait ataxia. She had profound vibration and proprioceptive loss in all extremities (lower extremities greater than upper extremities). She also had asymmetric reduction in pinprick sensation in her hands and feet distally. Muscle tone was normal. She had minimal distal weakness involving her toes and upper extremities. Her deep tendon reflexes were reduced in the upper limbs and absent in the lower limbs. Toes were downgoing to plantar stimulation. Cranial nerve, cerebellar, and mental status examinations were normal. Diagnoses considered at the time are shown in Table 40.1.

TESTING

Magnetic resonance imaging of the brain and entire spine showed no evidence of brain, spinal cord, or nerve root abnormalities. Nerve conduction studies demonstrated asymmetric, sensory-predominant, axonal peripheral neuropathy with absent left median and ulnar sensory responses and relatively preserved (reduced) right median and ulnar sensory responses. Bilateral sural sensory responses were absent (Figure 40.1A). Motor responses were relatively preserved. Cerebrospinal fluid (CSF) analysis showed mildly increased

Table 40.1 | DIFFERENTIAL DIAGNOSIS FOR THE CASE PATIENT

POSSIBLE DIAGNOSES	SUGGESTIVE OF ALTERNATIVE DIAGNOSIS
Sjögren sensory ganglionopathy	NA
Paraneoplastic sensory neuronopathy	No history of unintentional weight loss, no significant gastrointestinal tract dysmotility
Neuronopathy associated with vitamin B$_6$ toxicity	No history of multivitamin or pyridoxine supplementation
Chemotherapy-induced sensory neuronopathy (eg, cisplatin)	No history of cancer or chemotherapy use
CISP	Presence of sicca symptoms, severe burning pain
Multifocal CIDP (Lewis-Sumner syndrome)	No significant motor involvement, severe burning pain
Migrant sensory neuropathy (Wartenberg migrant sensory neuritis)	Lack of relapsing and remitting course
Myelopathy affecting dorsal column	No sensory level, no bowel or bladder symptoms
Fibromyalgia	Asymmetrical sensory abnormalities on examination, absent/reduced DTRs

Abbreviations: CIDP, chronic inflammatory demyelinating polyradiculoneuropathy; CISP, chronic immune sensory polyradiculopathy; DTR, deep tendon reflexes; NA, not applicable.

A

Nerve	Type	Record site	Side	Amp	CV	Distal Lat
Median	Sensory	Dig 2	R	4	49	3.8
Median	Sensory	Dig 2	L	NR	NR	NR
Ulnar	Sensory	Dig 5	R	6	40	3.4
Ulnar	Sensory	Dig 5	L	NR	NR	NR
Sural	Sensory	Ankle	R	NR	NR	NR
Sural	Sensory	Ankle	L	NR	NR	NR

B

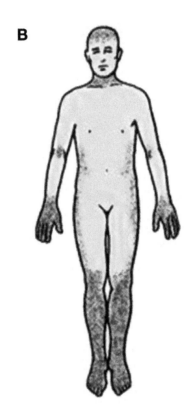

Figure 40.1 **Test Results for Case Patient.**
A, Sensory nerve conduction studies show asymmetric, axonal, sensory-predominant neuropathy. Amp indicates amplitude; CV, conduction velocity; Dig, digit; L, left; Lat, latency; NR, no response; R, right. B, Thermoregulatory sweat testing shows anhidrosis over the trunk and proximal extremities (yellow) and hypohidrosis over the forehead and distal extremities (purple) suggesting involvement of sudomotor sympathetic dysfunction.

protein concentration of 48 mg/dL (reference range, ≤35 mg/dL), normal blood cell count (2 cells/μL; reference range, ≤5 cells/μL), normal immunoglobulin G index, normal synthesis rate, and 5 CSF-restricted oligoclonal bands. CSF cytologic analysis was negative for malignant cells. Thermoregulatory sweat testing showed anhidrosis involving the proximal limbs and the trunk and hypohidrosis of the forehead and distal extremities (Figure 40.1B). Serum laboratory investigations identified an increased erythrocyte sedimentation rate of 38 mm/h (reference range, <29 mm/h). Serologic testing was remarkable for positive antinuclear antibody (1:80), rheumatoid factor (33 IU/mL; reference range, <15 IU/mL),

and Sjögren syndrome-A antibody (anti-Ro) (>8 U; reference range, <1.0 U). Serum and CSF evaluations for paraneoplastic antibodies including antineuronal nuclear antibody type 1 (anti-Hu), anti–collapsin-response mediator protein 5, Purkinje cell cytoplasmic antibody type 2, antiamphiphysin, and antineuronal nuclear antibody type 3 were negative. Screening for syphilis and Lyme disease was negative. Vitamin E, vitamin B_6, vitamin B_{12}, vitamin B_1, thyrotropin, and hemoglobin A_{1c} were within normal ranges. Serum protein electrophoresis results were unremarkable. Chest computed tomography showed a nonspecific solitary nodule (7 mm) in the right upper lobe but was otherwise normal.

DIAGNOSIS

The patient was diagnosed with Sjögren sensory ganglionopathy (or neuronopathy).

MANAGEMENT

The patient received a 12-week course of intravenous methylprednisolone, starting with 1 g/d for 3 days, followed by 1 g weekly for 5 weeks, followed by 1 g every other week for 6 weeks. She was also started on mycophenolate mofetil 500 mg twice daily, orally. Two weeks later, the mycophenolate mofetil dose was increased to 1,000 mg twice daily. At follow-up 4 months later, she reported improvement in neuropathic pain, but the sensory loss and ataxia continued to be treatment refractory.

DISCUSSION

The presence of sicca symptoms (dry eyes and mouth), polyarthralgias, morning stiffness, and anti-Ro antibody seropositivity were supportive of a Sjögren syndrome diagnosis. Sjögren syndrome has been associated with various neuropathic presentations, including sensory ganglionopathy, symmetric sensorimotor polyneuropathy, trigeminal neuralgia, small fiber neuropathy, multiple cranial neuropathy, autonomic neuropathies, and multiple mononeuropathies. Sensory ganglionopathy in Sjögren syndrome usually presents with asymmetrical sensory loss, neuropathic pain, sensory ataxia, and sometimes pseudoathetosis, which were presenting features in this case patient. Chronic immune sensory polyradiculopathy (CISP) can also have similar presenting signs and symptoms. However, patients with CISP usually have normal sensory nerve conduction studies because the immune-mediated pathogenesis is limited to sensory roots.

The dorsal root ganglion (DRG) is supplied by fenestrated capillaries that lack the typical blood-nerve barrier, which may be a potential factor making them more vulnerable to immune-mediated damage. In Sjögren sensory ganglionopathy, histopathologic analysis of the DRG has shown CD8+ lymphocytic infiltration and reduction of DRG neurons, supportive of cytotoxic T-cell–mediated pathogenesis. Immunotherapies commonly used for these patients include intravenous methylprednisolone, intravenous immunoglobulin, mycophenolate mofetil, azathioprine, or methotrexate. Even though the nonneuropathic symptoms, such as sicca syndrome or polyarthralgias, are readily responsive to immunotherapies, the ganglionopathy has a more refractory course. In previous case series of Sjögren sensory ganglionopathy with sensory ataxia, less than one-fourth of patients treated with immunotherapy had response. However, those receiving immunotherapies earlier in their disease course (<1 year after symptom onset) are more likely to have neurologic improvements.

KEY POINTS

- Sjögren syndrome is associated with varied neuropathy phenotypes, including sensory ganglionopathy, symmetric sensorimotor or sensory polyneuropathy, polyradiculoneuropathy, cranial neuropathies, multiple mononeuropathies, small fiber neuropathy, and autonomic neuropathy.

- Subacute progression, asymmetrical sensory loss, sensory ataxia, and relative sparing of motor nerves on electrodiagnostic studies are features supportive of a sensory ganglionopathy diagnosis.

- In Sjögren sensory ganglionopathy, DRG histopathologic analysis has shown CD8+ lymphocytic infiltration, supportive of cytotoxic T-cell–mediated pathogenesis.

- Most cases of Sjögren sensory ganglionopathy have a refractory course, especially for patients with delayed initiation of immunotherapy.

ASCENDING PAINFUL PARESTHESIAS, PROGRESSIVE ATAXIA, AND BILATERAL FOOT DROP

Rocio Vazquez Do Campo, MD, and Divyanshu Dubey, MBBS

CASE PRESENTATION

HISTORY AND EXAMINATION

A 63-year-old woman with a 40-pack-year cigarette smoking history had development of ascending paresthesias with lancinating and stabbing pain in all extremities. The symptoms began asymmetrically in the left leg and progressed to involve the right leg and both hands over 2 months. In subsequent weeks, she noticed progressive bilateral leg weakness, gait instability, and new numbness in the left middle back. Within 4 months of symptom onset, she had recurrent falls and required the use of a cane and eventually a walker. She had 18.2 kg (40 pounds) of weight loss over 12 months. She had no autonomic symptoms or bladder or bowel dysfunction.

Examination 1 year after symptom onset showed an emaciated, ill-appearing woman. On neurologic examination, she had marked gait ataxia with profound proprioceptive loss in all extremities. She had asymmetrically reduced pinprick sensation distal to the left thigh, right knee, and both forearms, as well as bilateral middle thoracic dermatomes. Muscle tone was normal. She had bilateral foot drop (worse on the left) and mild weakness in bilateral hamstring and intrinsic hand

muscles. Her deep tendon reflexes were globally absent. Toes were mute to plantar stimulation. Cranial nerve, cerebellar, and mental status examinations were normal. Diagnoses considered at the time are shown in Table 41.1.

TESTING

Magnetic resonance imaging (MRI) of the entire spine demonstrated subtle increased T2 signal in the posterior columns extending along cervical and thoracic segments and patchy gadolinium enhancement of the cervical and lumbosacral nerve roots (Figure 41.1). Electrodiagnostic testing demonstrated a length-dependent axonal sensorimotor peripheral neuropathy. Cerebrospinal fluid (CSF) analysis showed an increased protein concentration of 68 mg/dL (reference range, ≤35 mg/dL), 9 CSF-restricted oligoclonal bands, increased immunoglobulin G (IgG) index and synthesis rate, and normal blood cell count (1 cell/μL). CSF cytologic analysis was negative for malignant cells. Serum laboratory investigations showed normal complete blood cell count; normal levels of hemoglobin A_{1c}, vitamin B_{12}, copper, vitamin E, methylmalonic acid, homocysteine, thyrotropin, creatinine, angiotensin-converting enzyme, and C-reactive protein; and

Table 41.1 | DIFFERENTIAL DIAGNOSIS FOR THE CASE PATIENT

POSSIBLE DIAGNOSES	PERTINENT NEGATIVES
Chronic inflammatory demyelinating polyradiculoneuropathy	Usually painless, no weight loss, often motor-predominant symptoms
Mononeuropathy multiplex (systemic vasculitides)	Usually systemic symptoms (fever, malaise) or organ involvement (skin, lung, or kidneys), often motor-predominant symptoms
Metabolic-nutritional (vitamin B_{12}, copper, vitamin E) deficiencies	Usually symmetric symptoms, hyperreflexia, history of malabsorption, gastric bypass, or pernicious anemia
Infectious myelopathy or myeloneuropathy (HIV, human T-lymphotropic virus 1)	Other myelopathic features (spasticity, hyperreflexia, bladder, bowel), risk factors (travel history, unprotected sex)
Neurosarcoidosis	Often cranial neuropathies
Neurolymphomatosis	Often cranial neuropathies, other systemic symptoms (fever, night sweats), palpable lymph nodes
POEMS syndrome (*p*olyneuropathy, *o*rganomegaly, *e*ndocrinopathy, *M* component, *s*kin changes)	Often organomegaly, endocrinopathy, skin changes, edema, papilledema, motor-predominant symptoms

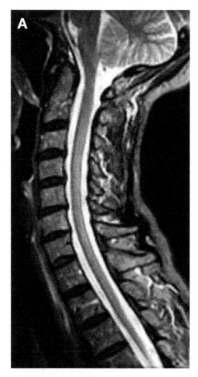

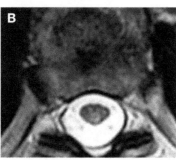

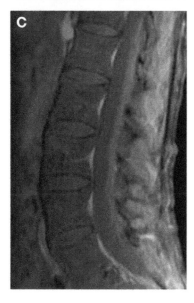

Figure 41.1 Magnetic Resonance Imaging (MRI) Findings for the Case Patient.
A, Sagittal, T2-weighted, short tau, inversion recovery MRI of the cervical spine shows subtle increased signal in the dorsal columns extending along cervical segments and the visualized portion of the thoracic spinal cord. B, Axial, T2-weighted, fast spin echo MRI of the cervical spine demonstrates subtle increased signal of the dorsal columns. C, Gadolinium-enhanced, sagittal, T1-weighted MRI of the lumbar spine shows enhancement of the lumbosacral nerve roots after gadolinium administration.

normal findings for serum and urine protein electrophoresis, erythrocyte sedimentation rate, anti–double-stranded DNA antibodies, complement C3 and C4, connective tissue cascade, extractable nuclear antigen, and antineutrophil cytoplasmic antibodies. Screenings for syphilis, Lyme disease, HIV, and human lymphotropic virus 1 and 2 were negative.

Paraneoplastic antibody evaluation showed high titers of collapsin-response mediator protein 5 (CRMP5)-IgG autoantibodies in the serum (1:491,520 [reference range, <1:240]) and CSF (1:512 [reference range, <1:2]). Prior cancer screening with mammography, colonoscopy, and computed tomography of the chest, abdomen, and pelvis had been unrevealing. Whole-body ¹⁸F-fludeoxyglucose–positron emission tomography (FDG-PET) indicated multiple hypermetabolic mediastinal and hilar lymph nodes without suspicious pulmonary lesions. Biopsy of a mediastinal lymph node was consistent with small cell lung carcinoma.

DIAGNOSIS

The patient was diagnosed with CRMP5-IgG paraneoplastic myeloneuropathy associated with small cell carcinoma of the lung.

MANAGEMENT

The patient received a trial of 5 days of 1 g/d intravenous methylprednisolone (IVMP) followed by chemotherapy with etoposide and cisplatin, along with chest and prophylactic brain radiotherapy. She achieved a short period of clinical stabilization and mild improvement in gait and limb ataxia for 2 to 3 months coinciding with regression of the thoracic lymphadenopathy. Subsequently, her ataxia and bilateral leg weakness worsened, and repeated electrodiagnostic evaluation demonstrated further reduction in summated motor and sensory amplitude responses and new denervation changes in proximal limb muscles. A second round of immunotherapy with IVMP or intravenous immunoglobulin (IVIG) on a weekly basis was considered, but the patient experienced several complications, including a traumatic hip fracture and radiation-induced esophageal stricture requiring stent placement, so treatment was delayed. Her clinical condition rapidly deteriorated, and she became severely malnourished and bedridden, dying 12 weeks later, 2 years after symptom onset.

DISCUSSION

CRMP5-IgG antibodies have been associated with asymmetric, painful polyradiculoneuropathy with coexisting myelopathy, often in the setting of thymoma or small cell lung cancer. Paraneoplastic myeloneuropathies have also been described with amphiphysin-IgG and antineuronal nuclear antibody type 1 (ANNA-1; anti-Hu), but seronegative cases also exist. Some aspects of the clinical history, such as heavy smoking, unexplained weight loss, subacute onset, asymmetric sensorimotor deficits, severe neuropathic pain, and relative refractoriness to immunotherapies can be important clues to a paraneoplastic cause. The diagnosis can be challenging; imaging and electrodiagnostic studies assist with precise localization because neuropathy may mask some of the myelopathic features on examination. Typical MRI findings include enlargement with or without enhancement of the nerve roots and symmetric, tract-specific signal changes with or without contrast enhancement involving longitudinally extensive segments of the lateral columns, dorsal columns, or central gray matter. Imaging studies may also be normal or show subtle abnormalities; therefore, careful evaluation is important. Axonal features with signs of active denervation in proximal and distal myotomes are common on electrodiagnostic testing.

The management of paraneoplastic neurologic syndromes involves detection and treatment of the underlying cancer, coordinated with immunotherapy. Common first-line immunotherapies in this setting are short courses of high-dose IVMP, IVIG, or plasma exchange. Longer immunosuppression trials of 6 or 12 weeks of IVIG or IVMP are also used. The combination of oncologic treatment and immunotherapy may lead to neurologic improvement, although the response is often variable and incomplete. After neurologic stabilization is achieved, and if cancer is in remission, a steroid-sparing agent, such as azathioprine, mycophenolate mofetil, rituximab, or cyclophosphamide, can be considered as IVMP or IVIG is maintained or tapered.

Ongoing cancer surveillance, including whole-body FDG-PET, is recommended if initial oncologic evaluation is unrevealing and the autoantibody detected is strongly associated with cancer. In some cases, despite extensive evaluation, the underlying cancer is not found until autopsy. Data regarding prognosis are limited, but in our experience some patients achieve clinical stabilization, especially with high-dose IVMP and cyclophosphamide combined with cancer-directed therapies. Unfortunately, a considerable proportion of patients have progressive decline, as this case patient did.

KEY POINTS

- Paraneoplastic myeloneuropathies are relatively rare paraneoplastic syndromes often associated with small cell lung cancer, thymoma, breast cancer, or testicular germ cell tumors.

- Amphiphysin, CRMP5, and ANNA-1 are the most commonly identified neural autoantibodies, but seronegative cases also exist.

- Subacute progressive and asymmetric sensorimotor deficits, severe neuropathic pain, and unexplained weight loss provide important diagnostic clues.

- Longitudinally extensive, symmetric, tract-specific MRI findings and features of axonal polyradiculoneuropathy on electrodiagnostic testing are supportive of the diagnosis.

- Recovery is usually limited despite combined use of immunotherapies and cancer-directed treatments.

PAINLESS, SYMMETRIC, ASCENDING WEAKNESS AND SENSORY LOSS

Christopher J. Klein, MD

CASE PRESENTATION

HISTORY AND EXAMINATION

A 60-year-old man sought care for painless, symmetric, ascending weakness and sensory loss affecting the lower, greater than upper, extremities, progressing over 3 weeks with associated orthostatism. He reported no recent travel, fever, weight loss, immunizations, or diarrheal or other illnesses. While supine, his blood pressure was 125/95 mm Hg and pulse was 75 beats/min, and on standing, at 1 minute, blood pressure and pulse were 89/70 mm Hg and 75 beats/min, with symptomatic light-headedness. He was diffusely areflexic and had symmetric weakness, distal greater than proximal, with normal bulbar strength (Medical Research Council strength grading scale), 0 out of 5 ankle dorsal and plantar flexion, 3 out of 5 hip flexion and knee extension and flexion, 3 out of 5 intrinsic hand muscles, and 4 out of

5 shoulder abduction. Muscle atrophy was not appreciated, and fasciculations were absent.

Sensory examination revealed pan-sensory loss (vibration, pinprick, light touch) at the feet and hands. Hoffmann, Babinski, and Chaddock signs were negative. His gait was unsteady with prominent steppage. He was unable to climb stairs, kneel, or arise without assistance. Pertinent medical and social history included a spinal fusion at C5-T1, a 10-pack-year smoking history discontinued 15 years earlier, and congestive heart failure, New York Heart Association class III (unable to walk 30 meters comfortably) with an intracardiac defibrillator for ventricular fibrillation, and taking carvedilol and furosemide. He was not diabetic (recent hemoglobin A_{1c} value, 5.2%), and he had also screened negative for monoclonal proteins by immunofixation. Diagnoses considered at the time are shown in Table 42.1.

Table 42.1 DIFFERENTIAL DIAGNOSIS FOR THE CASE PATIENT

POSSIBLE DIAGNOSES	PERTINENT NEGATIVES
Anterior spinal artery ischemia or structural myelopathy	Autonomic symptoms; sensory findings; progression over 48 hours
Idiopathic subacute polyradiculoneuropathy (GBS vs AMAN)	No viral prodrome or immunization; no diarrheal illness (*Campylobacter jejuni*-AMAN); progression past 10 days; absence of pain
Chronic inflammatory demyelinating polyneuropathy	Presence of dysautonomia
Infectious neuropathy (cytomegalovirus, Epstein-Barr virus, West Nile virus, Lyme disease)	No infectious prodrome; not immunosuppressed; winter onset relevant to West Nile virus and Lyme disease
Infiltrative B- or T-cell lymphoma	No B symptoms; absence of pain; no history of lymphoma
Antiamphiphysin neuropathy	Male sex; no pain; no stiff-person component
Anti-CRMP5 neuropathy	No asymmetry; presence of dysautonomia; absence of pain
Amyloidosis (AL-amyloidosis or familial TTR amyloidosis)	Rapid course; absent monoclonal protein or family history; cognitive involvement

Abbreviations: AL, immunoglobulin light-chain; AMAN, acute motor axonal neuropathy; CRMP5, collapsin-response mediator protein 5; GBS, Guillain-Barré syndrome; TTR, transthyretin.

Needle electromyography and nerve conduction studies showed a severe axonal sensory-motor polyneuropathy with proximal involvement, suggesting polyradicular colocalization. Cerebrospinal fluid (CSF) obtained during unremarkable spinal myelography, for exclusion of spinal compression, showed normal and abnormal findings: total nucleated cells, 3/μL (reference range, <4/μL); glucose, 87 mg/dL (<60% of plasma glucose; reference range, 70-140 mg/dL); and protein, 326 mg/dL (reference range, 0-35 mg/dL). CSF polymerase chain reaction testing for cytomegalovirus and Epstein-Barr virus was negative. Sural nerve biopsy showed marked active axonal injury without significant inflammatory infiltrates (Figure 42.1A and B). Expanded autoimmune neuroimmunologic testing by indirect immunofluorescence staining of mouse neural tissues identified the classic pattern for antineuronal nuclear antibody type 1 (ANNA-1)–immunoglobulin G (IgG), also known as anti-Hu, with an end point dilution of 1:1.6×10^6 (Figure 42.1C). This was confirmed positive by Western blot. Pertinent negative immunologic test results included autoantibody testing for ganglioside GM1-immunoglobulin M (IgM) and GD1a-IgM, Western blot for antiamphiphysin- and collapsin-response mediator protein 5 (CRMP5)-IgG, and immunoprecipitation assays for voltage-gated calcium channel autoantibodies (N and PQ types). Chest radiography and computed tomography showed a consolidation and volume loss in the left lower lobe without identifiable mass.

DIAGNOSIS

The patient was diagnosed with paraneoplastic axonal sensory-motor polyneuropathy in the setting of ANNA-1-IgG positivity and likely small cell lung carcinoma (SCLC).

Before completion of the autoantibody evaluation, acute motor axonal neuropathy (AMAN) was thought to be the most likely diagnosis, and the patient was treated with plasma exchange for 4 days. He continued to worsen and was transferred to the intensive care unit with new shortness of breath. Escalated therapy with intravenous immunoglobulin 2,000 mg/kg total did not help. He then had development of urinary retention (400 mL post void), bulbar weakness, confusion, and flail limbs in all extremities. On identification of ANNA-1-IgG, he was then treated with intravenous methylprednisolone 1 g for 3 days, but his condition still worsened. Bronchoscopy and positron emission tomography were planned to investigate for occult cancer, but given his worsening and treatment-refractory neuropathy with preexisting end-stage heart failure, the patient and his family opted for comfort measures. His defibrillator was turned off, and he died 20 days after first coming to the hospital. At autopsy, SCLC of the left lung was identified without bronchial mass or metastasis (Figure 42.1D). Neural tissues had diffuse microglial activation, with scattered microglial nodules and prominent perivascular chronic lymphocytic infiltrates (Figure 42.1E).

DISCUSSION

ANNA-1-IgG autoimmunity was first reported in 1965 by Wilkinson and Zeromski in Glasgow, Scotland. Patients had sensory neuropathy with nonmetastatic cancer and dorsal ganglia degeneration at autopsy. In 1985, Graus and colleagues at Memorial Sloan Kettering Cancer Center in New York refined the immunologic discovery, which assisted in the identification of Hu-RNA binding proteins (35-40 kDa) as

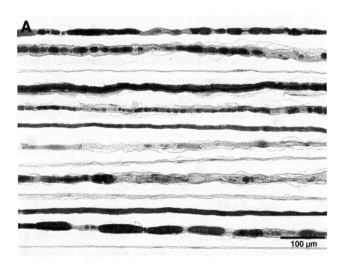

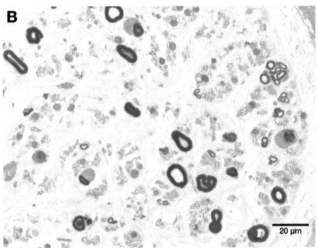

Figure 42.1 **Immunologic and Histopathologic Findings for the Case Patient.**
A, Sural nerve teased fibers show prominent axonal degeneration without demyelination (osmium stain). B, Semithin sections of sural nerve show markedly reduced fiber density without inflammation (methylene blue stain). C, Indirect immunofluorescence pattern of antineuronal nuclear antibody type 1–immunoglobulin G staining of mouse neural tissues shows nuclear-predominant staining sparing the nucleolus in Purkinje cells (PC), dentate neurons (DN), and myenteric plexus (MP). D, At autopsy, analysis of lung tissue shows small cell lung cancer isolated to the left lower lobe (hematoxylin-eosin stain). E, Characteristic lymphocytic perivascular infiltrates with microglial activation are seen in the cervical cord (and were also present in thoracic spinal cord, neocortex, subcortical nuclei, brainstem, and dorsal root ganglia) (hematoxylin-eosin stain).

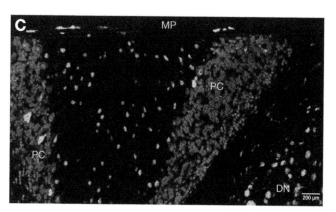

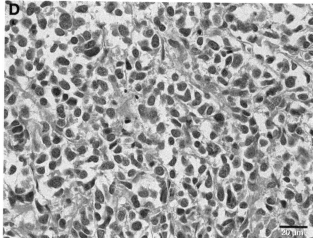

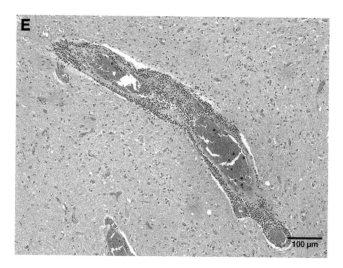

Figure 21.1 **Continued**

antigenic targets. ANNA-1-IgG (anti-Hu) autoantibodies serve as an important biomarker for SCLC in patients with subacute-onset neurologic symptoms and a history of smoking. Neuropathy is the most common neurologic presentation, but the neurologic phenotypes have expanded since the original descriptions to include cerebellar, cognitive, and spinal cord involvement, termed *paraneoplastic encephalomyelitis* and/or *paraneoplastic sensory neuronopathy*. In 1998 at Mayo Clinic, expanded neuropathy phenotypes from 162 patients were described to include the frequencies of neuropathy types: sensory > mixed motor and sensory > autonomic > cranial neuropathies (commonly VIII with hearing loss) > motor predominant, including motor neuronopathy. Of those with dysautonomia, findings of gastroparesis, esophageal achalasia, and pseudo-obstruction were all seen. All patients (100%) in this largest neuropathy series were documented to have coexisting cognitive decline, with or without seizures.

Patients with ANNA-1-IgG are often seen in urgent hospital referral. Distinction from Guillain-Barré syndrome (GBS) is important. The presence of coexisting myelopathic features and encephalopathy can aid in the diagnosis, but

those features are not always present at onset. Autoantibody evaluation should include not only ANNA-1-IgG but also CRMP5- and amphiphysin-IgGs. All of these autoimmune disorders can present similarly, with the latter 2 more commonly accompanied by pain, asymmetry, and, less commonly, autonomic symptoms. Albuminocytologic disassociation on CSF testing is common to both GBS and forms of paraneoplastic neuropathy, but most patients with GBS will have demyelination identified, with slowed motor nerve conductions, delayed or absent F-wave responses, prolonged R1 blink reflexes, or demyelinated teased fibers on nerve biopsy. In the differential diagnosis for patients with GBS with an axonal phenotype and diarrheal illness, *Campylobacter jejuni* AMAN is common. Serologic testing for ganglioside GM1- or GD1a-IgM autoantibodies will help identify 90% of patients with AMAN. Both acute inflammatory demyelinating polyneuropathy and AMAN have shortened clinical courses with early initiation of intravenous immunoglobulin or plasma exchange. In contrast, patients with ANNA-1-IgG generally have progression despite immunotherapy. The detection of ANNA-1-IgG autoantibodies should lead to an aggressive search for pulmonary or extrapulmonary SCLC, which may assist in initiation of appropriate cancer therapies and improved survival compared with patients with SCLC without neurologic presentations.

KEY POINTS

- ANNA-1-IgG paraneoplastic autoimmunity can mimic axonal GBS, and antibody testing can assist in making the diagnosis.

- Patients thought to have GBS with cognitive or myelopathic findings should be considered for paraneoplastic disorders including ANNA-1, CRMP5, and amphiphysin autoimmunity. CRMP5-IgG and amphiphysin-IgG are less commonly accompanied by dysautonomia and are typically associated with more pain.

- Patients with ANNA-1-IgG may be resistant to immunotherapy, although early cancer diagnosis and treatment may bring about neurologic stabilization and cancer cure.

DIFFICULT-TO-TREAT POLYRADICULONEUROPATHY

Marcus V. R. Pinto, MD, MS, and P. James B. Dyck, MD

CASE PRESENTATION

HISTORY AND EXAMINATION

A 51-year-old healthy man sought care for a 6-month history of progressive, distal, lower extremity weakness, imbalance, and numbness in the feet. He reported no upper extremity, urinary, bladder, or autonomic symptoms. Neurologic examination showed a steppage gait, upper and lower extremity weakness, distal greater than proximal, absent tendon reflexes, and large fiber–predominant sensation loss in the feet. Nerve conduction studies showed marked temporal dispersion and slowed conductions. Conduction velocity was 16 m/s peroneal, 18 m/s tibial, and 27 m/s ulnar. Cerebrospinal fluid (CSF) analysis showed an increased protein concentration of 87 mg/dL (reference range, 0-35 mg/dL), 1 white blood cell/μL (reference range, 0-5/μL), and normal glucose level. Lumbar spine magnetic resonance imaging (MRI) showed enlargement and enhancement of the nerve roots in the cauda equina, along with hypointensity in lumbar vertebral bodies, which suggested an infiltrative bone marrow process. Extensive testing of blood, urine, and fat aspirate was unrevealing.

He underwent right sural nerve biopsy that showed an inflammatory demyelinating process. The patient was diagnosed with chronic inflammatory demyelinating polyradiculoneuropathy (CIDP) and started on 0.4 g/kg of intravenous immunoglobulin (IVIG) twice per week for 6 weeks, followed by weekly infusions for 6 more weeks. Unfortunately, he was markedly worse at 12-week follow-up, with severe proximal and distal weakness and requiring the use of a walker.

TESTING

The diagnosis of CIDP was revisited. Radiographic bone survey was normal. Monoclonal gammopathy again was not found in the serum or urine. Fat pad aspiration was repeated and was negative for amyloid. Lumbar spine MRI again showed enhancement of the nerve roots. Bone marrow biopsy results were normal. Repeated CSF analysis was negative for findings of malignancy.

Because of concern for neurolymphomatosis, a proximal fascicular nerve biopsy of the right sciatic nerve was performed. It showed the hallmark pathologic features of CIDP: endoneurial inflammation and signs of long-standing demyelination and remyelination with stacks on Schwann cell processes (*onion bulbs*) (Figure 43.1).

DIAGNOSIS

The diagnosis of CIDP was confirmed.

MANAGEMENT

IVIG was stopped, and the patient was started on an aggressive plasma exchange regimen: twice per week for 6 weeks, and then weekly for 6 more weeks. He had modest improvement, and weekly 1-g intravenous methylprednisolone (IVMP) was added to weekly plasma exchange for 6 months. Azathioprine 2 mg/kg per day was also started. The patient continued to improve, and plasma exchange and IVMP infusions were spaced to every 10 days. He remained on this regimen for 2 years, when both treatments were spaced to every 2 weeks. Over the next year, the IVMP dose was reduced to 500 mg and then 250 mg every 2 weeks. After 2 more years, he was weaned off plasma exchange and IVMP. His condition remained stable, and at the last follow-up, 11 years after the beginning of his symptoms, he was walking independently, the disease was still in remission, and azathioprine was stopped. He remains well completely off immunotherapy.

DISCUSSION

CIDP was described and named by Peter J. Dyck at Mayo Clinic in 1975. It is one of the more common immune-mediated peripheral neuropathies and affects 1.0 to 8.9 persons per 100,000. It is a fairly symmetric peripheral neuropathy that usually presents with proximal and distal weakness, imbalance, and large fiber sensory dysfunction. CSF analysis shows albuminocytologic dissociation in 80% to 95% of those with typical CIDP. Different from Guillain-Barré syndrome, findings of facial weakness, autonomic dysfunction, and

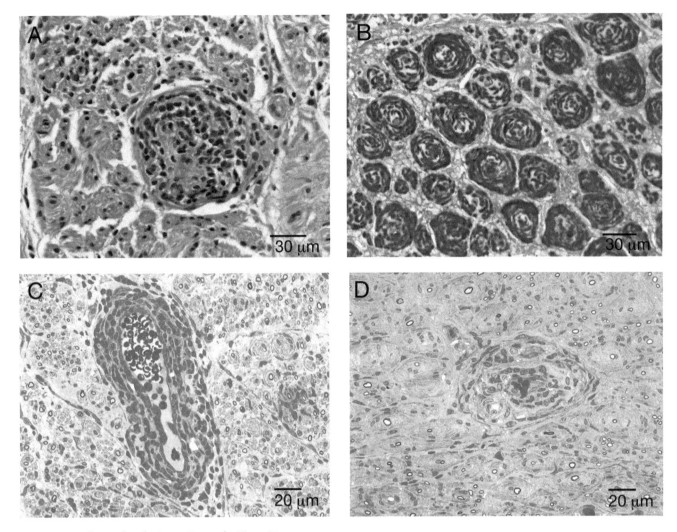

Figure 43.1 Findings of Right Sciatic Fascicular Nerve Biopsy.
A, Paraffin-embedded cross-section shows a moderate-sized endoneurial perivascular collection of mononuclear cells (hematoxylin-eosin). B, Immunohistochemical staining for S100 demonstrates onion bulb formations of various sizes. C, Semithin epoxy-embedded section of the same area shown in panel A highlights the diffuse onion bulb formations, a severe loss of large myelinated fibers, and the inflammatory collection. D, Semithin epoxy-embedded section shows onion bulbs intermixed with normal small myelinated nerve fibers and a small endoneurial perivascular inflammatory collection.

precipitant factors are uncommon. For the diagnosis of CIDP, patients must have symptoms for more than 8 weeks, proximal and distal weakness, decreased or absent tendon reflexes, and sensory loss on examination. Demyelinating findings on nerve conduction studies are almost always present, especially of temporal dispersion, conduction blocks, or both. The most common cause of misdiagnosis of CIDP is misinterpretation of mildly slowed nerve conduction velocities due to axonal loss as demyelinating.

Although a distal phenotype of CIDP (distal acquired demyelinating symmetric, or DADS, neuropathy) has been described, we emphasize the importance of proximal and distal weakness for an accurate diagnosis of CIDP. The most important CIDP mimickers are POEMS syndrome (*p*olyneuropathy, *o*rganomegaly, *e*ndocrinopathy, *M* component, *s*kin changes), amyloid neuropathy, vasculitic neuropathies, paraneoplastic syndromes, inherited neuropathy, and lymphoma. Serum and urine immunofixation, vascular endothelial growth factor measurement, bone skeletal survey, fat pad aspiration, and peripheral nerve MRI are usually important

for making the diagnosis. Three treatments are US Food and Drug Administration approved for CIDP: IVIG, corticosteroids, and plasma exchange. Table 43.1 outlines the available immunotherapies for CIDP. IVIG is the most commonly used first-line treatment. Its efficacy has been proved by several randomized clinical trials, and the most common regimen used starts with 2 g/kg divided over 5 days, followed by a 1-g/kg infusion every 3 weeks.

As with the patient described here, however, we at Mayo Clinic use a different regimen. In severe cases, IVIG is started at 0.4 g/kg per day twice a week for 6 weeks and then 0.4 g/kg per day once a week for 6 more weeks. The patient should be reevaluated with neurologic examination and, ideally, nerve conduction studies after the 12-week trial. If partial improvement has occurred, 1 g IVMP weekly is usually combined with IVIG for 12 more weeks, at which time the patient must be reevaluated. Usually, 70% of patients with CIDP respond to IVIG. If patients, such as the case patient, are unresponsive to IVIG, the diagnosis should be meticulously revisited. If the patient really has CIDP and their condition does not

Table 43.1 | IMMUNOTHERAPY OPTIONS FOR CIDP

TREATMENT	REGIMEN
First-line therapy	
Intravenous immunoglobulin	2 g/kg over 5 days, followed by 1 g/kg every 3 weeks OR 0.4 g/kg twice a week for 6 weeks followed by 0.4 g/kg weekly for 6 weeks; reevaluation at 12 weeks for dose adjustment
Subcutaneous immunoglobulin	Maintenance therapy only: 0.2 g/kg weekly
Corticosteroids	
Prednisone (oral)	1 mg/kg, adjusted after 4-8 weeks based on clinical response
Dexamethasone (oral)	40 mg/d for 4 days every 4 weeks; dose adjustment based on clinical response
IVMP	500 or 1,000 mg weekly
Plasma exchange	6 times every other day, followed by 1 exchange every 3 weeks OR 2 times per week for 6 weeks, followed by once weekly for 6 more weeks; reevaluation at 12 weeks for therapy adjustment
Second-line therapy	
Rituximab (IV)	Two 1-g infusions, given 2 weeks apart OR 375 mg/m² weekly for 4 weeks; redosing depends on severity, effectiveness, or relapse
Cyclophosphamide (IV)	1,000 mg/m² monthly for 6 months OR 50 mg/kg for 4 days
Steroid-sparing agents	
Azathioprine (oral)	2-3 mg/kg per day
Mycophenolate mofetil (oral)	2,000-3,000 mg/d

Abbreviations: CIDP, chronic inflammatory demyelinating polyradiculoneuropathy; IV, intravenous; IVMP, intravenous methylprednisolone.

improve or worsens with the first IVIG regimen, the patient's therapy is switched to plasma exchange for 12 weeks, sometimes combined with weekly IVMP infusions. A patient who has no response to IVIG, corticosteroids, or plasma exchange is unlikely to have CIDP. Recent studies have shown that patients with neurofascin-155–immunoglobulin G or contactin-1 autoimmunity, who have a demyelinating neuropathy similar to CIDP, usually do not respond well to IVIG or corticosteroids but may respond very well to rituximab or plasma exchange.

After positive response to a 12-week trial, the agent dose (IVIG or IVMP) should be reduced. The reduction is individualized to each patient, but we usually space IVIG infusions to every 2 weeks for 4 months, at which point the patient should be evaluated again. Subcutaneous immunoglobulin

is also efficacious and well tolerated for CIDP maintenance therapy. Some patients continue IVIG for their entire lives. For others, mycophenolate mofetil or azathioprine must be added because of relapses during IVIG weaning or as steroid-sparing agents.

KEY POINTS

- CIDP is one of the most common immune-mediated peripheral neuropathies.

- CIDP usually responds well to IVIG; unresponsiveness warrants revisiting the diagnosis.

- A combination of IVIG, plasma exchange, and corticosteroids may be needed in refractory CIDP cases.

AUTOIMMUNE PERIPHERAL NERVOUS SYSTEM HYPEREXCITABILITY

Christopher J. Klein, MD

CASE PRESENTATION

HISTORY AND EXAMINATION

A 25-year-old man was seen for assessment of progressive pain. He had a distant history of Guillain-Barré syndrome (GBS) at age 8 years, at which time he had symmetrical proximal and distal weakness of the upper and lower extremities with loss of ambulation. No facial weakness, dysarthria, dysphagia, ptosis, diplopia, or respiratory weakness occurred. Findings of cerebrospinal fluid analysis were believed to be consistent with GBS, and he was initially wheelchair confined before returning to ambulation 1 year later. At age 17 years, he began having pain in his extremities with associated continuous muscle twitching, initially in the calves and progressing to his thighs, hands, arms, and chest. The face was not affected. He had no prodromal infectious or vaccination triggers. The pain was initially mild, but within 5 years, at age 22 years, an episode of severe pain developed (10 of 10 on analog pain scale, previously 2 of 10) associated with worse twitching, which led to hospitalization.

At his initial evaluation at Mayo Clinic (age 25 years), there was touch hypersensitivity of the muscles and skin. He had no weakness or cognitive involvement, although the pain made it difficult for him to concentrate. His creatine kinase value was 1,700 U/L (reference range, 38-308 U/L), which improved with hydration to 300 to 600 U/L, but pain and muscle twitching persisted. Diagnoses considered at the time are shown in Table 44.1.

TESTING

On examination, he had diffuse extremity and truncal fasciculations and myokymia (◐ Video 44.1) and reported 8 out of 10 pain in not only the areas of twitching but also other areas of his extremities and trunk. He was cognitively normal. Strength, reflexes, and sensation were normal, except for residual ankle weakness from his previous GBS episode. On neurophysiologic testing, fibular and tibial motor compound muscle action potentials were decreased in amplitude, with normal ulnar and median motor responses. The sural, median, and ulnar sensory action potentials were normal. Repetitive stimulation of tibialis anterior and proximal muscles at 2 Hz was normal. Needle electromyography (EMG) of muscles proximally and distally showed diffuse spontaneous firing of muscles ranging in frequency from 100 to 500 Hz with waxing and waning characteristics, typical of complex repetitive discharges, neuromyotonia, myotonia, and myokymia (◐ Video 44.2). Motor unit duration varied (5-25 milliseconds).

These findings were thought to be consistent with a primary hyperexcitable disorder of muscles with a superimposed old polyradiculoneuropathy and possibly a myopathy. Biopsy of the right triceps was unrevealing for a cause. Expanded autoimmune neuroimmunologic testing of serum identified immunoglobulin G (IgG)-directed cerebellar molecular staining consistent with voltage-gated potassium channel (VGKC) autoantibodies. Radioimmunoprecipitation assay identified VGKC-IgGs. Pertinent negative testing included thyrotropin, electrolyte concentrations of calcium and magnesium,

Table 44.1 | **DIFFERENTIAL DIAGNOSIS FOR THE CASE PATIENT**

POSSIBLE DIAGNOSES	EXCEPTIONAL FINDINGS
Recurrent GBS or CIDP	**Absent new weakness, CK >1,000 U/L**
Serotonin syndrome	**No serotonin medications, no fever**
Stiff-person spectrum disorder	**No spasticity**
Infectious myositis	**No history of travel or HIV infection**
Genetic neuromyotonia	**No family history, diffuse twitching, no cold induction, no periodic paralysis events**
Electrolyte disturbance (calcium, magnesium)	**Cramping is typical, increased CK, prominent fasciculations as seen**

Abbreviations: CIDP, chronic inflammatory demyelinating polyradiculoneuropathy; CK, creatine kinase; GBS, Guillain-Barré syndrome.

and genetic testing for paramyotonia (*CACNA1S*, *CLCN1*, *KCNE3*, *KCNJ18*, *KCNJ2*, and *SCN4A*). Additional immunoprecipitation assays for calcium channel autoantibodies (voltage-gated calcium channel, N and PQ types) and enzyme-linked immunosorbent assay for glutamic acid decarboxylase 65-kDa isoform were also negative. The VGKC-IgG positivity led to reflex testing for contactin-associated protein 2 (CASPR2)-IgG and leucine-rich, glioma-inactivated protein 1 (LGI1)-IgG by cell-based assay. CASPR2-IgG autoantibodies were positive. Computed tomography of the chest with contrast was performed to exclude thymoma, and lymphadenopathy was identified, for which axillary lymph node biopsy demonstrated nonspecific inflammation.

DIAGNOSIS

The patient was clinically diagnosed with CASPR2-IgG–positive Isaacs syndrome.

MANAGEMENT

A trial of high-dose gabapentin was attempted, with only mild benefits. Next, intravenous immunoglobulin (IVIG) 0.4 g/kg every 3 weeks was initiated, which led to remarkable pain improvement and quiescence of muscle twitching. Pain and muscle activity would return 1 month after each infusion. Within 1 year after his first evaluation in our department, diabetes developed, and he was hospitalized with a glucose level of 400 mg/dL requiring initiation of insulin. His condition is now managed variably with IVIG (for painful flare-ups) and scheduled daily gabapentin.

DISCUSSION

The immune system has long been recognized to help regulate pain via non-IgG–mediated mechanisms. Specifically, cytokines decrease the nociceptive nerve fiber thresholds and are released after diverse tissue insults (eg, mechanical, chemical, thermal). This allows for speeded healing by increased blood flow and protection of the region by pain guarding mechanisms. It is now recognized that, in rare cases, IgG-mediated autoimmunity can lead to otherwise idiopathic pain disorders.

The idea of autoimmune IgG-mediated nociceptive pain was first described with VGKC-complex IgG-mediated disease. This work stemmed from earlier observations that patients could have muscle hyperexcitability and VGKC-IgG antibodies, as described in Isaacs syndrome (acquired neuromyotonia with hyperhidrosis) and Morvan syndrome (neuromyotonia, dysautonomia, limbic encephalitis, and sleep disturbance). Those patients, similar to the case patient described here, had muscle fasciculations and pain beyond areas of clinical muscle activity with EMG hyperexcitability, including myokymia (repetitive, regular firing bursts of

motor units, 20-80 Hz), cramp discharges, and neuromyotonia (rapid firing of long, continuous firing motor units, 150-300 Hz). Subsequently, in-depth immunologic experiments identified CASPR2 and LGI1 as the primary antigen targets within the VGKC-IgG complex. Patients with Isaacs syndrome most commonly have CASPR2-IgG autoimmunity, as with this case patient.

Other neurologic manifestations often coexist with pain in affected patients, including limbic encephalitis, seizures, faciobrachial dystonic seizures (LGI1-IgG specific), paroxysmal dizzy spells, and dysautonomia with gastric dysmotility. Cancer is uncommon, but when found, thymoma is most common, occurring in CASPR2 autoimmunity (2%) or dual LGI1-IgG and CASPR2-IgG seropositivity (22%). Small nociceptive fiber hyperexcitability can be identified by thermoregulatory sweat testing (early sweat production), quantitative sudomotor axon reflex testing (quantitated hyperhidrosis), or computer-assisted sensory examination, system IV (heat pain, hyperalgesia). In one study, approximately 21% of 256 patients with LGI1-IgG or CASPR2-IgG seropositivity had neuropathic pain. On EMG, 24% of LGI1-IgG–positive patients and 75% of CASPR2-IgG–positive patients had cramps (involuntary motor unit firing in a large area of muscle up to 150 Hz, typically painful), fasciculations, myokymia (continuous bursts of 2-10 motor unit potentials firing at 40-60 Hz), or neuromyotonia (motor unit potentials firing at 100-300 Hz, often with varying amplitude). Importantly, most patients with these autoantibodies have diffuse central nervous system involvement, and immunotherapy may help prevent progression to cognitive decline.

Younger age of onset and the presence of CASPR2-IgG are more commonly associated with peripheral pain and muscle hyperexcitability rather than a central nervous system presentation. Patients typically benefit from immunotherapy, including corticosteroids, IVIG, and others, with most needing long-term monitoring and treatment.

KEY POINTS

- Idiopathic (or occasionally paraneoplastic) autoimmune pain disorders can result from nerve and muscle hyperexcitability through IgG-mediated autoimmunity to CASPR2 or LGI1 membrane proteins in neural tissues.

- Computed tomography of the chest should be performed to exclude thymoma, which is most common if both CASPR2-IgG and LGI1-IgG autoantibodies are present.

- Patients with CASPR2-IgG– and LGI1-IgG–mediated autoimmune pain can benefit from both membrane-stabilizing drugs (eg, gabapentin, carbamazepine) and immunotherapy, which should be strongly considered because symptoms can expand to include encephalitis.

ORTHOSTATISM, CONSTIPATION, AND EARLY SATIETY

Kamal Shouman, MD, and Eduardo E. Benarroch, MD

CASE PRESENTATION

HISTORY AND EXAMINATION

A 65-year-old right-handed woman with a history of Graves disease, status post radioactive iodine therapy, and a biopsy-proven benign calcified breast nodule sought care for evaluation of multiple symptoms ongoing for 8 years.

She had constipation for 8 years, which was heralded by 48 hours of fecal urgency. She had also experienced intermittent diarrhea for the previous year. She was diagnosed with irritable bowel syndrome and had mild relief from laxatives. Her weight remained stable until 1½ years earlier, and she had lost 6.8 kg (15 lb) unintentionally. She noted that she would prefer to eat smaller and more frequent meals, although she did not notice prominent nausea, vomiting, or dysphagia.

For the previous 3 years, the patient had experienced multiple urinary symptoms including hesitancy, urgency, incontinence, and retention. She was diagnosed with a cystocele, the correction of which did not help.

Also for 3 years, she had noted difficulty focusing her eyes when moving from a dark to a well-lit environment, or vice versa. More recently, she had become more sensitive to light and wore sunglasses most of the time.

She also reported orthostatic light-headedness for 1½ years, which worsened on exposure to a hot environment. She had 6 syncopal episodes. She was treated with fludrocortisone and midodrine, with some relief. She had experienced sicca symptoms (dry eyes and dry mouth) for 6 months. She reported no problems with coordination, balance, muscle rigidity, or tremor. Neurologic examination showed abnormally dilated pupils with prominently sluggish constriction in response to light, but the examination was otherwise normal.

Diagnoses considered at the time included autoimmune autonomic ganglionopathy (AAG), immune-mediated autonomic and sensory neuropathy, autonomic neuropathy in the setting of Sjögren syndrome, nonautoimmune autonomic neuropathy (eg, amyloidosis, diabetes), and pure autonomic failure.

TESTING

Autonomic reflex screening indicated patchy postganglionic sympathetic sudomotor, marked cardiovagal, and cardiovascular adrenergic failure, with neurogenic orthostatic hypotension (Figure 45.1A). Thermoregulatory sweat testing showed 82% anhidrosis (Figure 45.2A). A nuclear medicine gastric-emptying study indicated delayed gastric emptying and colonic hypomotility and normal small-bowel transit. ^{18}F-Fludeoxyglucose–positron emission tomography was negative for malignancy. Serum testing was markedly positive for ganglionic (alpha 3) acetylcholine receptor autoantibodies, at 5.89 nmol/L (reference range, ≤0.02 nmol/L).

DIAGNOSIS

The patient was diagnosed with AAG.

MANAGEMENT

The patient received intravenous immunoglobulin (IVIG) 0.4 g/kg administered daily for 3 days, followed by once-weekly infusions for 12 weeks. She returned 5 months later and reported 80% improvement in all of her symptoms, and neurologic examination showed normal pupillary response to light. Repeated autonomic reflex screening indicated considerable improvement of her adrenergic function (Figure 45.1B), and thermoregulatory sweat testing showed an even more impressive improvement of her sudomotor function, with anhidrosis of only 3% (Figure 45.2B). Her postganglionic sympathetic sudomotor and cardiovagal function remained impaired. Repeated nuclear medicine gastric-emptying tests revealed normalization of colonic transit, but gastric emptying remained mildly delayed. She was maintained on IVIG at 0.4 g/kg every 3 weeks, which was later tapered after azathioprine was started (2.5 mg/kg per

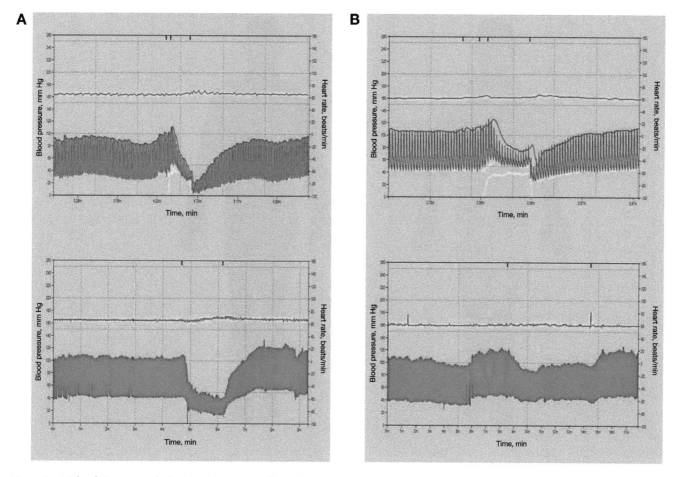

Figure 45.1 **Blood Pressure and Head-Up Tilt Test Findings for Case Patient.**
A, Findings of blood pressure response (red) to Valsalva maneuver (top) and head-up tilt test (bottom) before treatment. B, Findings of blood pressure response to Valsalva maneuver (top) and head-up tilt test (bottom) after treatment. Green traces indicate heart rate.

day). Her ganglionic (alpha 3) acetylcholine receptor auto-antibody level eventually decreased to 3.69 nmol/L and then to 1.99 nmol/L.

DISCUSSION

AAG usually presents subacutely, much like other autoimmune neurologic diseases. However, the case of this patient demonstrates that AAG may be suspected, and treatment may be effective, in patients with a more chronic temporal profile. Typical features of this disorder are the impaired pupillary reaction to light and prominent sicca symptoms, indicating prominent cranial parasympathetic (cholinergic) impairment. Also consistent with this diagnosis are the prominent gastrointestinal tract symptoms. Prominent cholinergic failure helps distinguish AAG from peripheral autonomic neuropathy or neurodegenerative disorders such as pure autonomic failure.

The patient's history of Graves disease emphasizes the importance of obtaining a comprehensive medical history, searching for diagnostic clues of autoimmunity in the patient's background. Ganglionic acetylcholine receptor antibody levels correlate with disease severity. Antibody levels greater than 1.00 nmol/L are highly specific for AAG.

Other biomarkers of autoimmune autonomic neuropathy (likely targeting peripheral and ganglionic antigens) include antineuronal nuclear antibody type 1 (anti-Hu), collapsin-response mediator protein 5–immunoglobulin G, and calcium channel antibodies (P/Q and N type). The latter serologic context (positive calcium channel antibodies) often occurs in patients with dysautonomia accompanying Lambert-Eaton syndrome. A paraneoplastic cause (usually accompanied by small cell carcinoma) should be considered in these patients. Occasionally, patients with a profile classically supportive of myasthenia gravis (positivity for muscle acetylcholine receptor binding, modulating, and striational antibodies) may have an autoimmune dysautonomia. The possibility of thymoma should be investigated in those patients. Contactin-associated protein 2 autoimmunity may present with autonomic hyperactivity (excessive salivation, hyperhidrosis, lacrimation, tachycardia, and gastrointestinal tract and urinary symptoms), alone or accompanied by insomnia, peripheral nervous system hyperexcitability, and encephalitis (Morvan syndrome). Thymoma should be sought in these patients, as well. Autonomic storms may accompany N-methyl-D-aspartate receptor autoimmune encephalitis. Seronegative

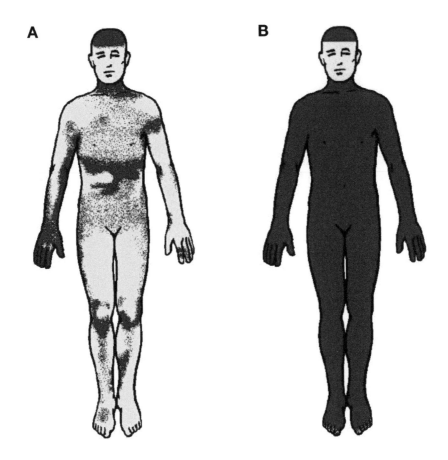

Figure 45.2 Thermoregulatory Sweat Testing (TST) Findings for Case Patient.
Results of TST before (A) and 3½ months after (B) immunotherapy show marked improvement, from anhidrosis of 82% before to 3% after. (Sweating indicated by purple areas.)

AAG should be suspected in the absence of antibody positivity, especially if the patient has classic subacute presentation and a history of autoimmunity.

Acute treatment options in AAG include corticosteroids, IVIG, and plasma exchange. Steroid-sparing or infusion-sparing agents for longer-term treatment include azathioprine and mycophenolate mofetil. The improvement of symptoms in this case patient and some objective measures of autonomic failure, such as thermoregulatory response, with immunotherapy, are consistent with an autoimmune cause. Her antibody values also decreased over time, which correlates less well with clinical outcome than objective measures of autonomic function. Abnormalities in objective indices of autonomic function (postganglionic sudomotor and cardiovagal) may be persistent despite improvement of symptoms. In some other patients treated for a prolonged period, the tests may normalize also. Some patients require several years of treatment to induce and maintain remission.

KEY POINTS

- AAG is a potentially treatable cause of autonomic failure.

- Female sex, subacute onset, impaired pupil reactivity, and prominent gastrointestinal tract symptoms should increase suspicion for AAG.

- Patient-reported symptoms and specific findings of neurologic examination, autonomic reflex screening, and thermoregulatory sweat testing are useful markers of response to immunotherapy.

- Early diagnosis and treatment is important for decreasing long-term disability.

CONSTIPATION AND SYNCOPE

Michelle F. Devine, MD, and Sean J. Pittock, MD

CASE PRESENTATION

HISTORY AND EXAMINATION

A 43-year-old woman sought care for 8 years of severe constipation associated with syncopal episodes while straining on the toilet. Her constipation later alternated with explosive diarrhea. In addition, chronic left-sided abdominal pain and severe bloating developed after eating. There was no association of the abdominal pain with certain foods or bowel movement. She was diagnosed with irritable bowel syndrome on the basis of the chronic abdominal pain and constipation.

Six years after the initial onset of symptoms, nausea, bloating, and intractable vomiting developed. Symptoms were exacerbated by food and, on occasion, were partially relieved with vomiting. There was no change in symptoms with bowel movements. She had multiple episodes of bilious, undigested emesis per day. Trials of antiemetics and motility agents provided no substantial relief. She adopted a liquid diet, avoided solid foods, and eventually had a gastrostomy tube placed. She lost at least 15.9 kg (35 lb) over 2 years.

On her evaluation in our department, review of systems was significant for generalized fatigue and a burning sensation in her hands and feet. She did not report dry eyes, dry mouth, skin lesions, hematologic abnormalities, dizzy spells, palpitations, or bladder dysfunction. Her medical history was pertinent for Graves disease previously treated with remote thyroid radioablation, and she was now taking thyroid hormone replacement therapy. Neurologic examination findings were normal except for unreactive pupillary light reflexes.

TESTING

A gastrointestinal tract (GI) transit study was performed, which showed persistently delayed colonic transit with mildly delayed gastric emptying (Table 46.1). Autonomic reflex screening showed diffuse postganglionic sympathetic sudomotor, severe cardiovagal, and severe cardiovascular adrenergic impairment. Thermoregulatory sweat testing (TST) showed diffuse anhidrosis (Figure 46.1A).

Laboratory evaluations showed normal complete blood cell count, erythrocyte sedimentation rate, and levels of C-reactive protein, albumin, vitamin D, hemoglobin A_{1c}, and thyroid hormones. Creatinine value was mildly increased at 1.3 mg/dL (reference range, 0.6-1.1 mg/dL). Heavy metal screening and urine drug screening were unremarkable.

Serum evaluation for neural autoantibodies associated with paraneoplastic or autoimmune dysautonomia was negative for antineuronal nuclear autoantibody type 1 (ANNA-1; anti-Hu), Purkinje cell cytoplasmic antibody type 2 (PCA-2; MAP1B antibody), collapsin-response mediator protein 5 (CRMP5)–immunoglobulin G (IgG), and

Table 46.1 GASTROINTESTINAL TRANSIT STUDIES FOR THE CASE PATIENT

TIME FRAME	GASTRIC EMPTYING AT 4 H, %[a]	COLONIC TRANSIT AT 24 H, GC[a]
Initial evaluation	77 (reference range, 84-98)	0.9 (reference range, 1.6-3.8)
After first IVIG trial	83 (reference range, 84-98)	2.5 (reference range, 1.6-3.8)
Relapse	76 (reference range, 81-100)	1.0 (reference range, 1.4-3.6)
After repeated IVIG for relapse	92 (reference range, 81-100)	2.8 (reference range, 1.4-3.6)

Abbreviations: GC, geometric center; IVIG, intravenous immunoglobulin.

[a] Reference ranges were changed by the testing laboratory between the patient's initial evaluation and relapse.

dipeptidyl-peptidase-like protein-6 (DPPX)-IgG. The serum was strongly positive for ganglionic (alpha 3) acetylcholine receptor (α3-AChR)-IgG at 3.69 nmol/L (reference range, <0.02 nmol/L).

On cancer screening including positron emission tomography–computed tomography, no malignancy was detected.

DIAGNOSIS

The findings strongly suggested an autonomic autoimmune polyganglionopathy, with autoimmune gastrointestinal dysmotility (AGID) as the predominant phenotype.

MANAGEMENT

Given the concern for an autoimmune dysautonomia, a 12-week trial of intravenous immunoglobulin (IVIG) was recommended. She received IVIG 0.4 g/kg daily for 3 days, followed by 0.4 g/kg once weekly for 11 weeks. With this IVIG trial, she had complete resolution of her previous constipation, nausea, and vomiting. She regained 22.7 kg (50 lb) within 15 weeks. Her gastrostomy tube was removed. Repeated GI transit studies approached normal findings (Table 46.1). Repeated autonomic testing and TST showed substantial improvement (Figure 46.1B).

Over several months, the IVIG dose was tapered. The patient remained asymptomatic for 8 years on long-term immunosuppression with azathioprine 75 mg twice daily

(150 mg/d), after which time, despite compliance with azathioprine, she had a recurrence of her previous symptoms. Repeated GI transit studies again showed delayed GI emptying (Table 46.1). Another 12-week IVIG course controlled her symptoms, with normalization of GI transit studies (Table 46.1).

DISCUSSION

AGID can manifest as either hypomotility or hypermotility but most often presents as gastroparesis or pseudo-obstruction. Symptoms include nausea, vomiting, bloating, early satiety, diarrhea, constipation, and involuntary weight loss. It can be idiopathic or paraneoplastic. Risk factors for idiopathic cases include personal or family histories of autoimmunity.

Patients with predominantly GI symptoms (without or with only minimal other signs or symptoms of dysautonomia) are often initially misdiagnosed as having irritable bowel syndrome. Other causes of dysautonomia could also be considered, including amyloid neuropathy, diabetic neuropathy, and multiple system atrophy, but other significant findings are usually detected on examination or diagnostic testing with these conditions.

GI dysmotility can be associated with several neural-specific antibodies. Patients with antibodies targeting α3-AChR, at titers greater than 1.0 nmol/L, typically have subacute-onset diffuse autonomic failure, with symptoms of dry eyes, dry mouth, orthostatic hypotension, and anhidrosis.

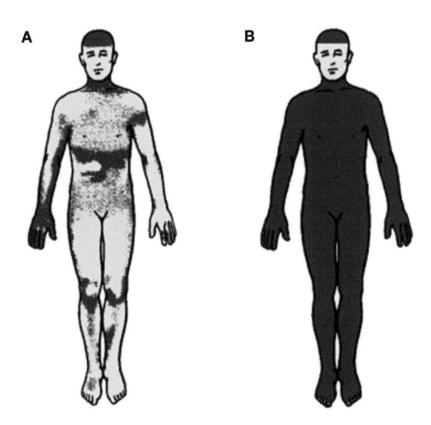

Figure 46.1 Thermoregulatory Sweat Testing (TST) Findings for the Case Patient.
TST shows diffuse anhidrosis before immunosuppression (A) and marked improvement after immunosuppression therapy (B). Purple indicates areas of sweating.

Up to 70% of cases will have GI hypomotility, and in some cases the GI dysmotility may be the presenting symptom, but the autonomic dysfunction is usually not limited to the enteric nervous system. ANNA-1 or PCA-2 can be detected in patients with small cell carcinoma; ANNA-1 can be detected in patients with pediatric neuroblastoma or thymoma, up to 30% of whom will have a paraneoplastic GI dysmotility. This typically responds poorly to immunotherapy. Patients with DPPX autoimmunity commonly have initial symptoms of GI hypermotility with profound diarrhea and weight loss that evolves into a multifocal central nervous system disorder.

Evaluations will usually show abnormalities in GI transit studies and/or GI manometry. Transit studies generally show multifocal abnormalities with involvement of at least 2 of the stomach, small bowel, and colon. Patients taking antikinetic agents, such as opioids, must discontinue these before motility testing. Findings on TST and autonomic testing can also be supportive and may indicate a more diffuse disorder of the autonomic nervous system. Serologic testing should include assessment for organ-specific autoantibodies (eg, neural antibodies [α3-AChR-IgG, ANNA-1, CRMP5-IgG, and DPPX-IgG]) and non–organ-specific autoantibodies (eg, Sjögren syndrome [SS-A and -B antibodies]; systemic lupus erythematosus [anti-dsDNA]) known to be associated with autonomic involvement. If the neural antibody profile is predictive of underlying malignancy, then appropriate cancer screening is warranted. Positron emission tomography can be considered if there is high suspicion for cancer.

Treatment includes symptomatic management with antiemetics, prokinetic agents, and/or cholinesterase inhibitors. After exclusion of alternative diagnoses, patients with severe, refractory symptoms can be considered for a trial of immunotherapy, even if they are seronegative for related neural-specific antibodies. It is imperative that objective testing be performed before a trial of immunotherapy and that no other therapies are initiated during the trial. The patient can be defined as an *immunotherapy responder* if they have substantial objective improvement. A favorable response to a 6- to 12-week immunosuppression trial can support the diagnosis of AGID.

KEY POINTS

- AGID can result in either hypomotility or hypermotility.

- AGID can be idiopathic or paraneoplastic.

- AGID is rarely isolated and most commonly associated with other signs and symptoms of autonomic failure such as orthostatic hypotension or small fiber dysfunction.

- Neural antibodies associated with AGID and autoimmune/paraneoplastic dysautonomias include α3-AChR-IgG, ANNA-1 (anti-Hu), CRMP5-IgG, PCA-2 (MAP1B-IgG), and DPPX-IgG.

- A favorable response to a 6- to 12-week immunosuppression trial can support the diagnosis of suspected AGID.

BULBAR-PREDOMINANT WEAKNESS

Jennifer A. Tracy, MD, and Vanda A. Lennon, MD, PhD

CASE PRESENTATION

HISTORY AND EXAMINATION

A 61-year-old White man, a nonsmoker with a medical history of hypertension and hypercholesterolemia, sought care for recurrent episodes of dysarthria for about 1 year. This symptom was more common after prolonged speaking. Six months before his evaluation he had significant slurring of his speech after talking for 3½ hours at work about a new project. This led to emergency evaluation and hospital admission, where concern was raised for stroke. Magnetic resonance imaging of the brain showed normal findings, and his speech normalized by the following morning. However, his symptoms were thought to represent a transient ischemic attack, and he was started on aspirin and a statin medication.

Despite these interventions, the episodes continued to recur. He also experienced intermittent binocular double vision 11 months before evaluation, which did not improve with new eyeglasses, and a sensation that chewing and swallowing was more effortful. He reported no focal weakness but noted that his arms and legs felt "heavy" at times. All these symptoms tended to occur later in the day or after exertion. He disclosed no orthopnea, dyspnea, numbness, radicular symptoms, or bladder or bowel incontinence. He had not started any new medications or supplements around the time of symptom onset.

Neurologic examination was remarkable for binocular double vision with prolonged gaze upward or to the far right. Facial strength and speech were normal. Neck flexor and extensor strength and limb strength were normal. He could squat and rise 5 times but with difficulty by the 5th attempt. He had no fatigable weakness in his upper extremities. Deep tendon reflexes and sensory examination were normal.

The patient's symptoms suggested myasthenia gravis (MG). The differential diagnosis for autoimmune MG, particularly with prominent ocular and facial muscle involvement, can include central nervous system disorders (eg, stroke), motor neuron disease (eg, amyotrophic lateral sclerosis), and myopathy (eg, oculopharyngeal muscular dystrophy, faducioscapulohumeral muscular dystrophy, mitochondrial myopathy, and some congenital myopathies). The Miller-Fisher variant of Guillain-Barré syndrome can also mimic the presentation of MG. However, fluctuations of weakness and fatigable weakness are hallmarks that localize this disorder to the neuromuscular junction. Having established neuromuscular junction localization, a genetic myasthenic syndrome (usually, but not invariably, distinguished by age of onset) and infectious causes (eg, botulism) must be considered. Certain medications can compromise neuromuscular transmission and can unmask subclinical MG (eg, neomycin and some other aminoglycoside antibiotics). In addition, MG has been associated with the use of immune checkpoint inhibitor therapies for cancer. Thus, a careful interrogation of the medical history and medications is important.

TESTING

Serologic evaluation showed positivity for acetylcholine receptor (AChR)-binding antibody (5.05 nmol/L; reference range, 0.00-0.02 nmol/L) and AChR-modulating antibody (100% AChR loss; reference range, 0%-20% loss). Striated muscle antibody was also positive at a titer of 1:15,360 (reference range, <1:120). Values for complete blood cell count, routine blood chemistry studies, alanine aminotransferase, aspartate aminotransferase, antinuclear antibody, creatine kinase, and rheumatologic markers were unremarkable. Thiopurine S-methyltransferase activity was low (tested on a precautionary basis to avoid myelosuppression associated with use of azathioprine).

Standard nerve conduction studies showed normal findings. Repetitive stimulation studies at 2 Hz showed a decrement of 21% in the right facial nerve, which partially improved to 16% decrement after exercise. There was no significant amplitude decrement in the right spinal accessory or ulnar nerves. Routine needle examination showed motor unit variation in the right orbicularis oculi but no myopathic changes. Single-fiber electromyography (EMG) showed increased jitter in the right orbicularis oculi. There were no myopathic changes on routine needle examination.

Chest computed tomography showed scattered tiny pulmonary nodules but no evidence of thymoma or other neoplasm.

DIAGNOSIS

The clinical diagnosis was autoimmune generalized MG, seropositive for AChR antibody, without evident thymoma or other neoplasm.

MANAGEMENT

The patient was initially treated with oral pyridostigmine, 60 mg 3 times a day, with some symptomatic benefit, but gastrointestinal adverse effects limited dosing increase. Oral prednisone was then initiated, at 10 mg daily; symptoms resolved when the dose was titrated to 40 mg daily. Calcium and vitamin D supplements, as well as *Pneumocystis* prophylactic therapy, were initiated concurrently. Because the prednisone dose could not be lowered to less than 30 mg/d, mycophenolate mofetil was added as a steroid-sparing agent. On thoracic surgery consultation, thymectomy was recommended.

DISCUSSION

Autoimmune MG is a disorder of impaired neuromuscular transmission caused by immunoglobulin G (IgG)-mediated attack on a critical component of the AChR signaling complex in the muscle's postsynaptic membrane. The most commonly identified antibodies, detected in 85% of patients with generalized MG, target the nicotinic AChR. This form of MG, with nicotinic AChR antibodies, is the only one known to occur in a paraneoplastic context. Muscle-specific tyrosine kinase (MuSK)-IgG is detected in 5% of patients with MG. Its pattern of muscle weakness (generally predominantly facial-bulbar, with propensity to atrophy) is often clinically different from that of AChR-IgG MG; histologic findings of the thymus are normal, and thymectomy is not advised. Approximately 10% of patients with generalized MG lack both AChR-IgG and MuSK-IgG antibodies. Seronegativity is encountered most frequently if immunosuppressant therapy has commenced. In nonimmunosuppressed patients, seronegativity may be transient in the first year of symptoms; thus, repeated serologic evaluation after 12 months is helpful. Rare cases initially thought to be seronegative have been reported to have low-density lipoprotein receptor-related protein 4 antibodies. In patients without evidence of neural autoantibodies but who meet clinical, EMG, and pharmacologic criteria for MG, a diagnosis of autoimmune MG is supported if other organ-specific autoantibodies are detected (eg, thyroid, gastric parietal cell, or glutamic acid decarboxylase 65-kDa isoform–IgG), or if there is a personal or family history of autoimmune disorders (eg, thyroiditis, type 1 diabetes, pernicious anemia, or systemic lupus erythematosus).

MG may manifest in a pure ocular form with clinical findings limited to ptosis or diplopia (15%); about 40% of those patients lack detectable AChR-complex autoantibodies.

However, patients with generalized MG usually have ocular symptoms at onset, and most patients who initially have ocular-restricted symptoms will have development of generalized weakness within 2 years of symptom onset. Generalized MG is characterized by diffuse fatigable weakness and, commonly, ptosis, binocular diplopia, dysarthria, dysphagia, and limb weakness. Respiratory involvement can be severe. Patients may experience myasthenic crises, with severe bulbar or respiratory involvement, requiring hospitalization and often ventilatory support. A syndrome of transient neonatal MG occurs in a small minority of babies (≈10%-15%) born to mothers who have MG. This reflects transplacental passage of pathogenic AChR-complex IgG. The baby's weakness may be observed at birth or soon after, which may manifest as poor sucking and respiratory difficulties. In rare cases, the maternal IgG is predominantly reactive with fetal muscle-type AChR. Those mothers may lack evidence of MG, and in severe cases the baby is born with arthrogryposis or is stillborn.

The first-line management strategy for autoimmune MG starts with an oral acetylcholinesterase inhibitor, to increase the availability of acetylcholine at the neuromuscular synapse. Patients with MuSK-IgG MG, however, often respond poorly to these agents. Symptom control usually requires supplementary strategies to lower circulating antibody levels. Prednisone remains a first-line agent, with variable doses required for disease control. In some cases, high-dose prednisone is instituted early in the course of disease, but notably, a minority of patients can have early worsening of symptoms on high-dose prednisone, so in many cases, low-dose prednisone is started with upward titration. Once adequate symptom control is achieved, standard of care is to gradually lower the corticosteroid dose to the minimum dose needed to maintain strength. Several oral steroid-sparing agents are efficacious for long-term management of MG symptoms; azathioprine is the most commonly used agent. Mycophenolate mofetil is often used, particularly for patients whose blood thiopurine S-methyltransferase activity is low.

Intravenous immunoglobulin and plasma exchange are effective treatment strategies in many cases, but given the expense and more invasive modes of administration, these are usually reserved for myasthenic crises (with severe progressive bulbar and/or respiratory decline). Another therapeutic option, rituximab (a B-lymphocyte–depleting monoclonal IgG), is used increasingly for MG, particularly in MuSK-IgG–positive cases. In AChR-IgG–positive cases with identified thymoma, tumor resection is necessary. A recent large trial of thymectomy in adult patients with nonthymomatous AChR-IgG–positive generalized MG showed significantly greater improvement in strength and reduced corticosteroid requirements in patients with thymectomy.

Many medications negatively affect neuromuscular transmission and should be avoided, if possible, in patients with MG. These include, but are not limited to, several classes of antibiotics, including aminoglycosides, macrolides, and quinolones. The Myasthenia Gravis Foundation of America website provides a useful summary of potentially risky medications as a reference for clinicians and patients.

KEY POINTS

- Autoimmune MG is a disorder characterized by fatigable weakness, usually with some bulbar component, caused by IgG-mediated damage to components of the AChR complex in the postsynaptic membrane of skeletal muscle.

- Serologic tests for AChR antibodies are positive in approximately 85% of patients with generalized MG and 60% of patients with ocular MG; MuSK-IgG is positive in about 40% of patients who have AChR-IgG–negative generalized MG.

- Electrophysiologic testing is important for disease confirmation—repetitive stimulation studies of motor nerves innervating weak muscles are first-line tests. Single-fiber EMG of a clinically affected muscle is also useful but usually reserved for cases in which repetitive stimulation studies are not clearly diagnostic in patients for whom clinical suspicion for MG is high.

- Most patients are immunotherapy responsive; thymectomy is a beneficial procedure to improve clinical outcome and decrease immunotherapy requirements in selected patients with AChR-IgG–positive MG.

DIFFICULTY CLIMBING THE STAIRS

Anastasia Zekeridou, MD, PhD, and Vanda A. Lennon, MD, PhD

CASE PRESENTATION

HISTORY AND EXAMINATION

A 72-year-old woman with a history of rheumatoid arthritis (stable without treatment) and chronic obstructive pulmonary disease secondary to 50 pack-years' smoking sought care for a 3-month history of progressive difficulty walking on uneven terrain and climbing stairs. In the 2 preceding weeks, she also noted difficulty standing up from a seated position. She reported no sensory symptoms but recently noticed dry mouth and new-onset constipation with decreased appetite.

The neurologic examination indicated bilateral symmetric, moderate weakness in the proximal lower extremities (including hip flexion, abduction, and adduction, as well as knee flexion and extension) and subtle weakness in the proximal upper extremities. Muscle bulk and tone were normal. Deep tendon reflexes were hypoactive in the upper extremities and absent in the lower extremities. Sustained quadriceps activation resulted in augmentation of patellar reflexes. The rest of the neurologic examination was normal. On the basis of the 3-month evolution of proximal weakness and hyporeflexia/areflexia with no sensory involvement, several diagnoses were considered (Table 48.1).

TESTING

Electromyography (EMG) showed diffusely low-amplitude compound muscle action potential (CMAP) responses to single-nerve stimuli at rest, with normal sensory nerve action potentials. Studies of the ulnar and femoral motor nerves demonstrated a decrement to low-frequency repetitive stimulation (12%) and substantial postexercise facilitation (200%) and decrement repair (Figure 48.1).

Magnetic resonance imaging of the neuraxis was normal. Serum testing showed normal creatine kinase value and negative metabolic and other inflammatory and infectious indices. The serum was positive for cyclic citrullinated peptide antibody, rheumatoid factor, and P/Q-type voltage-gated calcium channel (VGCC) antibody (0.24 nmol/L; reference range, ≤0.02 nmol/L). Other neural-specific autoantibodies were negative, including SOX1 (sex-determining region Y-box 1)–immunoglobulin G. Computed tomography (CT) of the chest showed subcarinal and right hilar lymphadenopathy without evidence of a primary lesion, with avidity on ^{18}F-fludeoxyglucose–positron emission tomography (PET)/CT. Transbronchial fine-needle aspiration biopsy of the lymph node revealed small cell lung carcinoma (SCLC).

Table 48.1 | **DIFFERENTIAL DIAGNOSIS FOR THE CASE PATIENT**

POSSIBLE DIAGNOSES	PERTINENT NEGATIVES
Myasthenia gravis	No ocular/bulbar symptoms; postexercise facilitation of tendon reflexes
Myopathy (inflammatory or inclusion body myositis)	No pain; postexercise facilitation of tendon reflexes; autonomic symptoms
Guillain-Barré syndrome, chronic inflammatory demyelinating polyradiculoneuropathy	No sensory symptoms; no pain; postexercise facilitation of tendon reflexes
Motor neuron disease	No atrophy; no hyperreflexia, spasticity, or fasciculations
Multifocal motor neuropathy with conduction blocks	Symmetric distribution; postexercise facilitation of tendon reflexes
Lumbar canal stenosis with neurogenic claudication	No pain; no sensory symptoms; postexercise facilitation of tendon reflexes
Myelopathy	No sensory symptoms; no hyperreflexia or spasticity

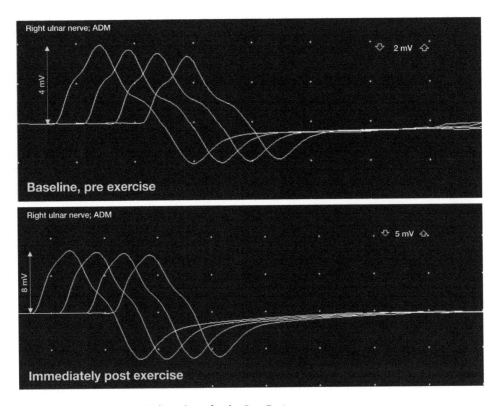

Figure 48.1 Nerve Conduction (Electromyography) Findings for the Case Patient.
Right ulnar nerve low-frequency repetitive stimulation (2 Hz) demonstrates, at baseline, a low-amplitude compound muscle action potential and a 12% decrement (top) with significant postexercise facilitation (200%) and decrement repair (bottom). ADM indicates abductor digiti minimi.

DIAGNOSIS

The patient was diagnosed with Lambert-Eaton myasthenic syndrome (LEMS) and SCLC.

MANAGEMENT

Concurrent chemotherapy (etoposide and carboplatin) and radiation were administered for the SCLC, with some improvement of the patient's weakness. The patient had no history of seizure or cardiac dysrhythmias (normal electrocardiography findings), so symptomatic treatment for LEMS was initiated. Pyridostigmine was not tolerated because of severe nausea. Therapy with 3,4-diaminopyridine (3,4-DAP [amifampridine] 40 mg/d) improved the patient's weakness, but her daily activities were limited by persistent, moderate, lower extremity weakness. Oral prednisone and intravenous methylprednisolone were not tolerated. The weakness objectively improved with intravenous immunoglobulin (IVIG) therapy at 0.4 g/kg for 3 days, then once weekly for 6 weeks; intervals between infusions were progressively increased to once monthly. Two years later, the patient was maintained on 3,4-DAP and monthly IVIG, with minimal persistent weakness and no evidence of cancer recurrence.

DISCUSSION

LEMS was first described at Mayo Clinic in 1956 as a "myasthenic syndrome associated with malignant tumors" that had characteristic electromyographic findings, later shown to be presynaptic by microelectrophysiologic testing. Mayo Clinic and English investigators subsequently showed an autoimmune basis for this presynaptic impairment of neuromuscular transmission and identified autoantibodies to the P/Q-type VGCC as the disorder's diagnostic marker. Injection of patients' immunoglobulins into experimental mice decreases acetylcholine release from motor nerve terminals.

A clinical diagnosis of LEMS is based on history, neurologic examination findings, electrophysiologic characteristics, and detection of VGCC-immunoglobulin G in a patient's serum. The usual presentation is of proximal muscle weakness and mild autonomic symptoms (dry eyes, skin, and mouth, erectile dysfunction). More pronounced autonomic symptoms such as gastrointestinal tract hypomotility (present in this patient), orthostasis, and bladder-voiding problems are far more common in paraneoplastic cases and may suggest a coexisting autoimmune dysautonomia. The neurologic examination in patients with LEMS shows decreased or absent tendon reflexes. EMG representative of a presynaptic disorder typically shows low-amplitude CMAPs with mild initial decrement at low-frequency repetitive stimulation and a more than 100% increase in CMAP amplitude from baseline (facilitation) during high-frequency repetitive stimulation (50 Hz) or directly after voluntary sustained muscle contraction (Figure 48.1). Exercise is better tolerated by the patient than high-frequency electrical stimulation during the EMG examination; the facilitation is of short duration.

About 50% of LEMS cases are paraneoplastic, with SCLC accounting for the vast majority of identified cancers. A new diagnosis of LEMS mandates a comprehensive search for cancer, at least in adult cases, including whole-body PET/CT for patients with negative findings of first-line screening by conventional imaging. An extrapulmonary small cell carcinoma should also be considered (eg, skin [Merkel cell], tongue, cervix, breast, ovary, or prostate). If a cancer other than SCLC is found, the search for a less obvious coexisting SCLC should continue, and cancer screening should be repeated at intervals in high-risk persons (older patients or with known cancer risk factors). LEMS has been associated with improved survival in patients with SCLC. Cerebellar ataxia, another syndromic manifestation of P/Q-type VGCC autoimmunity, can accompany LEMS.

The goal of symptomatic treatment is to increase acetylcholine release from motor terminals (ie, with 3,4-DAP) or reduce its destruction by inhibiting acetylcholinesterase in the synaptic cleft (ie, with pyridostigmine). 3,4-DAP is generally well tolerated but is contraindicated in patients with seizures (increases seizure frequency, especially in higher doses). Treatment in paraneoplastic cases includes cancer therapy in addition to immunotherapy. Plasma exchange is efficient and should be considered in severe cases. Corticosteroids and IVIG are also used in patients who have weakness that does not adequately respond to symptomatic treatment. Depending on the patient's neurologic and oncologic status, long-term immunosuppression might be necessary, such as azathioprine or mycophenolate mofetil. The B-cell–depleting therapeutic monoclonal antibody rituximab has also been efficacious in some cases.

KEY POINTS

- LEMS is an autoimmune presynaptic disorder of neuromuscular transmission that is thought to be caused by P/Q-type VGCC autoantibodies.

- LEMS presents with proximal weakness and usually mild dysautonomia.

- Diagnosis is based on clinical presentation, electromyographic findings consistent with a presynaptic defect, and detection of P/Q-type VGCC autoantibodies in the serum.

- LEMS is paraneoplastic in half of cases; SCLC is the most common cancer involved.

- Symptomatic treatments include acetylcholinesterase inhibitors and 3,4-DAP.

- Treatment includes cancer therapy when a tumor is identified, along with immunotherapy (eg, corticosteroids, plasma exchange, or IVIG). Long-term immunotherapy may be necessary (eg, azathioprine, rituximab, or other agents).

RAPIDLY PROGRESSIVE PROXIMAL WEAKNESS

Teerin Liewluck, MD, and Margherita Milone, MD, PhD

CASE PRESENTATION

HISTORY AND EXAMINATION

A 53-year-old previously healthy woman had development of subacute-onset muscle weakness resulting in difficulty climbing stairs, rising from a chair, and reaching over her shoulders. She reported no dysphagia, dysarthria, dyspnea, or diplopia. She also disclosed no rash, joint pain, or urine discoloration. She had no history of statin exposure. There was no family history of neuromuscular disorders, early cataracts, cardiac arrhythmia, or cardiomyopathy. Two months of treatment with prednisone 60 mg/d before the current evaluation had resulted in no clinical improvement. Neurologic examination indicated moderate neck flexor, shoulder, and hip girdle muscle weakness, with sparing of cranial muscles. There was no action- or percussion-induced myotonia. Sensory examination findings and tendon reflexes were normal.

TESTING

Results of nerve conduction studies were normal. Needle electromyography showed short-duration, low-amplitude, and complex motor unit potentials, predominantly affecting proximal muscles, associated with fibrillation potentials and myotonic discharges in proximal and axial muscles. Her creatine kinase (CK) level was increased at 5,460 IU/L (reference range, <176 IU/L). Biopsy of the left quadriceps (Figure 49.1) showed variation in muscle fiber size, a moderate increase in internalized nuclei, fiber splitting, and scattered necrotic and regenerating fibers. Inflammatory changes were absent. There was a mild increase in perimysial fibrous and fatty connective tissue. Myositis-specific and myositis-associated antibodies, including signal recognition particle (SRP) antibodies, were negative. 3-Hydroxy-3-methylglutaryl–coenzyme A reductase (HMGCR) antibodies were strongly positive (>200 U; reference range, <20 U). Electrocardiography, echocardiography, and pulmonary function test findings were normal. No cancer was indicated by positron emission tomography, mammography, pelvic ultrasonography, or esophagogastroduodenoscopy.

DIAGNOSIS

The patient was diagnosed with HMGCR antibody–positive necrotizing autoimmune myopathy (NAM).

MANAGEMENT

The patient received intravenous immunoglobulin (IVIG) 2 g/kg of ideal body weight in 5 divided doses each month and mycophenolate mofetil 1,000 mg twice a day (2,000 mg/d) while continuing prednisone 60 mg/d. The CK level was 3,154 IU/L after 2 weeks. Complete blood cell count was assessed to monitor for potential mycophenolate mofetil toxicity. Prednisone was tapered gradually after 2 months. Five months after beginning the above treatment, she had only mild residual weakness of the hip girdle muscles. CK level was then 635 IU/L, and HMGCR antibodies were 75 U. The IVIG frequency was gradually reduced. At 1-year follow-up, she had no weakness, and her CK value was normal while she

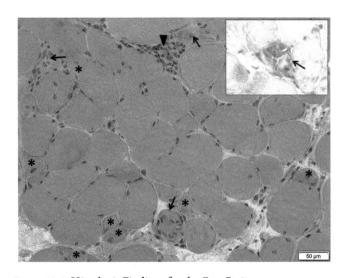

Figure 49.1 **Histologic Findings for the Case Patient.**
Hematoxylin and eosin–stained section shows scattered necrotic (arrows) and regenerating (asterisks) fibers. Only a few mononuclear cells are seen at a single perivascular site in the perimysium (arrowhead) adjacent to a necrotic fiber. Inset, Acid phosphatase–stained section highlights macrophages invading necrotic fibers (red).

continued taking prednisone 5 mg/d, mycophenolate mofetil 1,000 mg twice a day, and IVIG 2 g/kg every 6 weeks.

DISCUSSION

NAM, or immune-mediated necrotizing myopathy, is a subtype of immune-mediated myopathy, clinically characterized by subacute, progressive, proximal limb weakness and persistently increased CK level. Pathologically, it is characterized by myonecrosis with minimal or no inflammation. The weakness affects lower greater than upper limbs, but distal, axial, bulbar, or respiratory muscle involvement occurs in 30% to 40% of patients. NAM generally affects adults but can also manifest in children. It can be associated with statin exposure (35%), cancer (10%), or connective tissue diseases (5%). One-third of patients with NAM have myalgia. In a Mayo Clinic cohort, 60% of patients had abnormal echocardiography findings, most commonly diastolic dysfunction, but often occurring in the setting of preexisting cardiac diseases or hypertension. Immunotherapy-responsive cardiomyopathy as an initial presentation of NAM has been described.

Early recruiting, short-duration, and low-amplitude motor unit potentials associated with fibrillation potentials are universally present in all patients. Myotonic discharges without clinical myotonia are observed in half of patients, especially those with prior statin exposure regardless of HMGCR antibody positivity. The myopathologic findings are nonspecific. Necrotic fibers on biopsy, in the absence of inflammation, are nonspecific and may occur in any active myopathy, including muscular dystrophies and rhabdomyolysis. In most cases, NAM can be distinguished from muscular dystrophies. Indeed, patients with muscular dystrophies typically have a more insidious onset of weakness and more fibrous or fatty replacement of myofibers on muscle biopsy, compared with patients with NAM. Occasionally, however, NAM can show a slowly progressive course or increased connective tissue elements on biopsy, mimicking muscular dystrophies. Although sarcolemmal expression of major histocompatibility complex class I immunoreactivity is considered a pathologic hallmark of immune-mediated myopathies, it can also occur in muscular dystrophies. Compared with rhabdomyolysis, which has a more acute onset, increased CK value and weakness persist in untreated NAM but improve with time in rhabdomyolysis. Contrary to rhabdomyolysis, necrotic fibers appear in various stages of the degenerating process in NAM.

About 60% of patients with NAM are seropositive for either SRP (25%) or HMGCR (35%) immunoglobulin G autoantibodies. Among those with NAM associated with statin exposure, approximately 70% to 85% are HMGCR antibody positive. One-third of patients positive for HMGCR antibodies are statin naïve. In HMGCR antibody–positive patients with prior statin exposure, discontinuation of the statin does not halt the progression of weakness. Titers of both antibodies correlate with CK levels and severity of weakness. NAM has a paraneoplastic cause in 10% to 15% of patients, especially seronegative or HMGCR antibody–positive patients. Therefore, cancer screening is recommended. Most cancers are discovered within 3 years of the diagnosis of NAM.

NAM generally requires aggressive immunotherapy. High-dose corticosteroid monotherapy is often insufficient, and most patients require at least 2 immunotherapeutic agents. Early treatment within the first 3 months of onset predicts a favorable outcome. Patients typically respond well to IVIG. IVIG has been successfully used as monotherapy in a few HMGCR antibody–positive patients. SRP antibody–positive patients with NAM who are refractory to conventional immunotherapy may respond to rituximab. The relapse rate is high during medication dose reduction or discontinuation.

Recently, necrotizing myopathy has emerged as a catastrophic immune-related adverse event in cancer patients treated with immune checkpoint inhibitors. Such patients typically have proximal weakness but, in contrast to NAM in general, often have extraocular muscle involvement as a result of either the myopathy itself or coexisting myasthenia gravis.

KEY POINTS

- NAM is a clinicoseropathologic diagnosis.

- Antibodies to HMGCR or SRP are present in about 60% of patients with NAM. HMGCR autoimmunity may occur with or without prior statin exposure.

- Cancer screening is recommended in seronegative or HMGCR antibody–positive patients.

- Corticosteroid monotherapy is often not sufficient, and patients typically require at least 2 or even 3 immunotherapeutic agents. Early and aggressive pharmacologic treatment predicts a favorable outcome.

PROGRESSIVE WEAKNESS AND RASH

Margherita Milone, MD, PhD, and Teerin Liewluck, MD

CASE PRESENTATION

HISTORY AND EXAMINATION

A 47-year-old man with hypercholesterolemia managed with atorvastatin sought care for a 4-month history of progressive, proximal upper limb weakness and myalgia, followed by dysphagia, difficulty climbing stairs, and facial rash. He reported no visual symptoms, dyspnea, or urine discoloration. Discontinuation of atorvastatin was of no benefit. There was no family history of muscle weakness. Neurologic examination showed moderate weakness of the neck flexor muscles, shoulder girdle muscles, and finger extensors, and mild weakness of hip flexor and ankle dorsiflexor muscles. The rest of the neurologic examination was normal. He had a heliotrope rash and Gottron sign (a flat red rash over the back of the fingers, elbows, or knees). No contractures or dysmorphic features were observed.

In considering the differential diagnosis, the proximal weakness, normal tendon reflexes, and lack of sensory abnormalities suggested a myopathy or a defect of neuromuscular transmission and made a neurogenic process unlikely. The rash and lack of ocular involvement favored a myopathy but pointed away from statin-associated necrotizing autoimmune myopathy (NAM); the progression of the weakness, despite statin discontinuation, argued against statin toxicity. In addition, the combined clinical course and rash suggested an immune-mediated, not a genetic, cause.

TESTING

Serum testing showed an increased creatine kinase (CK) level (851 U/L; reference range, <308 U/L). Needle electromyography showed myopathic changes with fibrillation potentials in proximal and axial muscles. Nerve conduction studies and 2-Hz repetitive nerve stimulation were normal. Biopsy of the deltoid demonstrated a perifascicular pathologic process, including muscle fiber atrophy, and perivascular inflammatory exudate in the perimysium (Figure 50.1A-C). Immunocytochemical studies showed patchy loss of intramuscular capillaries, some of which had complement (C5b9)

deposition, and sarcoplasmic expression of myxovirus resistance protein A, mainly in the perifascicular regions (Figure 50.1D). Immunologic testing was positive for autoantibodies to nuclear matrix protein 2 and negative for 3-hydroxy-3-methylglutaryl–coenzyme A reductase antibodies. Video swallow studies showed oropharyngeal dysphagia. Pulmonary function tests indicated mildly decreased maximal respiratory pressures but normal diffusing lung capacity for carbon monoxide. Positron emission tomography, testicular ultrasonography, and colonoscopy indicated no malignancy.

DIAGNOSIS

The findings were consistent with a diagnosis of dermatomyositis (DM).

MANAGEMENT

The patient was started on oral prednisone 60 mg/d and azathioprine 2.5 mg/kg per day in 2 divided doses, after checking for adequate thiopurine methyltransferase activity. Liver function tests and complete blood cell count with differential were assessed to monitor for potential azathioprine toxicity. Because of the development of insomnia and mood disturbance, prednisone was quickly tapered. Intravenous immunoglobulin 2 g/kg of ideal body weight was given monthly for 3 months, and then every other month for 2 months. Follow-up examination revealed mild weakness of the shoulder girdle muscles after 4 months of immunotherapy, and normal strength and CK value 8 months later, while on azathioprine monotherapy.

DISCUSSION

DM is an idiopathic inflammatory myopathy (IIM). IIM is a group of autoimmune muscle diseases that includes DM, polymyositis (PM), inclusion body myositis (IBM), NAM (or immune-mediated necrotizing myopathy), and overlap myositis, including antisynthetase syndrome. Although classified as an IIM, NAM exhibits little or no inflammation on muscle biopsy (see Case 49). PM is a controversial

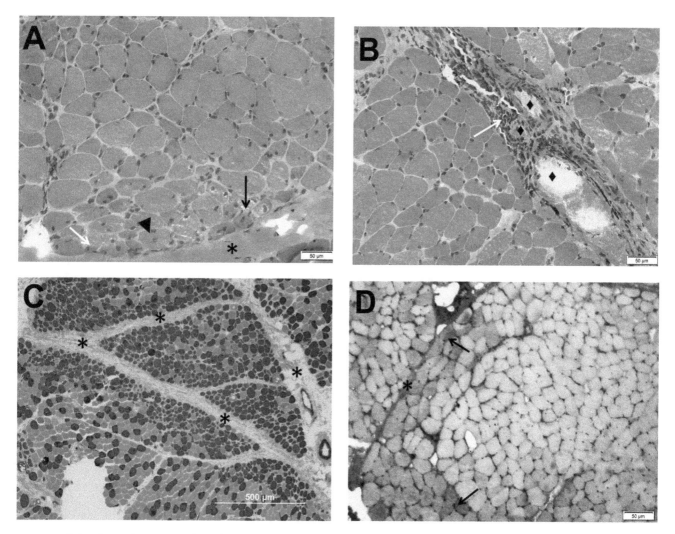

Figure 50.1 **Deltoid Muscle Biopsy Findings for the Case Patient.**

A and B, Hematoxylin and eosin–stained sections show structural abnormalities preferentially distributed in the perifascicular regions (A; asterisk marks perimysium) and consisting of muscle fiber atrophy (white arrow), regenerating fibers (black arrow), and internalized nuclei (arrowhead); the inflammatory exudate (B, arrow) is concentrated at perivascular sites (black diamonds indicate blood vessels) in the perimysium. C, ATPase–reacted section at pH 4.2 highlights the perifascicular distribution of the atrophic fibers (asterisks mark perimysium). D, Sarcoplasmic expression of myxovirus resistance protein A (MxA) is observed in the perifascicular regions where fibers stain darker (arrows, anti-MxA stain; asterisk marks perimysium).

entity because many patients initially diagnosed with PM are later diagnosed with IBM or overlap myositis. Most IIM types manifest with proximal and symmetric, subacute or chronic muscle weakness. IBM instead presents with quadriceps and finger flexor weakness, which is often asymmetric. Dysphagia is frequent in IIM. IIM can have extramuscular involvement, such as skin, lung (interstitial lung disease), or joint involvement. Pathognomonic DM skin involvement includes heliotrope rash, Gottron sign, and Gottron papules (red, often scaly, bumps overlying the knuckles of the fingers), although other skin changes can occur. The rash may precede or follow the muscle weakness in DM. Cardiac involvement is uncommon. Among the various IIMs, DM has the highest risk of associated cancer, which is found in 10% to 20% of patients within 2 years before or 3 years after the myositis onset. Older age and more severe skin disease accompany the highest risk of cancer.

CK values are often increased. Whereas patients with NAM have CK values in the thousands of units per liter,

patients with DM or IBM tend to have lower or even normal CK levels.

Electromyography shows myopathic changes consisting of early recruiting, short-duration/low-amplitude motor unit potentials, fibrillation potentials, and positive sharp waves.

Several autoantibodies have been identified in IIM. Those recognizing nuclear matrix protein 2, transcriptional intermediary factor-1γ, melanoma differentiation-associated protein 5, and small ubiquitin-like modifier activating enzyme are specific for DM, with the first 2 associated with a higher cancer risk. Antibodies against aminoacyl transfer RNA synthetase, including anti-Jo1, are detected in antisynthetase syndrome. Antibodies to cytosolic 5′-nucleotidase 1A are a serologic marker of IBM, although nonspecific and not sufficient for diagnosis.

Myopathologic findings vary among the different IIMs. DM is notable for predominantly perifascicular pathology and perivascular inflammation (Figure 50.1). Myxovirus resistance protein A sarcoplasmic expression is the most sensitive pathologic test for DM and seems to distinguish DM from antisynthetase syndrome, which can sometimes have perifascicular pathologic findings mimicking DM. The canonical pathologic features of IBM are autoaggressive inflammatory reaction (inflammatory cells attacking non-necrotic muscle fibers), rimmed vacuoles, and congophilic inclusions. Similar to IBM, PM shows autoaggressive inflammation but lacks rimmed vacuoles and congophilic inclusions.

There are no consensus-based treatment guidelines for IIM. With the exception of IBM, for which no effective drug is available, pharmacologic treatment of IIMs usually consists of a combination of corticosteroids and a steroid-sparing immunosuppressant agent, such as azathioprine or mycophenolate mofetil. Tacrolimus, cyclosporine, cyclophosphamide, and rituximab are optional drugs but should not be used as first-line therapy. Intravenous immunoglobulin can be used as first-line treatment, often in combination with an immunosuppressant drug, or as a second-line drug. Methotrexate should be used with caution, or avoided if there is potential risk of interstitial lung disease, because of its potential pulmonary toxicity.

KEY POINTS

- IIMs are immune-mediated myopathies characterized by muscle weakness and inflammation on muscle biopsy, with the exception of NAM in which inflammation is often lacking.

- Clinical history and findings are crucial for diagnosis and distinction from inherited myopathies.

- Combined serologic testing and muscle biopsy are the diagnostic standard tests.

- Immunotherapy is effective for treatment of most IIMs, with the exception of IBM.

"RESTLESSNESS" AFTER CANCER DIAGNOSIS AND TREATMENT

Anastasia Zekeridou, MD, PhD

CASE PRESENTATION

HISTORY AND EXAMINATION

A 76-year-old woman with no prior medical history sought care for unintentional weight loss, hematuria, and fatigue. She was diagnosed with plurimetastatic renal cell carcinoma. After resection of the primary tumor and metastases, she was treated with pembrolizumab, an immune checkpoint inhibitor (ICI) targeting programmed cell death protein 1 (PD-1). Three months after her cancer immunotherapy was initiated, the patient experienced involuntary tongue and face movements with dysphagia and weight loss. She was also described as "restless." Almost 1 year after neurologic symptom onset, she had generalized dystonia/dyskinesias, more prominent in the orofacial/mandibular and neck regions and proximal upper extremities, along with some choreiform movements. At that point, the patient was in cancer remission with ongoing ICI treatment.

The patient had subacute onset of hyperkinetic movements in the context of ICI therapy for a recently diagnosed cancer. The differential diagnosis for hyperkinetic movement disorders in this age group includes neurodegenerative disorders, genetic diseases, metabolic disorders, paraneoplastic or other disorders, and drug/toxin exposures. The patient had no prior exposure to dopamine receptor–blocking agents. Structural basal ganglia lesions can be responsible, including basal ganglia calcifications. Genetic diseases such as levodopa-responsive dystonia seemed improbable given the patient's age. Wilson disease, which can manifest with dystonia, is often accompanied by tremor and parkinsonism. The lack of parkinsonism in this patient also made parkinsonian syndromes unlikely. The main presentation in this patient was dystonic movements that were in a distribution similar to Meige syndrome. Even though chorea was not the main presentation, Huntington disease could also be considered. The subacute disease onset, in the presence of cancer and ICI treatment, indicated a paraneoplastic neurologic syndrome or an autoimmune complication of ICI treatment, as seen in patients with collapsin-response mediator protein 5–immunoglobulin G (IgG) basal ganglionitis or phosphodiesterase 10A (PDE10A)-IgG autoimmunity.

TESTING

Blood testing was unremarkable, including findings of complete blood cell count and morphology, kidney function, and levels of electrolytes, liver enzymes, thyroid hormones, vitamin B_{12}, ceruloplasmin, and copper, as well as infectious workup with HIV and syphilis testing. Brain magnetic resonance imaging showed basal ganglia T2/fluid-attenuated inversion recovery hyperintensities without gadolinium enhancement. Cerebrospinal fluid (CSF) testing showed normal white blood cell count, slightly increased protein concentration (44 mg/dL; reference range, <35 mg/dL), and 8 CSF-restricted oligoclonal bands. Serum and CSF testing for neural autoantibodies showed IgG immunoreactivity in a mouse tissue indirect immunofluorescence assay, predominantly staining the basal ganglia. The IgG was subsequently identified to bind to PDE10A. Whole-body positron emission tomography/computed tomography after 1 year of cancer immunotherapy showed cancer remission.

DIAGNOSIS

The patient was diagnosed with paraneoplastic PDE10A-IgG autoimmunity manifesting as hyperkinetic movement disorder triggered by ICI treatment.

MANAGEMENT

Given the patient's cancer remission, the ICI treatment was discontinued. She was treated with high-dose intravenous corticosteroids (methylprednisolone 1 g/d for 3 days, followed by weekly for 11 weeks), with improvement of her hyperkinetic movement disorder but persistence of some dystonic movements. Further treatment with oral prednisone at 1 mg/kg and plasma exchange, 5 treatments every other day, did not produce further improvement. The patient was treated

Table 51.1 | NEUROLOGIC COMPLICATIONS OF IMMUNE CHECKPOINT INHIBITOR CANCER IMMUNOTHERAPY

CNS DISORDERS	NEUROMUSCULAR DISORDERS
Meningitis	Muscle
Encephalitis/encephalopathy (limbic, brainstem, posterior reversible encephalopathy, other)	Inflammatory myopathy
Hyperkinetic movement disorders	Neuromuscular junction
Cerebellar ataxia	Myasthenia gravis
Multiple sclerosis	Lambert-Eaton myasthenic syndrome
Optic neuritis	Peripheral nerve
Myelitis	Guillain-Barré syndrome/chronic inflammatory demyelinating polyradiculoneuropathy
Granulomatous inflammation (neurosarcoidosis, Tolosa-Hunt syndrome)	Axonal and demyelinating neuropathies (eg, sensory neuronopathy, mononeuritis/multiple cranial neuropathies, vasculitic neuropathy)
CNS vasculitis	Autonomic and enteric neuropathy
Other	Plexopathy
Hypophysitis	Polyradiculoneuropathy
Retinopathy	Parsonage-Turner syndrome/neuralgic amyotrophy

Abbreviation: CNS, central nervous system.

symptomatically with onabotulinumtoxinA injections and tetrabenazine, which ameliorated her dystonic movements. Three years after her cancer diagnosis, she was alive and in cancer remission with minimal residual movements.

DISCUSSION

ICIs are monoclonal antibodies targeting "stop signs" of the immune response, which lead to enhanced endogenous responses, including those against cancer. Autoimmune complications are consequences of the enhanced immunity and can affect all organs, including the nervous system. The neurologic manifestations vary (Table 51.1), and even though they are rare overall, neuromuscular complications are twice as common as central nervous system complications. Classic central nervous system autoimmune/paraneoplastic neurologic syndromes such as limbic encephalitis and cerebellar ataxia are seen, but unusual presentations and novel autoantibodies are often discovered, as in this case patient. New-onset demyelination and aggravation of preexisting demyelination, including in the brain and the spinal cord, have also been described. Patients with ICI-related myopathy often have a myasthenialike phenotype with involvement of the ocular muscles. Patients with ICI-related myopathy and myasthenia gravis require cardiology workup, including cardiac enzymes, electrocardiography, and, depending on the results, echocardiography because cardiomyopathy is often seen in these patients.

The neurologic manifestations are seen with all categories of ICIs (targeting cytotoxic T-lymphocyte-associated protein 4, the PD-1/PD-L1 [programmed cell death ligand 1] pathway, or combination treatment) and most often occur in the first 1 to 3 months after ICI treatment, even though they have also been described after ICI cessation. These complications can arise in patients with any treated cancer, such as melanoma or renal cell carcinoma, and not only in those traditionally associated with paraneoplastic neurologic syndromes such as small cell lung cancer and thymoma. When ICI reactions are suspected, workup should be according to the neurologic phenotype and may include imaging, electromyography, spinal fluid evaluation, and neural autoantibody profiles.

The overall management of ICI-related autoimmune complications depends on their severity. In most cases, except in patients with minor symptoms, the ICIs are temporarily or permanently discontinued. The first line of treatment is high-dose corticosteroids, either oral or intravenous, which often leads to improvement, especially in cases of peripheral nervous system involvement. The duration of the treatment depends on the results. In patients who do not improve with corticosteroids or have severe disease, plasma-exchange, intravenous immunoglobulin, or cyclophosphamide can be considered. Long-term immunosuppression is ideally avoided because of the risk of aggravating the underlying cancer but might be necessary in patients with relapsing neurologic disease. ICI rechallenge should be considered on an individual basis. In patients with preexisting paraneoplastic neurologic autoimmunity, ICI treatment should be used with caution and only if absolutely necessary.

KEY POINTS

- Neurologic complications of ICIs can affect any level of the neuraxis and can be seen with all ICI treatments and all cancers.

- These complications often appear in the first few months of ICI treatment.

- In cases of myositis and myasthenia gravis, workup for cardiomyopathy should be undertaken.

- ICI suspension or permanent discontinuation and use of corticosteroids are the first line of treatment. Escalation to plasma exchange, intravenous immunoglobulin, or cyclophosphamide might be necessary depending on the severity of the complication, as well as the response to initial treatment.

- Long-term immunosuppression is ideally avoided because of the risk of aggravating the underlying cancer, but it might be necessary in patients with relapsing neurologic disease.

SUDDEN ONSET OF DIPLOPIA AND A SKELETAL MUSCLE ANTIBODY

John R. Mills, PhD

CASE PRESENTATION

HISTORY AND EXAMINATION

A 62-year-old man with a history of migraine came to the emergency department with sudden onset of horizontal diplopia and, subsequently, bilateral ptosis. At the time of the event he had no vertigo, focal weakness, numbness, tingling, or headache. He noted feeling unsteady when walking. He reported that the diplopia worsened throughout the day. He had no history of seizures, meningitis, encephalitis, uveitis, iritis, deep vein thrombosis, pulmonary embolism, coronary artery disease, or hyperlipidemia. He had no history of diabetes. He had a history of hepatitis C infection. He had some vision loss in his left eye, which was thought to relate to a retinopathy. He disclosed that he had a history of cold feet and had notably high arches. No other neurologic symptoms were reported. He had a pacemaker because of syncope attributed to sick sinus syndrome.

On examination, the patient had slight intermittent ptosis on the left and reported vertical diplopia, mainly on leftward gaze. He had some asymmetric forehead weakness and mild weakness in the arms and legs. No significant fatigable component was noted on examination. Ophthalmologic assessment found no evidence of ptosis or orbicularis fatigue on sustained lid closure. However, orbicularis oculi weakness was noted. Diagnoses considered at the time are shown in Table 52.1.

TESTING

Computed tomography (CT) angiography of the head and neck were ruled negative for intracranial stenosis, occlusions, or aneurysms. CT of the head indicated a tiny lacunar infarct in the right caudate head but was otherwise normal. Magnetic resonance imaging of the brain identified a tiny, periaqueductal, enhancing abnormality in the right midbrain that was thought to be likely ischemic, but there was some concern for a demyelinating or inflammatory lesion. Cerebrospinal fluid evaluation indicated an increased protein concentration (55 mg/dL; reference range, ≤35 mg/dL) but normal immunoglobulin G findings, blood cell counts, and oligoclonal bands. Serologic evaluation for myasthenia gravis was negative for acetylcholine receptor (binding and modulating) and muscle-specific tyrosine kinase antibodies, but striational antibodies were positive at a titer of 1:240 (reference value, <1:120).

Nerve conduction studies of the facial and accessory nerves were normal without evidence of decrement. Single-fiber electromyography (EMG) of the orbicularis oculi was normal. The patient had no response to edrophonium (Tensilon). Serum protein studies indicated the presence of polyclonal hypergammaglobulinemia (2.2 g/dL; reference range, 0.6-1.6 g/dL). The patient was negative for the presence of cryoglobulins. Workup for vasculitis was negative, including negative serologic findings for anti–myeloperoxidase/proteinase 3 antibodies. Random glucose testing was within

---

Table 52.1 | DIFFERENTIAL DIAGNOSIS FOR THE CASE PATIENT

POSSIBLE DIAGNOSES	EXCLUSIONARY FINDINGS
Inherent strabismus worsened by migraine	Has weakness outside simple strabismus
PCOM aneurysm bleeding with oculomotor nerve palsy	Pupil dilation is not seen, which is typical
Brainstem stroke	No crossed body signs, no dysphagia, no dysarthria
Neuromuscular junction dysfunction	Absence of fatigable weakness
Brain tumor	Acute onset
Diabetic oculomotor nerve palsy	Patient is not diabetic
Hepatitis C–associated vasculitis	Atypical without arm or leg mononeuritis

Abbreviation: PCOM, posterior communicating artery.

the normal range (97 mg/dL). CT of the chest to rule out thymoma (because of the slightly increased striational antibodies) was negative.

DIAGNOSIS

Myasthenia gravis was effectively ruled out by the clinical evaluation, electrophysiologic studies, and laboratory studies. Given the hyperacute time course, the patient's clinical disorder was most probably explained by an ischemic stroke that affected the oculomotor nuclei regions causing ptosis and ophthalmoparesis.

MANAGEMENT

On follow-up, the patient was discovered to have a patent foramen ovale (PFO). Whether the PFO was a contributing factor to the stroke is uncertain. The recurrence rate in this setting is thought to be low relative to other causes of stroke. Ultimately it was decided to not close the PFO and to maintain the patient on clopidogrel and adult low-dose aspirin.

DISCUSSION

The onset of diplopia is typically sudden, but this occurs exclusively with vascular pathologic processes. Diplopia that appears intermittently with diurnal variation suggests the possibility of a neuromuscular junction disease such as myasthenia gravis. In this case patient, the classic features of myasthenia gravis were lacking, including, most importantly, bedside fatigable weakness. Of all tests, single-fiber EMG has the best sensitivity (97%) but is not entirely specific. For example, it cannot distinguish oculomotor weakness from mitochondrial disease or oculopharyngeal dystrophy, and not all electromyographers perform the test given the extent of technical expertise required. Given these factors and the need for an urgent diagnosis with myasthenia gravis, it is typical for serologic myasthenia gravis testing to be ordered simultaneously with neurophysiologic testing. This frequently leads to results that require careful interpretation in the proper clinical context.

A comprehensive evaluation includes testing for antibodies against the acetylcholine receptor, both binding and modulating, as well as for antibodies against muscle-specific tyrosine kinase and, often, striated muscle antigens (striational antibody). The latter is included in comprehensive evaluations given the risk of thymoma in patients with myasthenia gravis. In paraneoplastic serologic evaluations, isolated low-titer striational antibodies provide little guidance. In cases of thymic neoplasia, the median titer of striational antibody is 10-fold higher than in nonthymic neoplasia cases. The overall positive predictive value of a positive striational antibody result (any titer) is only 7% for predicting thymoma. As in this case patient, a low-titer striational antibody (1:240) in isolation, in the absence of a high pretest probability of myasthenia gravis, has low positive predictive value for thymoma. In the absence of other indicators, the yield of chest CT is low.

Although each autoantibody and its associated titer have specific clinical performance characteristics to consider, in general, low-titer antibodies should always be viewed conservatively, particularly outside of the correct clinical context. Diagnostic cutoffs are set by laboratories to ensure an acceptable balance between the risk of missing true cases of disease and generating positive results in patients lacking the disease. Antibody assays often do not provide the best of both worlds, and one or the other must be sacrificed. In the case of striational antibodies, the cutoff favors clinical sensitivity. It is critical for the physician interpreting the test result to be informed of a particular assay's clinical performance at the diagnostic cutoff.

KEY POINTS

- Low-titer autoantibodies, near cutoffs, often have lower clinical specificity.

- Low-titer autoantibodies in the context of low clinical suspicion are of limited clinical utility.

- Low-titer striational antibodies in isolation have low positive predictive value for the presence of thymoma.

- Single-fiber EMG has a very high negative predictive value but is not entirely specific.

SECTION III

OTHER INFLAMMATORY CNS DISORDERS AND NEUROIMMUNOLOGIC MIMICS

DIPLOPIA, ORBITAL PAIN, AND VISION LOSS IN A MIDDLE-AGED WOMAN

Lauren M. Webb, and Eoin P. Flanagan, MB, BCh

CASE PRESENTATION

HISTORY AND EXAMINATION

A 59-year-old woman with type 2 diabetes had development of fluctuating, binocular, painless diplopia. A few months later she experienced headache, orbital pain, facial numbness, and progressive vision loss in the left eye. Her left eye vision worsened over the subsequent 2 months. Magnetic resonance imaging (MRI) of the brain and orbit showed bilateral optic nerve enhancement. She started treatment with empiric intravenous corticosteroids for presumed optic neuritis, which resulted in transient improvement. Subsequently, her vision worsened to no light perception in the left eye, and despite monthly intravenous corticosteroids, she had fluctuating vision loss in the right eye.

She was referred to our department 1 year after symptom onset and 5 months after complete vision loss in the left eye. Her neurologic examination at that time indicated left optic disc pallor, a left relative afferent pupillary defect, no light perception in the left eye, and normal vision and examination findings in the right eye. Her neurologic and ophthalmologic examinations were otherwise normal.

Diagnoses considered at the time are shown in Table 53.1. Although toxic (eg, methanol), metabolic (eg, mitochondrial), nutritional (eg, vitamin B$_{12}$ deficiency), or genetic (eg, Leber hereditary optic neuropathy) diseases can result in optic neuropathy, these are typically not associated with optic nerve enhancement, so they were excluded from the differential diagnosis for this patient.

TESTING

The serum was negative for autoantibodies to aquaporin-4 and myelin oligodendrocyte glycoprotein. Cerebrospinal fluid (CSF) evaluation was performed because the patient's fluctuating diplopia and facial numbness suggested involvement of multiple cranial nerves. The CSF showed 133 white blood cells/μL (reference range, 0-5/μL) with 82% lymphocytes, increased protein concentration of 55 mg/dL (reference range, 0-35 mg/dL), and negative oligoclonal bands and cytologic findings. Chest computed tomography (CT) was negative for hilar adenopathy. Whole-body ^{18}F-fludeoxyglucose-positron emission tomography (PET)

Table 53.1 | **DIFFERENTIAL DIAGNOSIS OF OPTIC NEUROPATHY WITH OPTIC NERVE ENHANCEMENT ON MAGNETIC RESONANCE IMAGING**

DISEASE TYPE	SPECIFIC DIAGNOSIS
Inflammatory central nervous system demyelinating disease	Multiple sclerosis
	Aquaporin-4-IgG–seropositive neuromyelitis optica spectrum disorder
	Myelin oligodendrocyte glycoprotein-IgG–associated disorder
	Acute disseminated encephalomyelitis
	Idiopathic
Other inflammatory diseases	Sarcoidosis
	IgG4-related disease
	Rheumatologic disorders (eg, systemic lupus erythematosus)
	Paraneoplastic autoimmune diseases
Infectious	Bacterial
	Mycobacterium tuberculosis
	Treponema pallidum
	Borrelia burgdorferi (Lyme disease)
	Bartonella spp.
	Fungal
	Mucor (in the setting of diabetes)
	Cryptococcus spp.
	Parasitic
	Toxoplasma gondii
	Viral
	Cytomegalovirus
	Varicella-zoster virus
	(Any infectious cause of meningitis can be associated with optic neuropathy)
Neoplastic	Lymphoma
	Glioma
	Meningioma
	Metastasis

Abbreviation: IgG, immunoglobulin G.

was normal, without abnormalities concerning for an underlying tumor, systemic sarcoidosis, or immunoglobulin G (IgG)4-related disease. Paraneoplastic autoantibodies were negative, including those for collapsin-response mediator protein 5. Levels of angiotensin-converting enzyme, antinuclear antibody, Sjögren syndrome-A antibody (anti-Ro), Sjögren syndrome-B antibody (anti-La), antineutrophil cytoplasmic antibody, and rheumatoid factor were all negative or within normal limits. Tests for tuberculosis, *Bartonella*, *Borrelia*, and *Toxoplasma* were all negative. Infectious agents in the CSF, including cryptococcal antigen, were negative, as were the VDRL test and polymerase chain reaction for cytomegalovirus and varicella-zoster virus.

Repeated brain MRI 1 year after symptom onset showed persistent bilateral (left > right) optic nerve enhancement (Figure 53.1A and B) along with oculomotor nerve (Figure 53.1B) and left midbrain enhancement.

Given her prominent bilateral enhancement of the optic nerves with complete loss of left eye vision and fluctuating

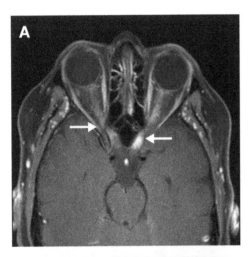

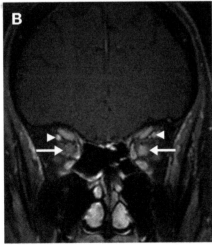

Figure 53.1 **Magnetic Resonance Imaging Findings for the Case Patient.**
Postgadolinium T1-weighted axial (A) and coronal (B) images of the brain show bilateral enhancement of the optic nerve, more on the left than right (arrows), with oculomotor nerve enhancement also notable (B, arrowheads) 1 year after onset of symptoms.

right eye vision, we recommended left optic nerve biopsy to obtain the diagnosis and attempt to preserve vision in the threatened right eye. Because the patient had no light perception in the left eye for 5 months, with significant pallor of the optic nerve, it was unlikely that she had salvageable left eye vision. Furthermore, there was concern for lymphomatous infiltration of the optic nerve, because lymphoma can transiently respond to corticosteroids. Confirmation of a lymphoma diagnosis would be critical for initiation of specific chemotherapy. The pathologic analysis identified noncaseating granulomas.

DIAGNOSIS

The finding of noncaseating granulomas was consistent with neurosarcoidosis infiltrating the left optic nerve.

MANAGEMENT

The patient was treated with intravenous methylprednisolone, 1 g/d for 5 days, followed by prolonged, high-dose, oral corticosteroids (1 mg/kg per day) along with corticosteroid prophylaxis of calcium, vitamin D, a proton-pump inhibitor, and dapsone for *Pneumocystis* prophylaxis (trimethoprimsulfamethoxazole could not be used because of sulfa allergy). Thereafter, she was lost to follow-up.

DISCUSSION

Sarcoidosis is a systemic disease of unknown cause that can occur anywhere in the body but most commonly involves the lungs. The pathologic hallmark of sarcoidosis is noncaseating granulomas. Interestingly, our patient had no history of systemic sarcoidosis, and her chest CT and whole-body PET findings were negative for hilar lymphadenopathy or increased glucose uptake; thus, there were no extraneurologic sites to biopsy. The optic nerve is the most common cranial nerve involved in neurosarcoidosis radiologically and the second most common cranial nerve to cause clinical symptoms after the facial nerve. Up to 5% of patients with neurosarcoidosis have involvement of the optic nerve, chiasm, or tract. Compared with demyelinating causes of optic neuritis, sarcoid optic neuropathy is less frequently associated with orbital pain but similarly presents with abnormal pupillary responses, as well as decreased visual acuity and color vision. Sarcoid optic neuropathy symptoms most commonly develop subacutely over days to weeks. Optic disc edema is often visible early in sarcoid optic neuropathy and evolves to optic disc pallor with prolonged damage from inflammation. It is common for other brain regions to be involved, including other cranial nerves.

Current criteria for a definitive neurosarcoidosis diagnosis require a finding of noncaseating granulomas on central nervous system (CNS) biopsy, with clinical, MRI, and CSF manifestations consistent with sarcoidosis. Involving any part of the CNS, neurosarcoidosis may mimic many other neurologic diseases. Thus, the noncaseating granulomas were critical to determining the diagnosis in the case patient. Neurologists may face a clinical conundrum when CNS biopsy could injure neural tissue. Optic nerve biopsy, for example, may provide a definitive diagnosis but risks permanent vision loss, the very function that the physician attempts to preserve. Thus, the neurosarcoidosis diagnosis is considered *probable* if there are clinical, MRI, and CSF manifestations consistent with neurosarcoidosis in the setting of systemic, extraneural sarcoidosis.

Neurosarcoidosis typically responds to prolonged high-dose corticosteroids, but intermittent intravenous corticosteroids (as in this case) are frequently ineffective. Disease severity and corticosteroid adverse effects often necessitate the use of other immunosuppressive agents and biologic immunotherapies (eg, infliximab). Steroid-sparing agents (eg, methotrexate) can be considered in patients who have relapse on corticosteroid taper or can be used in conjunction with high-dose corticosteroids to reduce the risk of recurrence.

KEY POINTS

- The optic nerve is the second most common cranial nerve clinically affected by sarcoidosis after the facial nerve.

- Obtaining a neurosarcoidosis diagnosis can be difficult when there are no extraneurologic sites to biopsy, which necessitates biopsy of neural tissue to achieve a diagnosis.

- High-dose intravenous corticosteroids, followed by prolonged high-dose oral corticosteroids for many months with a slow taper, is the mainstay of treatment for neurosarcoidosis. Patients treated with intermittent intravenous corticosteroids often have disease breakthrough.

A YOUNG MAN WITH VISUAL FIELD LOSS, DECREASED HEARING, AND CONFUSION

M. Tariq Bhatti, MD, Eric R. Eggenberger, DO, Marie D. Acierno, MD, and John J. Chen, MD, PhD

CASE PRESENTATION

HISTORY AND EXAMINATION

A previously healthy 27-year-old man noted imbalance and staggering when walking. One week later, vertigo, nausea, vomiting, and mild fever developed. This was initially presumed to be due to an inner ear infection, and antibiotics were prescribed. Several weeks later, he began experiencing intermittent left face and arm numbness, as well as bilateral hearing loss and tinnitus. Audiography indicated low-frequency hearing loss in both ears, left worse than right. One month later, he reported headaches and neck stiffness, and his family noticed that he was moody, easily aggravated, and confused, with slow mentation. Diagnoses considered at the time are shown in Table 54.1.

TESTING

Magnetic resonance imaging (MRI) showed patchy, nodular, leptomeningeal enhancement involving both cerebral hemispheres and the posterior fossa, with scattered hyperintense T2 signal changes of the internal capsule and prominent abnormal signal changes in the corpus callosum. Serum studies for infectious, paraneoplastic, and inflammatory conditions were all normal or negative. Cerebrospinal fluid analysis was remarkable for a markedly increased protein concentration (164 mg/dL; reference range, ≤35 mg/dL) and 5 white blood cells/µL (100% lymphocytes). Eye examination showed 20/20 vision in both eyes with a superior visual field defect in the right eye. Retinal whitening was noted in the vascular distribution of the inferotemporal arcade. Intravenous fluorescein angiography (IVFA) showed delayed filling in this region consistent with a branch retinal artery occlusion (BRAO) and scattered areas of arteriolar wall hyperfluorescence (Figure 54.1).

Table 54.1 | **DIFFERENTIAL DIAGNOSIS FOR THE CASE PATIENT**

POSSIBLE DIAGNOSES	EXAMPLES
Inflammatory demyelinating central nervous system disease	• Multiple sclerosis • Acute disseminated encephalomyelitis • Neuromyelitis optica spectrum disorder
Cerebrovascular disease	• Stroke • Transient ischemic attack • CADASIL (cerebral autosomal dominant arteriopathy with subcortical infarcts and leukoencephalopathy)
Autoimmune disease	• Primary central nervous system vasculitis • Paraneoplastic encephalitis • Polyarteritis nodosa • Granulomatosis with polyangiitis • Systemic lupus erythematosus • Sarcoidosis • Sjögren syndrome • Behçet disease • Antiphospholipid antibody syndrome • Cogan syndrome • Susac syndrome
Infectious central nervous system disease	• Lyme disease • Syphilis • Tuberculosis • Viral encephalitis
Neoplastic central nervous system disease	• Lymphoma • Metastases
Miscellaneous	• Migraine • Mitochondrial disease (ie, MELAS [mitochondrial encephalomyopathy, lactic acidosis, and stroke-like episodes]) • Meniere disease • Psychiatric disorders

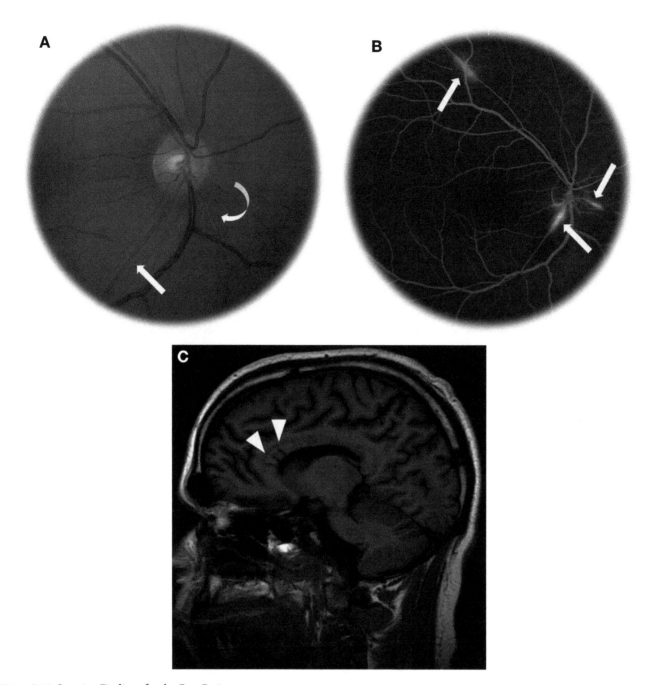

Figure 54.1 **Imaging Findings for the Case Patient.**

A, Fundus photography of the right eye shows a Gass plaque (straight arrow) and sclerotic vessels (curved arrow). B, Intravenous fluorescence angiography of the right eye shows retinal arteriolar wall hyperfluorescence (arrows). C, Sagittal, T1-weighted magnetic resonance imaging shows multiple central hypointense lesions (arrowheads) in the corpus callosum.

DIAGNOSIS

A diagnosis of Susac syndrome was made on the basis of the BRAO, MRI findings, and hearing deficit.

MANAGEMENT

Intravenous methylprednisolone (IVMP) at 1 g/d was given for 3 days, followed by 80 mg/d of oral prednisone, which resulted in substantial improvement in headaches and cognition. Cyclophosphamide was also started at the same time as IVMP. However, 3 months later during the prednisone taper,

a new visual field defect developed due to a BRAO in the left eye, which prompted initiation of intravenous immunoglobulin and transition from cyclophosphamide to rituximab. He had no recurrent BRAOs or other relapses of his underlying Susac syndrome on this treatment regimen.

DISCUSSION

Susac syndrome was initially described as a microangiopathy of the brain and retina. It is an idiopathic autoimmune disorder that primarily affects the brain, eye, and inner ear.

More recently, Susac syndrome has also been called RED-M (retinopathy-encephalopathy-deafness associated with microangiopathy) or SICRET syndrome (small infarctions of cochlear, retinal, and encephalic tissue). Although the exact etiopathogenesis is not known, Susac syndrome is believed to be a vasculopathy due to an immune-mediated endotheliopathy. Immunohistologic analysis, primarily from antemortem brain biopsies, have demonstrated microinfarction associated with arteriolar wall proliferation, scant lymphocytic infiltration, basement membrane reduplication, and, in some cases, complement deposition.

The incidence of Susac syndrome is not known. Although considered to be very rare, it is most likely underrecognized and underreported because of the potential overlap with and misdiagnosis as multiple sclerosis and other mimickers. There is a substantial sex predilection—80% of patients are female, with a median onset in the third decade of life.

The classic clinical triad of BRAO, sensorineural hearing loss (usually low frequency), and encephalopathy is present at onset in only 10% to 15% of patients. The majority of patients (85%) eventually have all 3 during the course of the disease, but until then the diagnosis can be challenging to establish.

The hallmark ocular manifestation of Susac syndrome is BRAO. However, other ocular signs are important in establishing the diagnosis:

- Retinal arterial wall plaques or Gass plaques can mimic the appearance of cholesterol emboli but are found in the mid-segment of the retinal vessel and not at bifurcation sites (Figure 54.1A). Retinal arterial wall plaques are believed to be a result of vessel wall damage leading to lipid extravasation and atheromatous formation. They are most often found during the acute phase of the disease and can resolve and reappear during the course of the disease.

- Arteriolar wall hyperfluorescence seen on IVFA can be present in the setting of a BRAO or in the absence of a BRAO (Figure 54.1B). Arteriolar wall hyperfluorescence in the absence of a BRAO or away from the site of a BRAO is considered a confirmatory sign of Susac syndrome. IVFA is an important test that should be performed during follow-up of a patient with Susac syndrome to monitor for active disease.

- Retinal arterioarterial collaterals are late findings seen in the retina of some patients and may be more commonly seen in Susac syndrome than other causes of BRAO.

- Ghost or sclerotic retinal vessels represent a prior vascular occlusion.

The sensorineural hearing loss is typically asymmetric and usually involves low or medium frequencies. In addition, patients may report vertigo and severe tinnitus.

Central nervous system (CNS) manifestations are broad and can result in severe neurologic consequences. Headache is a common symptom and often the first sign of the disease. Confusion, cognitive impairment, vertigo, seizures, dysarthria, and occasionally cranial nerve and cauda equina involvement may occur. Psychiatric issues such as dysphoria, psychosis, and paranoia can be prominent features in some patients.

Most patients with Susac syndrome, particularly those with CNS manifestations, have abnormalities on MRI. The classic MRI triad is white matter lesions, gray matter lesions, and leptomeningeal enhancement. Central corpus callosum lesions (hyperintense on T2-weighted and hypointense on T1-weighted sequences), described as spokes representing linear lesions and snow balls representing large round lesions, are best seen on sagittal images and are considered hallmark radiologic features of Susac syndrome (Figure 54.1C).

Currently, there are no specific diagnostic biomarkers for Susac syndrome. Endothelial cell antibodies have been identified in patients with Susac syndrome but lack sensitivity and specificity and therefore are not clinically useful at this time. Cerebrospinal fluid analysis can reveal mild pleocytosis with increased protein levels.

Although Susac syndrome is sometimes self-limited, more often it is a chronic relapsing disease, requiring ongoing treatment to reduce the risk of permanent sequelae. To date, there have been no randomized clinical trials for treatment of Susac syndrome, and current recommendations are based on case reports and clinical experience. In general, the initial treatment of Susac syndrome is with corticosteroids, either IVMP at 1 g/d for 3 to 5 days or oral prednisone at 1 mg/kg per day. Some experts advocate concomitant treatment with intravenous immunoglobulin at a loading dose of 2 g/kg per day for 3 days in the first month, followed by monthly infusions at 0.4 mg/kg per day for 6 months. Cyclophosphamide can be used in severe cases. The oral prednisone should be tapered slowly, typically over several months. Chronic immunotherapy agents, such as mycophenolate mofetil or azathioprine, are also often used in patients with relapsing disease.

Surveillance of clinical activity requires a multidisciplinary approach assessing the eye (eg, vision, visual field, and retina), hearing, and CNS function. In addition to MRI, IVFA is sensitive for detecting recurrent disease activity, even if the patient is asymptomatic, and can be used to monitor treatment response.

KEY POINTS

- The clinical triad for definitive diagnosis of Susac syndrome is BRAO, hearing loss, and encephalopathy.

- The characteristic MRI triad for identifying Susac syndrome is white matter lesions, gray matter lesions, and leptomeningeal enhancement.

- The distinctive MRI sign in Susac syndrome is central corpus callosum lesions.

- Initial treatment is with corticosteroids (IVMP or oral prednisone), with or without intravenous immunoglobulin for 3 to 6 months. Treatment with rituximab, mycophenolate mofetil, or azathioprine is used for patients with continued disease activity.

A WOMAN WITH PROGRESSIVE GAIT DIFFICULTY AND WHITE MATTER ABNORMALITIES

Adrian Budhram, MD, and Ralitza H. Gavrilova, MD

CASE PRESENTATION

HISTORY AND EXAMINATION

A 45-year-old right-handed woman was assessed in the neurology clinic for slowly progressive gait difficulty. Eight years earlier, she first noticed dragging of her right foot and stumbling on uneven surfaces. She also described difficulty bending the right knee and intermittent spasms of the right leg. She did not perceive any motor difficulty in the left leg or sensory abnormalities. She reported no involvement of the upper extremities, with the exception of bilateral, mild hand weakness when she was doing repetitive tasks such as using scissors. She reported increasing urinary urgency and frequency over the past 3 years. Her medical history was noncontributory, and her family history was negative for inherited neurologic disease. She had 3 living siblings with no neurologic symptoms and 1 brother who was stillborn.

Neurologic examination showed normal mental status and language assessment findings. Cranial nerve examination revealed bilateral optic disc pallor and nystagmus in lateral gaze. Upper extremity examination was remarkable for mild intention tremor bilaterally, greater on the right. Lower extremity examination was remarkable for moderate,

asymmetric, pyramidal weakness and spasticity, worse on the right, with abnormal plantar responses and high arches noted. There was decreased appreciation of cold sensation two-thirds of the way up the legs and absent appreciation of vibration to the hips bilaterally. Her gait was broad based and spastic, with circumduction of the right leg. Overall, her examination findings were suggestive of mainly corticospinal tract and dorsal column dysfunction, with mild cerebellar involvement. Diagnoses considered at the time are shown in Table 55.1.

TESTING

Magnetic resonance imaging (MRI) of the spinal cord showed continuous, relatively symmetric, T2 hyperintensity of the dorsal columns and, to a lesser extent, the lateral columns, as well as medullary pyramids (Figure 55.1 A and B). Brain MRI showed T2 hyperintensity in the corticospinal tracts bilaterally extending from the precentral gyrus through the corona radiata (Figure 55.1 C and D) and again seen in the pons. Additional findings included T2 hyperintensity scattered throughout the subcortical white matter of both cerebral hemispheres, within the posterior aspect of the corpus callosum, the intraparenchymal part of the trigeminal

Table 55.1 | **DIFFERENTIAL DIAGNOSIS FOR THE CASE PATIENT**

POSSIBLE DIAGNOSES	COMMENT
Compressive myelopathy	No spinal cord compression on MRI
Primary progressive multiple sclerosis	Spinal cord tract-specific signal change not typical
Paraneoplastic myelopathy	Long disease course, noninflammatory CSF not typical
Infectious myelopathy (HIV, human T-lymphotropic virus 1, syphilis)	Noninflammatory CSF, negative serologic findings not typical
Vitamin B_{12} deficiency	Extensive white matter change in brain not typical, normal vitamin B_{12} level
Copper deficiency	Extensive white matter change in brain not typical, normal copper level
Primary lateral sclerosis	Sensory involvement, extensive white matter change in brain not typical
Dural arteriovenous fistula	Spinal cord tract-specific signal change not typical
Hereditary spastic paraparesis	Extensive white matter change in brain not typical
Genetic leukodystrophy	Major diagnostic consideration

Abbreviations: CSF, cerebrospinal fluid; MRI, magnetic resonance imaging.

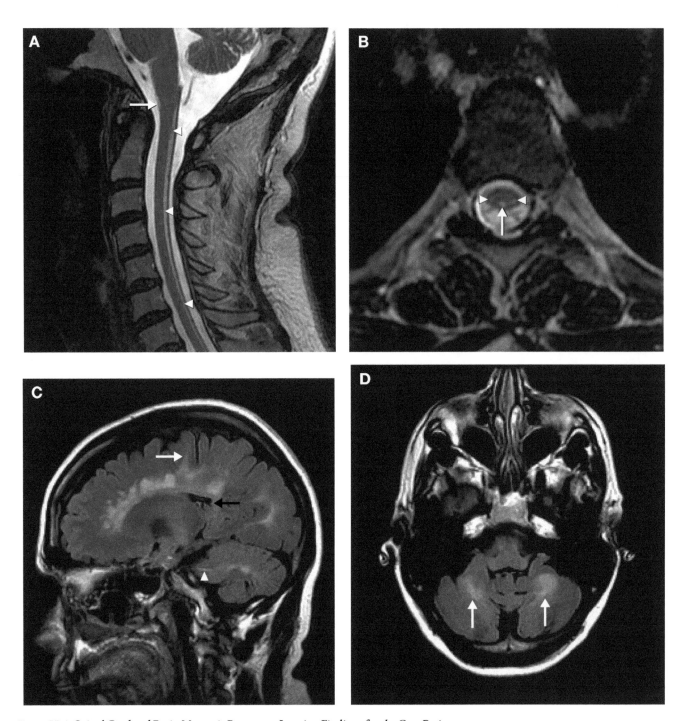

Figure 55.1 **Spinal Cord and Brain Magnetic Resonance Imaging Findings for the Case Patient.**
A, Sagittal, T2-weighted, cervicothoracic spinal cord imaging shows T2 hyperintensity of the medullary pyramids (white arrow), as well as longitudinally extensive T2 hyperintensity of the dorsal columns (arrowheads). B, Axial, T2-weighted, thoracic spinal cord imaging shows tract-specific T2 hyperintensity of the dorsal columns (white arrow) and to a lesser extent the lateral columns (arrowheads). C, Sagittal, T2-weighted, fluid-attenuated inversion recovery (FLAIR) brain imaging shows extensive patchy subcortical white matter T2 hyperintensities. Abnormal signal extending to the corona radiata from the precentral gyrus with sparing of U fibers is seen (white arrow). There is also T2 hyperintensity of the splenium of the corpus callosum (black arrow) and the intraparenchymal part of the trigeminal nerve (arrowhead). D, Axial, T2/FLAIR brain imaging shows T2 hyperintensity of the deep cerebellar white matter (white arrows).

nerve, and the deep cerebellar white matter. No gadolinium enhancement was seen. These extensive white matter abnormalities were interpreted by the radiologist as most likely long-standing, acquired, demyelinating disease, such as multiple sclerosis (MS). Laboratory investigations were negative for metabolic (vitamin B₁₂ and copper deficiency), infectious (HIV, human T-lymphotropic virus 1 and 2, and syphilis),

and autoimmune causes (serum and cerebrospinal fluid [CSF] paraneoplastic panel, including anti–collapsin-response mediator protein 5, antiamphiphysin, and antineuronal nuclear antibody type 1). Her CSF profile was noninflammatory, with a normal white blood cell count and no CSF-specific oligoclonal bands. Nerve conduction studies with electromyography were remarkable only for median neuropathies at both wrists, without evidence of a peripheral neuropathy or motor neuron disease.

Review of the patient's case by the MS clinic noted that the longitudinally extensive, tract-specific, T2 hyperintensity in the spinal cord was atypical for MS. In addition, the slowly progressive clinical course, absence of relapses typical of MS, and extensive, relatively symmetric, white matter abnormalities on MRI raised the possibility of a genetic leukodystrophy, despite the negative family history. Metabolic screening for the most common genetic leukodystrophies, including adrenoleukodystrophy, Krabbe disease, and metachromatic leukodystrophy were negative. Review of the MRI pattern of white matter abnormalities, however, led to specific clinical suspicion for leukoencephalopathy with brainstem and spinal cord involvement and lactate elevation (LBSL), an autosomal recessive condition due to *DARS2* (aspartyl-tRNA synthetase 2) gene sequence variation. Brain magnetic resonance spectroscopy did not show lactate peaks. Genetic testing findings were abnormal and showed compound heterozygous *DARS2* sequence variations.

DIAGNOSIS

The presence of *DARS2* sequence variations confirmed the diagnosis of LBSL.

MANAGEMENT

The patient was counseled that gradual progression of her gait difficulties could be expected, and symptomatic management was emphasized. Referral to the physical medicine and rehabilitation clinic was made for her gait difficulties, where stretching and strengthening exercises for the lower extremities were reviewed. A right ankle-foot orthosis was also prescribed to help with right foot dragging. The following year she reported increasing urinary urgency and several episodes of urge incontinence. She was then referred to the urology clinic, where an antimuscarinic agent was prescribed for neurogenic bladder.

DISCUSSION

LBSL is a leukodystrophy that most commonly presents clinically with spasticity, dorsal column dysfunction, cerebellar ataxia, and sometimes mild cognitive decline. LBSL classically has a childhood onset and therefore may not be included

in the differential diagnosis of chronic progressive white matter disease in adults. One of the major diagnostic considerations in adults with such a presentation is MS, particularly if there is no family history of neurologic disease to suggest a genetic cause. The slowly progressive disease course, lack of clinically discernible relapses, and white matter abnormalities in the brain may resemble progressive MS. However, symmetric white matter abnormalities, sparing of U fibers, absence of CSF-specific oligoclonal bands, and longitudinally extensive, tract-specific signal change in the spinal cord are clues that may suggest a genetic leukodystrophy.

Distinct patterns of neuroimaging abnormalities can indicate a specific leukodystrophy, as illustrated in this case patient. Neuroimaging criteria for LBSL have been developed, with 3 major criteria that must be fulfilled for MRI-based diagnosis: signal abnormalities in 1) the cerebral white matter that relatively spare the U fibers, 2) the dorsal columns and lateral corticospinal tracts of the spinal cord, and 3) the pyramids of the medulla oblongata. All these criteria were met in our case patient, along with several supportive criteria including signal abnormality of the splenium of the corpus callosum, the intraparenchymal part of the trigeminal nerve, and the deep cerebellar white matter. Lactate levels on magnetic resonance spectroscopy are typically increased, but this is not required for diagnosis and may be normal in adult-onset cases.

Genetic leukodystrophies should be included in the differential diagnosis for patients with relatively symmetric white matter abnormalities and slowly progressive neurologic decline, with close review of neuroimaging to help guide diagnostic testing.

KEY POINTS

- Leukodystrophies can present later in life and should be a diagnostic consideration in an adult with slowly progressive neurologic decline and white matter abnormalities.

- Symmetric cerebral white matter abnormalities, subcortical U-fiber sparing, and longitudinally extensive tract-specific signal abnormality in the spinal cord may suggest a leukodystrophy rather than MS.

- Specific neuroimaging patterns of white matter abnormality can help distinguish among leukodystrophies and guide genetic testing.

PROGRESSIVE ASYMMETRICAL LIMB IMPAIRMENT AND COGNITIVE DECLINE WITH LEUKOENCEPHALOPATHY

B. Mark Keegan, MD

CASE PRESENTATION

HISTORY AND EXAMINATION

A 41-year-old man sought care for progressive left-sided impairment over many months consistent with progressive left hemiapraxia and left hemiparesis and cognitive decline. He also exhibited features of the alien limb phenomenon, with the left arm grabbing things involuntarily. He had no prior medical disorders and no family history of significant neurologic disorders.

Neurologic evaluation indicated decreased cognitive status with impairments in orientation, construction, and delayed recall. Optic disc evaluation and eye movement evaluation were normal. He demonstrated a spastic upper motor neuron dysarthria and had frontal lobe release findings including a brisk jaw jerk, and bilateral grasp reflexes. He had a mild left hemiparesis in an upper motor neuron fashion and apraxia, of the left side predominantly. Diagnoses considered at the time are shown in Table 56.1.

TESTING

Initial evaluations with brain magnetic resonance imaging (MRI) showed evidence of bilateral, asymmetrical, severe white matter abnormalities, right greater than left hemisphere (Figure 56.1). There was no gadolinium enhancement. Cervical and thoracic spine MRI findings were normal. The MRI white matter abnormalities progressed over serial imaging. Cerebrospinal fluid (CSF) assessment was normal except for increased neuron-specific enolase value, without increased white blood cells, immunoglobulin G index, or unique CSF oligoclonal bands. Serologic and urine testing were entirely negative, including for inherited leukoencephalopathies, fatty acids, inherited mitochondrial disorders, cholesterol esterification, and amino acids. Genetic testing for spinocerebellar ataxia and CADASIL syndrome (cerebral autosomal dominant arteriopathy with subcortical infarcts and leukoencephalopathy) was negative.

A brain biopsy of the right hemispheric white matter showed marked axonal spheroids on hematoxylin and eosin staining, as well as on electron microscopy (Figure 56.2).

DIAGNOSIS

A diagnosis of sporadic, adult-onset, diffuse leukoencephalopathy with axonal spheroids was made.

Table 56.1 | **DIFFERENTIAL DIAGNOSIS FOR THE CASE PATIENT**

POSSIBLE DIAGNOSES	COMMENTS
MS	Normal neuroimaging of the spinal cord, lack of CSF inflammatory markers argue against MS
Adrenoleukodystrophy	Normal analysis of serum very-long-chain fatty acids, lack of family history, age of onset
Metachromatic leukodystrophy	Normal arylsulfatase A
Neuronal intranuclear inclusion disease	Clinical/subclinical EMG for peripheral neuropathy, minority have fever, headache (encephaliticlike episodes), MRI of brain shows cortical ribbon diffusion-weighted abnormalities (vs subcortical)
Adult-onset autosomal-dominant leukodystrophy	No family history, early autonomic dysfunction, or sensorineural hearing loss; presentation is more rapidly progressive without MRI evidence of symmetrical cerebellar abnormality

Abbreviations: CSF, cerebrospinal fluid; EMG, electromyography; MRI, magnetic resonance imaging; MS, multiple sclerosis.

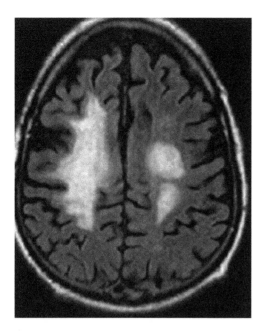

Figure 56.1 **Brain Magnetic Resonance Imaging Findings for the Case Patient.**
Axial fluid-attenuated inversion recovery imaging shows confluent, right greater than left, white matter hyperintensity.
(From Keegan BM, Giannini C, Parisi JE, Lucchinetti CF, Boeve BF, Josephs KA. Sporadic adult-onset leukoencephalopathy with neuroaxonal spheroids mimicking cerebral MS. Neurology. 2008 Mar 25;70[13 Pt 2]:1128-33. Epub 2008 Feb 20; used with permission.)

MANAGEMENT

There are no known treatments for diffuse leukoencephalopathy with axonal spheroids. Treatment is symptomatic only, directed by physical medicine and rehabilitation experts and cognitive experts. Continued rapid worsening of the patient's ambulatory dysfunction over months required increasing use of gait aids, including a cane and wheelchair. He had development of neurogenic bladder dysfunction and pseudobulbar-associated emotional incontinence. His condition progressed leading to death 29 months after onset of his neurologic dysfunction.

DISCUSSION

This case patient had common features of sporadic, adult-onset, diffuse leukoencephalopathy with axonal spheroids, with progressive neurologic degeneration typically over months to a few years, often with substantial asymmetry in presentation. This insidiously progressive central nervous system disease process with typical onset in young adulthood could suggest diseases such as progressive multiple sclerosis, degenerative central nervous system diseases, and other inherited leukoencephalopathies.

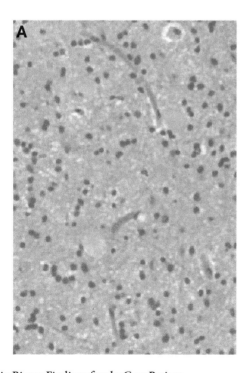
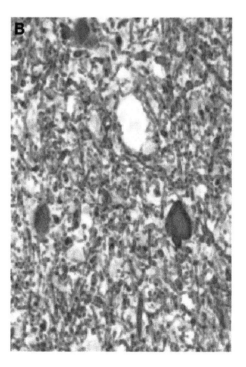

Figure 56.2 **Brain Biopsy Findings for the Case Patient.**
A, On hematoxylin and eosin staining, axonal spheroids are seen as pale eosinophilic globules. B, The pale eosinophilic globules are also apparent on neurofilament immunostain. C and D, Electron microscopy shows the white matter axonal spheroids (also seen in the inset [D] at higher magnification).
(From Keegan BM, Giannini C, Parisi JE, Lucchinetti CF, Boeve BF, Josephs KA. Sporadic adult-onset leukoencephalopathy with neuroaxonal spheroids mimicking cerebral MS. Neurology. 2008 Mar 25;70[13 Pt 2]:1128-33. Epub 2008 Feb 20; used with permission.)

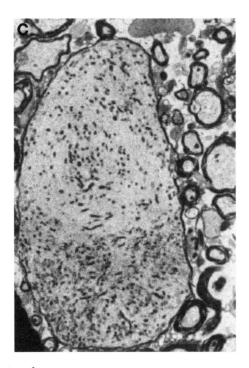
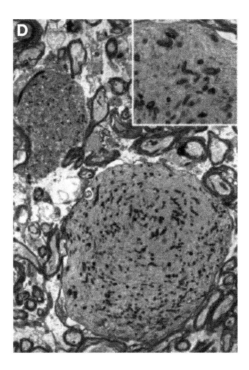

Figure 56.2 **Continued**

Neuroimaging findings show progressive leukoencephalopathy that is also often asymmetrical and without gadolinium enhancement. Some patients with rapid deterioration have evidence of restricted diffusion on diffusion-weighted MRI. Some patients will have calcification within the cortical regions on brain MRI and computed tomography. The cerebellar region is spared in most cases. In addition, MRI of the spinal cord shows that it is intact and unaffected, which may be helpful in distinguishing it from most cases of progressive multiple sclerosis in which spinal cord involvement is common.

The inherited form of diffuse leukoencephalopathy with axonal spheroids has been identified as being caused by sequence variations in the colony-stimulating factor 1 receptor gene. It is currently unclear how many cases of the sporadic form are associated with this genetic abnormality.

KEY POINTS

- Subacute and progressive cortical and subcortical impairment with leukoencephalopathy that is asymmetrical can suggest sporadic, adult-onset, diffuse leukoencephalopathy with axonal spheroids.

- The inherited form of diffuse leukoencephalopathy with axonal spheroids is caused by sequence variations in the colony-stimulating factor 1 receptor gene.

- Genetic testing, instead of brain biopsy, may be performed to diagnose this condition, if suspected.

A WOMAN WITH FEVER, CONFUSION, AND SEIZURES[a]

Michel Toledano, MD

CASE PRESENTATION

HISTORY AND EXAMINATION

A previously healthy 62-year-old woman from Minnesota sought care in late summer for a 4-day history of upper respiratory tract symptoms, intermittent fevers, headache, and a 1-day history of disorientation, word-finding difficulties, and unsteady gait. Upon arrival to the emergency department, she had a witnessed seizure and was intubated because of increased lethargy. Her temperature was 39.4 °C, but she was otherwise hemodynamically stable. Neurologic examination was limited because of the sedation, but she had normal ophthalmoscopic examination findings and antigravity strength in all 4 extremities. Her deep tendon reflexes were brisk, but plantar responses were flexor. She had no rash.

Findings for complete blood cell count, C-reactive protein, erythrocyte sedimentation rate, liver function tests, and chest radiography were unremarkable. Cerebrospinal fluid (CSF) analysis showed a normal glucose value, protein concentration of 82 mg/dL (reference range, ≤35 mg/dL), and mixed pleocytosis with 153 nucleated cells/μL (35% neutrophils, 38% lymphocytes, and 27% monocytes). She had been hiking recently, but her family reported that there were no tick exposures or mosquito bites. She had no history of alcohol or recreational drug use and no recent history of vaccination. Brain magnetic resonance imaging (MRI) showed areas of T2 fluid-attenuated inversion recovery hyperintensity involving primarily the left thalamus and basal ganglia without definitive gadolinium enhancement (Figure 57.1). HIV screen was negative.

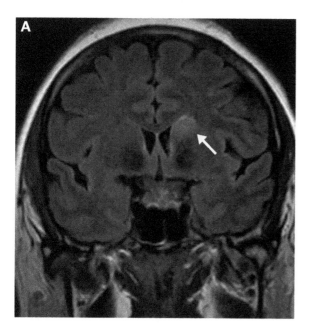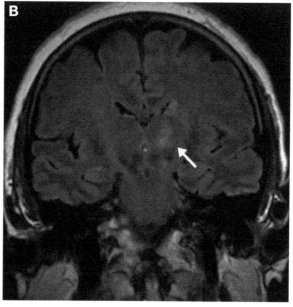

Figure 57.1 **Brain Magnetic Resonance Imaging Findings for the Case Patient.**
Increased T2/fluid-attenuated inversion recovery signal was seen in the left caudate nucleus (A, arrow) and thalamus (B, arrow).

[a] Portions previously published in Toledano M, Davies NWS. Infectious encephalitis: mimics and chameleons. Pract Neurol. 2019 Jun;19(3):225–37. Epub 2019 Mar 16; used with permission.

Table 57.1 DIFFERENTIAL DIAGNOSIS FOR THE CASE PATIENT

POSSIBLE DIAGNOSES	MITIGATING FACTORS
Immune-mediated process	
Acute disseminated encephalomyelitis	Rare in this age group
	No history of vaccination
	Short latency between viral prodromal stage and onset of neurologic symptoms
	No white matter lesions on MRI
Bickerstaff brainstem encephalitis	Marked CSF pleocytosis with polymorphonuclear predominance uncommon
	Absent brainstem findings
Anti–glial fibrillary acidic protein meningoencephalomyelitis	MRI does not show typical perivascular radial gadolinium enhancement in the white matter perpendicular to the ventricle
	No papilledema
Anti–*N*-methyl-D-aspartate receptor encephalitis	Rare in this age group
	No prominent psychiatric symptoms, autonomic dysfunction, or orofacial/limb dyskinesia
	Polymorphonuclear CSF is uncommon
Autoimmune limbic encephalitis	Acute onset
	No mesiotemporal signal change on MRI
	No memory changes or hallucinations
Infectious process	
Viral	
Herpes simplex virus	Brain MRI does not demonstrate classic changes in mesiotemporal structures, insular cortex, and orbitofrontal lobe
Varicella-zoster virus	Not immunocompromised
	Absent zoster rash
Human herpesvirus (HHV)-6, cytomegalovirus (CMV)	Not immunocompromised
	HHV-6 usually affects limbic structures
	CMV more commonly causes a meningoventriculitis or painful polyradiculitis
Enterovirus	Commonly causes meningitis, except in children or immunocompromised adults
Rabies	No history of animal bite
	No hydrophobia
Bacterial	
Rickettsia rickettsii (Rocky Mountain spotted fever), *Anaplasma phagocytophilum*, *Ehrlichia chaffeensis*	No rash
	No thrombocytopenia, jaundice, or increased liver enzymes
Listeria monocytogenes	No hypoglycorrhachia
	No brainstem findings

Abbreviations: CSF, cerebrospinal fluid; MRI, magnetic resonance imaging.

Diagnoses considered at the time are shown in Table 57.1. The initial presentation in this patient was consistent with a clinical diagnosis of encephalitis (fever, behavioral disturbances, focal neurologic deficits, and seizures). Although the acute onset, high fever, and presence of CSF polymorphonuclear cells suggested infection, a postinfectious, paraneoplastic, or idiopathic autoimmune encephalitis was also possible. Systemic infection, toxins, vasculitis, or inherited metabolic disorders are causes of acute encephalopathy, seizures, and fever, but they were considered unlikely in this case given the CSF and MRI findings.

TESTING

CSF Gram stain and bacterial cultures were negative, as was CSF polymerase chain reaction (PCR) testing for herpes simplex virus (HSV), varicella-zoster virus (VZV), and enterovirus. Both serum and CSF were positive for immunoglobulin M antibodies to West Nile virus (WNV). Neural-specific antibody panels in serum and CSF were negative.

DIAGNOSIS

The patient was diagnosed with WNV encephalitis.

MANAGEMENT

After the seizure, the patient was treated with levetiracetam, and empiric antimicrobials (vancomycin, ceftriaxone, ampicillin, and acyclovir) were started for acute meningoencephalitis, along with adjunctive dexamethasone (Figure 57.2). Continuous electroencephalography was obtained because of the persistent encephalopathy and showed no evidence of subclinical seizures. The dexamethasone was stopped after 2 doses because of low suspicion for pneumococcal meningitis, and the antibiotics were discontinued after results of serum and CSF

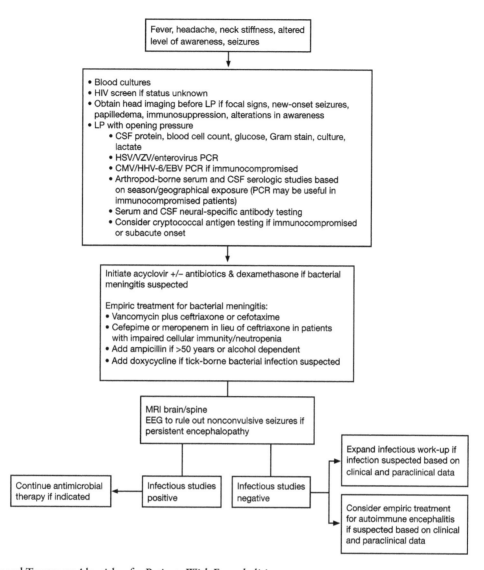

```
┌─────────────────────────────────────┐
│ Fever, headache, neck stiffness, altered │
│ level of awareness, seizures            │
└─────────────────────────────────────┘
```

- Blood cultures
- HIV screen if status unknown
- Obtain head imaging before LP if focal signs, new-onset seizures, papilledema, immunosuppression, alterations in awareness
- LP with opening pressure
  - CSF protein, blood cell count, glucose, Gram stain, culture, lactate
  - HSV/VZV/enterovirus PCR
  - CMV/HHV-6/EBV PCR if immunocompromised
  - Arthropod-borne serum and CSF serologic studies based on season/geographical exposure (PCR may be useful in immunocompromised patients)
  - Serum and CSF neural-specific antibody testing
  - Consider cryptococcal antigen testing if immunocompromised or subacute onset

Initiate acyclovir +/– antibiotics & dexamethasone if bacterial meningitis suspected

Empiric treatment for bacterial meningitis:
- Vancomycin plus ceftriaxone or cefotaxime
- Cefepime or meropenem in lieu of ceftriaxone in patients with impaired cellular immunity/neutropenia
- Add ampicillin if >50 years or alcohol dependent
- Add doxycycline if tick-borne bacterial infection suspected

MRI brain/spine
EEG to rule out nonconvulsive seizures if persistent encephalopathy

Continue antimicrobial therapy if indicated

Infectious studies positive

Infectious studies negative

Expand infectious work-up if infection suspected based on clinical and paraclinical data

Consider empiric treatment for autoimmune encephalitis if suspected based on clinical and paraclinical data

Figure 57.2 **Testing and Treatment Algorithm for Patients With Encephalitis.**
CMV indicates cytomegalovirus; CSF, cerebrospinal fluid; EBV, Epstein-Barr virus; EEG, electroencephalography; HHV-6, human herpesvirus-6; HSV, herpes simplex virus; LP, lumbar puncture; MRI, magnetic resonance imaging; PCR, polymerase chain reaction; VZV, varicella-zoster virus.

cultures were negative for bacteria (48 hours). Acyclovir was stopped after the PCR results were negative for HSV and VZV.

The patient was successfully extubated 3 days after admission. As her encephalopathy improved, she was noted to have parkinsonism, with abulia, hypomimia, and hypokinetic dysarthria, as well as flaccid left hemiparesis and areflexia. Spinal cord MRI findings were normal. Electromyography showed a diffuse subacute disorder of anterior horn cells, most profoundly affecting the left cervical myotomes. A trial of carbidopa/levodopa did not result in significant improvement of her abulia. Ultimately, despite gradual improvement in her right upper extremity function, she required placement in a skilled nursing facility owing to persistent cognitive and motor disability.

DISCUSSION

Viruses cause most cases of infectious encephalitis in immunocompetent hosts, but bacteria (especially intracellular organisms such as *Rickettsiae*), as well as fungi and parasites, can cause a similar clinical picture. Viral encephalitis can be sporadic, as

with HSV, or epidemic, as with some arthropod-borne viruses. Geography, season, and patient age, immunocompetence, and socioeconomic factors define the range of potential pathogens and should guide infectious workup. An HIV screen should be obtained in all patients with encephalitis because HIV predisposes patients to opportunistic infections and can itself cause meningoencephalitis during acute infection.

The pattern of neurologic involvement also provides important clues. HSV-1, the most common cause of sporadic encephalitis, preferentially affects the mesiotemporal, orbitofrontal, and insular regions. Deep gray matter involvement, sometimes resulting in parkinsonism, is more common with flavivirus infections, such as WNV. Brainstem encephalitis, characterized by cranial neuropathies, dysautonomia, and myoclonus, may be observed with certain arthropod-borne viruses, enteroviruses, as well as listeriosis and brucellosis. Encephalomyelitis presenting with acute flaccid paralysis can occur with enteroviruses such as enterovirus A71, as well as flaviviruses such as WNV. HSV-2, VZV, and cytomegalovirus infections can present with myeloradiculitis.

The CSF profile can help distinguish between different causes of encephalitis. Lymphocytic-predominant pleocytosis is typical of viral encephalitis, although polymorphonuclear cells may predominate early in the disease. Certain bacterial and mycobacterial infections such as listeriosis, brucellosis, and tuberculosis also show a lymphocytic predominance, but these are usually associated with higher protein level, hypoglycorrhachia, and increased CSF lactate concentration. The CSF profile of immune-mediated encephalitis mimics that of viral encephalitis, but neutrophilic predominance would be atypical. Acellular CSF (common in autoimmune encephalitis) is rare in infectious encephalitis, although it is possible early in the disease course or in immunosuppressed patients.

Arthropod-borne viruses (arboviruses) are transmitted to humans by the bite of a mosquito or tick. WNV, a flavivirus, is the leading cause of neuroinvasive arboviral disease in the continental United States. Other arboviruses such as Powassan, La Crosse, or St. Louis encephalitis virus can also cause neuroinvasive disease. In general, viremia is short lived with most of these viruses, and PCR of the serum and the CSF are insensitive diagnostic tests. Diagnosis is usually established by demonstrating the presence of immunoglobulin M antibodies in serum or CSF. Serologic tests, however, can be falsely negative in patients with congenital or acquired humoral deficiency (eg, patients on B-cell–depleting therapies such as rituximab), and PCR is usually needed to establish the diagnosis in these cases. Treatment is supportive care.

KEY POINTS

- Persistent high fever and neutrophilic-predominant pleocytosis favors infectious over autoimmune encephalitis.

- Viruses cause most cases of infectious encephalitis in immunocompetent hosts.

- HSV-1 is the most common cause of sporadic encephalitis.

- Serologic testing is more sensitive than PCR when evaluating patients with suspected arthropod-borne viral meningoencephalitis. PCR may be useful in immunocompromised patients, particularly those with congenital or acquired humoral immunodeficiency.

ENCEPHALOPATHY WITH ALTERNATING HEMISPHERIC MRI ABNORMALITIES

Andrew McKeon, MB, BCh, MD

CASE PRESENTATION

HISTORY AND EXAMINATION

A 21-year-old woman with a long-standing history of migraine sought care at her local provider for a 1-week history of confusion and mixing up her words. She then had a witnessed seizure, with dyscognitive features and secondary generalization. On hospitalization, electroencephalography (EEG) demonstrated left temporal theta slowing and sharp waves. Magnetic resonance imaging (MRI) showed patchy T2-signal abnormality, nonenhancing, in the left temporal region (only a report was available). General blood tests were normal or negative, including vitamin B_{12} and folate levels and thyroid function tests. Thyroid peroxidase antibodies were increased at 271 IU/mL (reference range, <9 IU/mL). A diagnosis of an autoimmune encephalopathy was made, and the patient was treated with phenytoin, levetiracetam, and high-dose corticosteroids (1,000 mg intravenous methylprednisolone daily for 5 days), followed by a slow oral prednisone taper. The patient improved cognitively but had considerable emotional lability and an increase in headache frequency and severity and, thus, sought a second opinion.

Neurologic examination at Mayo Clinic indicated an amnestic syndrome; she lost 3 of 4 points for 5-minute recall on the Kokmen short test of mental status. Her examination also indicated short stature compared with that of her parents. EEG and MRI findings at that time were normal. Thyroid peroxidase antibodies again were increased to 17.6 IU/mL, but thyrotropin value was normal. Neural serologic and cerebrospinal fluid (CSF) autoantibody evaluations were negative. Her CSF protein concentration was mildly increased at 47 mg/dL (reference range, ≤35 mg/dL). Blood cell counts, immunoglobulin G index, oligoclonal bands, and immunoglobulin G synthesis rate in the CSF were all within normal limits.

Because follow-up brain MRI and CSF findings were normal, further immunotherapy was not pursued, except for completion of the oral prednisone taper. Two months later, the patient's symptoms relapsed (she had a seizure with preceding aura of vision loss, cognitive symptoms, and headache), but new proximal upper and lower extremity weakness also developed. Repeated MRI showed T2/fluid-attenuated inversion recovery and diffusion-weighted T2-signal abnormality in the right posterior temporal lobe region, without restricted diffusion or enhancement (Figure 58.1). The patient was treated empirically with corticosteroids and azathioprine for presumed relapsing autoimmune encephalitis. The encephalopathy and seizures persisted.

Diagnoses considered at the time included autoimmune encephalopathy, although the radiologic appearance was not typical for acute disseminated encephalomyelitis, multiple sclerosis, or limbic encephalitis. The migratory radiologic abnormalities were considered atypical for abscess or neoplasia but potentially consistent with a mitochondrial disorder. The patient's mother (and other maternal relatives) were reported to be healthy without histories of diabetes, deafness, muscle weakness, neurologic symptoms, or cardiomyopathy. Taking other factors into account (migraine history, short stature, radiologic findings, and lack of response to immunotherapy), mitochondrial encephalopathy, lactic acidosis, and stroke-like episodes (MELAS syndrome) was considered.

TESTING

Blood was drawn for genetic testing. The patient died in her sleep a short time later, most likely in the context of sudden unexplained death in epilepsy.

DIAGNOSIS

Her genetic testing results became available 1 month later, which showed findings consistent with MELAS syndrome: heteroplasmic sequence variation m.3243A>G (tRNA Leu) and homoplasmic rare variant m.2294A>G (16S rRNA).

DISCUSSION

Encephalopathy or encephalitis of subacute onset with fluctuating course is not unique to autoimmune encephalitis. Common acquired metabolic disorders must be considered

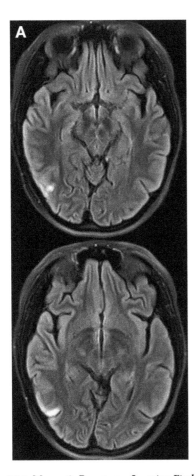 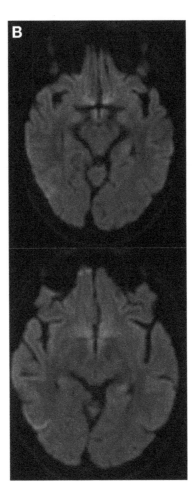 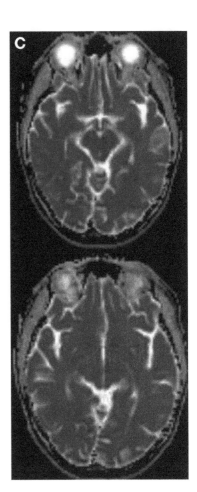

Figure 58.1 Magnetic Resonance Imaging Findings for the Case Patient.
Axial brain images at 2 levels (top and bottom) through the posterior temporal lobes. Images are A, T2/fluid-attenuated inversion recovery (FLAIR); B, diffusion-weighted imaging (DWI); and C, apparent diffusion coefficient imaging (ADC). Abnormal increased T2/FLAIR signal was observed in the posterior right temporal lobe, without true diffusion restriction (hyperintense on DWI, but not hypointense on ADC).

and excluded in all cases, such as deficiencies of vitamin B_{12} and folate, hypothyroidism, sepsis, and central nervous system–active medications. Herpes zoster encephalitis could result in seizures and neocortical temporal lobe abnormalities but would progress rapidly to necrosis and not remit spontaneously. Less common hereditary disorders should be considered in some cases, depending on patient age and presentation. These include inborn errors of metabolism, lysosomal storage disease, peroxisomal disorders, and mitochondrial cytopathies.

MELAS syndrome is a maternally inherited multisystem disorder caused by sequence variations in mitochondrial DNA. Stroke-like episodes are the hallmark of MELAS syndrome and may result in hemiparesis, hemianopia, or cortical blindness. Other common features include seizures (focal or generalized), recurrent migrainelike headaches, vomiting, short stature, hearing loss, and muscle weakness. Diverse tRNA sequence variations underlie MELAS syndrome, although 80% of cases are caused by m.3243A>G and 10% by m.3271T>C tRNA variation. Diagnostic clues may emanate from patient and family history, examination, increased lactate and pyruvate levels in plasma and CSF, and findings on brain MRI and magnetic resonance spectroscopy (evaluating

for a lactate peak), EEG, electromyography, and muscle biopsy (evaluating for ragged red fibers).

The stroke-like episodes that occur in patients with MELAS syndrome are characterized by an acute onset of neurologic symptoms with hyperintense lesions on diffusion-weighted brain MRI. These episodes are different from typical ischemic strokes and thus are called "stroke-like" for several reasons. The brain lesions do not respect vascular territories, and apparent diffusion coefficient on MRI is not decreased (as it would be in true infarction). Apparent diffusion coefficient is typically increased or has a mixed pattern. The acute MRI signal changes are not static and may migrate, fluctuate, or resolve quickly, atypical for ischemic stroke. Indeed, patients may have apparent, but misleading, responses to immunotherapy, most likely coinciding with spontaneous remissions typical of MELAS syndrome. Thyroid autoantibodies, in the right clinical context, may be a clue to an autoimmune diagnosis but are also common in the general healthy population.

MELAS syndrome usually manifests first in childhood after normal early development. A relapsing-remitting course is most common, with stroke-like episodes leading to progressive neurologic dysfunction and dementia. Variations in the DNA polymerase γ gene (*POLG*) have also been associated with stroke-like episodes in childhood or adulthood with predominant involvement of the occipital lobes.

- The differential diagnostic considerations for encephalopathy should be broad and not include only autoimmune disorders.

- Clues to MELAS syndrome include fluctuating, migrating, T2-signal abnormalities on brain MRI in the context of stroke-like episodes, as well as more generic features of encephalopathy.

- Blood genetic testing for mitochondrial DNA sequence variations is diagnostic. Testing for *POLG* (somatic DNA) variations should be considered if mitochondrial genetic testing is negative.

RAPID-ONSET HEMIBODY SENSORY LOSS, INCOORDINATION, AND MUSCLE JERKING

Andrew McKeon, MB, BCh, MD, and Nicholas L. Zalewski, MD

CASE PRESENTATION

HISTORY AND EXAMINATION

A 61-year-old woman with no pertinent medical history had progressive decline in multiple neurologic domains over the course of 2 months. Initially, she had development of progressive sensory loss in her left foot that subsequently spread up the left lower extremity and into the left upper extremity; this was accompanied by a sense of unsteadiness, with progression week by week. Later, jerky movements of the left leg occurred while she was lying supine and sometimes when walking, which resulted in falls. At times, her left hand would wander involuntarily. Later in the course of her symptoms, mild short-term memory loss was also noted by her husband. There was no family history of dementia. On examination including the Kokmen short test of mental status, she was unable to recall her home address, but findings were otherwise normal. She had mild gaze-evoked nystagmus and significant saccadic intrusion of smooth pursuits. A mild upper motor pattern of weakness, action myoclonus, hyperreflexia, and moderate loss of vibration was present on the left. Gait was markedly ataxic.

For the differential diagnosis, given the subacute onset and rapid progression of multiple neurologic symptoms, vascular, neoplastic, infectious, and autoimmune causes were initially considered. Succinct clinical localization of deficits was initially difficult, and magnetic resonance imaging (MRI) of the brain and spine (at 1 month) did not indicate any clear abnormalities to help focus the localization and differential diagnosis. Cerebrospinal fluid (CSF) testing was normal, including blood cell count, immunoglobulin G (IgG) index and synthesis rate, oligoclonal bands, and extended infectious workup.

Ultimately, clinical reevaluation showed new development of ideomotor apraxia, alien limb phenomenon, and tactile neglect of the left upper limb. With this progression of clinical findings, particularly the alien limb phenomenon, a component of the disorder was demonstrating localization in the right parietal cortex, whereas additional examination features (nystagmus, ataxia) supported cerebellar involvement.

Recognition of the alien limb phenomenon led to close consideration of the most common causes of this syndrome: corticobasal syndrome, stroke, and Creutzfeldt-Jakob disease (CJD). The rate of progression was atypical for corticobasal syndrome (a degenerative disorder caused by tau or Alzheimer pathology), and the patient did not have a clinical presentation or MRI findings consistent with a stroke. The multifocal cerebral localization, subacute decline, action myoclonus, and alien limb phenomenon raised strong suspicion for CJD. Further review with the patient and family revealed no family history of prion disease or risk factors for an acquired prion disease.

TESTING

Repeated MRI of the brain 2 months after illness onset showed right parietal cortical hyperintense signal on diffusion-weighted imaging (DWI) consistent with cortical ribboning (Figure 59.1), a common diagnostic finding early in the course of prion disease. Although characteristic of prion disease, similar imaging findings have been reported in autoimmune encephalitis (eg, autoantibodies to voltage-gated potassium channels or α-amino-3-hydroxy-5-methyl-4-isoxazolepropionic acid [AMPA] receptor) and in the postictal setting. However, the putamen and caudate nucleus also demonstrated subtle asymmetric DWI hyperintense signal, which in the clinicoradiologic context is highly specific for prion disease. Electroencephalography (EEG) showed frequent sharp wave discharges over right posterior temporal and left occipital head regions, along with frontal intermittent rhythmic delta slowing, consistent with encephalopathy (not otherwise specified). Autoimmune encephalopathy antibody evaluations in the serum and CSF were normal. Real-time quaking-induced conversion (RT-QuIC) testing of CSF was positive for misfolded prion proteins.

DIAGNOSIS

The positive RT-QuIC result confirmed a diagnosis of sporadic CJD (sCJD).

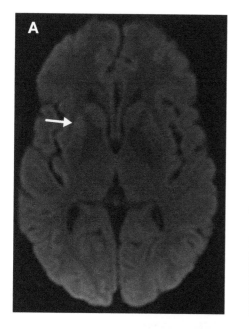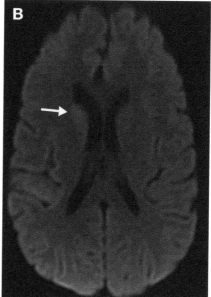

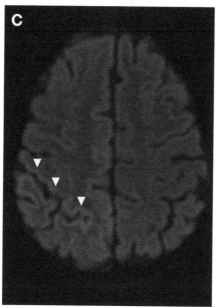

Figure 59.1 **Brain Magnetic Resonance Imaging Findings for the Case Patient.**
Axial diffusion-weighted imaging demonstrates subtle hyperintense signal in the right putamen (A, arrow), right caudate head (B, arrow), and right parietal cortex (C, arrowheads).

MANAGEMENT

The patient's treatment was palliative. Hospice services implemented a home palliation program. Clonazepam was prescribed to reduce myoclonus. The patient died 18 weeks after onset of her neurologic symptoms.

DISCUSSION

The differential diagnosis of a rapidly progressive multifocal neurologic syndrome includes many considerations but can be focused in complex situations by first confirming lesion localization and characterization with neuroimaging or other objective studies (eg, electromyography). However, if imaging findings are normal despite clear objective deficits localizing to a particular region of the central nervous system, several important questions should be considered: Is the imaging adequate? Has a small lesion(s) been missed? Is the localization correct? Is this an entity that can sometimes demonstrate normal imaging despite substantial deficits (autoimmune, neurodegenerative, toxic-metabolic, viral, functional)?

When the case patient had clear signs of cerebellar/brainstem involvement (gaze-evoked nystagmus with ataxia) with no clear explanatory imaging abnormality, a close review of these considerations was key. Close assessment for the left-sided sensory deficits required a detailed review of imaging by following the entire sensory pathway from the left-sided nerve roots to the postcentral gyrus, which ultimately showed cortical ribboning in the right parietal cortex. This diagnostic imaging finding was additionally corroborated by other right-sided parietal deficits (alien limb phenomenon, tactile neglect, action myoclonus). Cortical ribboning in a patient with sub-acute neurologic decline and cerebellar ataxia was strongly suggestive of CJD, which was ultimately confirmed with CSF RT-QuIC testing.

sCJD is a prion disease that typically presents as a rapidly progressive dementia with various accompanying focal cerebral neurologic deficits and eventually myoclonus. The peak age of onset is 55 to 75 years (median, 67 years). sCJD accounts for the majority of cases (≈90%), with an incidence of about 1 per million persons, but other forms of prion disease include genetic (genetic CJD, fatal familial insomnia, and Gerstmann-Sträussler-Scheinker syndrome) and acquired (Kuru, iatrogenic, variant CJD) causes. Although brain MRI in sCJD demonstrates diffusion restriction in cortical and/or deep gray matter with a sensitivity and specificity of approximately 90% to 95%, mimickers can have similar MRI abnormalities. Autoimmune encephalitides, particularly with antibodies targeting voltage-gated potassium channels (leucine-rich, glioma-inactivated protein 1–IgG and contactin-associated protein 2–IgG) and AMPA receptors, may show cortical ribboning on MRI (although without deep nuclear involvement) and, thus, should be excluded when considering a diagnosis of CJD. Occasionally, diffuse Lewy body disease and Alzheimer disease can present as rapidly progressive dementia, although the time frame of decline is longer than the 18 weeks our patient experienced. Positron tomography/computed tomography can be used to evaluate for patterns of brain metabolism characteristic of those 2 disorders.

Although increased levels of CSF 14-3-3 protein, neuron-specific enolase, and tau have primarily been used as diagnostic tests to support CJD in the past, the sensitivity and specificity of these tests are low, and the recent development and clinical use of CSF RT-QuIC testing has become the standard diagnostic test in the evaluation of CJD (≈90%-95% sensitive,

98% specific). Notably, the Centers for Disease Control and Prevention diagnostic criteria now include positive RT-QuIC findings in CSF or other tissues, along with a neuropsychiatric disorder, as consistent with a probable diagnosis of sCJD. However, components of the previous criteria are still used in the current criteria to make a probable diagnosis of sCJD; these include rapidly progressive dementia, 2 of 4 additional clinical features (myoclonus, visual or cerebellar dysfunction, pyramid dysfunction or extrapyramidal dysfunction, or akinetic mutism), a supportive finding on 1 or more tests (EEG with periodic sharp wave complexes, increased 14-3-3 protein level, MRI with typical hyperintensity pattern [T2/fluid-attenuated inversion recovery or DWI]), and no findings suggestive of an alternative diagnosis. The additional criteria especially help serve as a framework in patients with negative RT-QuIC testing and with strong clinical and radiographic suspicion for prion disease, because certain prion protein genotypes may be more frequently associated with normal RT-QuIC testing. Pathologic findings typical of CJD on brain biopsy or autopsy remain the standard for confirming diagnosis when necessary.

KEY POINTS

- The differential diagnosis for rapidly progressive dementia includes vascular, neoplastic, infectious, autoimmune, neurodegenerative, and prion diseases.

- A comprehensive evaluation for rapidly progressive cognitive decline includes brain MRI (including DWI), positron emission tomography/computed tomography of the brain, EEG, antibody testing of serum and CSF, and RT-QuIC testing of CSF.

- DWI (deep nuclear and cortical DWI changes) has high sensitivity and specificity for sCJD, but findings may be subtle early in the course. RT-QuIC prion testing of CSF is highly sensitive and specific to help confirm the suspected diagnosis.

A HISTORY OF SARCOIDOSIS AND A NEW BRAIN LESION

Andrew McKeon, MB, BCh, MD, and Julie E. Hammack, MD

CASE PRESENTATION

HISTORY AND EXAMINATION

A 59-year-old man with long-standing hypertension sought a second opinion for a left-sided posterior headache and aphasia of approximately 1 week's duration. The acuity of onset was unclear from the provided history. He had a mild fever at onset, which subsequently resolved. Eight months before neurologic symptom presentation, he was febrile with night sweats, 22.7-kg (50-lb) weight loss, arthralgias, dyspnea, and wheezing. Bronchoscopy and hilar lymph node biopsy showed noncaseating granulomatous inflammation consistent with pulmonary sarcoidosis. Remotely, as a teenager, given exposure to a family member with active pulmonary tuberculosis infection, he had a purified protein derivative skin test, which was positive; he received 6 months of isoniazid treatment. His father was suspected to have had heart disease and died in his sleep after 1 week of chest pain, but no autopsy proved this definitively. The patient's sister had proven hypertrophic cardiomyopathy (HCM). On examination, he was aphasic but had an otherwise normal neurologic examination.

Diagnostic considerations included central nervous system sarcoidosis, metastatic neoplasm, and stroke (secondary to vasculitis, embolic stroke, or venous infarction). Magnetic resonance angiography and venography of cerebral vessels showed negative findings. Because of the patient's history of sarcoidosis and the atypical clinicoradiologic presentation, brain biopsy was undertaken and showed evidence of subacute infarction, without evidence of vasculitis or sarcoidosis. Transthoracic echocardiography showed concentric left ventricular wall thickening consistent with HCM. Cardiac magnetic resonance imaging (MRI) indicated HCM, left ventricular apical thrombus, and left ventricular apical aneurysm.

TESTING

Brain MRI performed at hospital admission (1 week after symptom onset) showed extensive T2 signal abnormality in the left temporal neocortex, with vasogenic edema, and abnormal gyriform gadolinium enhancement (Figure 60.1A and 60.1B).

There was no restricted diffusion in the left temporal lobe on diffusion-weighted imaging (DWI), but an apparent diffusion coefficient (ADC) map showed a gyriform hypointense pattern (Figure 60.1C and 60.1D). Prior outside MRI obtained 1 day into the patient's symptoms showed similar findings on T2/fluid-attenuated inversion recovery and T1 postgadolinium images but also gyriform hyperintensity on DWI, with hypointensity on ADC map in the same region (Figure 60.1 E-H).

DIAGNOSIS

The patient was diagnosed with subacute cerebral infarction in the context of cardioembolic disease secondary to hereditary HCM.

MANAGEMENT

As a result of the findings and diagnosis, the patient received an implantable cardioverter-defibrillator and was treated with warfarin, aiming for an international normalized ratio of 2.0 to 3.0 to reduce the risk of recurrent cardioembolic disease.

DISCUSSION

The patient had a subacute ischemic stroke mimicking a brain mass radiologically. The acuity of symptom onset could have been a key clinical clue in this case but was absent from the patient history. Patients with stroke typically have hyperacute symptom onset (over seconds to minutes). Autoimmune and inflammatory central nervous system disease symptoms tend to have subacute evolution (over days to weeks) or might be chronic (over months). Radiologic findings of hypointensity on ADC map and, at least on his initial scan, corresponding hyperintensity on DWI, were additional salient findings, which prompted suspicion for stroke. Evaluating DWI (hyperintense or bright) and ADC (hypointense or dark) sequences, in addition to T2 and T1 postgadolinium images, can assist in evaluating for the possibility of subacute infarction. Ischemic strokes tend to be bright on DWI and dark on ADC (diffusion restriction). Brain abscesses may have a similar appearance on DWI and ADC but also demonstrate diffuse T2 hyperintensity and

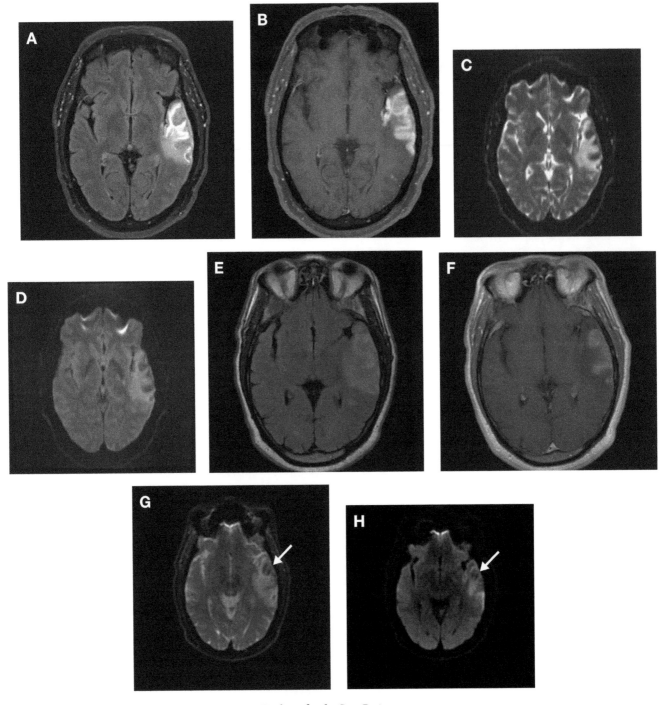

Figure 60.1 **Axial Brain Magnetic Resonance Imaging Findings for the Case Patient.**

A-D, Images obtained at hospital admission (approximately 1 week after symptom onset) showed (A) extensive left temporal neocortical T2/fluid-attenuated inversion recovery (FLAIR) hyperintensity, (B) postgadolinium T1 enhancement, and (C) gyriform hypointensity on apparent diffusion coefficient (ADC) map, but (D) no specific findings on diffusion-weighted imaging (DWI). E-H, Earlier imaging obtained at the outside hospital. At that time, imaging demonstrated similar findings on T2/FLAIR (E) and T1 postgadolinium images (F). The gyriform hypointensity on ADC map (G) and T2 hyperintensity on DWI imaging (H) were suspicious for stroke (arrows).

ring enhancement post gadolinium. Brain tumors tend to be bright on both DWI and ADC.

Because of the history of sarcoidosis and the masslike appearance of the left temporal abnormality radiologically, the patient underwent brain biopsy, which ultimately demonstrated ischemic findings alone at histologic examination.

KEY POINTS

- A subacute infarct can mimic brain mass lesions, including inflammatory diagnoses.

- Close attention to the onset of clinical symptoms and ADC and DWI images can aid in diagnosis.

HEADACHE AND HEMIPARESIS IN MIDDLE AGE

Catalina Sanchez Alvarez, MD, and Kenneth J. Warrington, MD

CASE PRESENTATION

HISTORY AND EXAMINATION

A 53-year-old man with a medical history of hypertension, hyperlipidemia, and a remote, cryptogenic, multifocal, posterior circulation ischemic stroke, came to the emergency department with 1 day of vertigo, ataxic gait, nausea, occipital headache, and painless binocular diplopia. Symptoms were present upon awakening on the day of presentation and progressed throughout the day.

While he was in the emergency department, his blood pressure was 130/80 mm Hg, heart rate was 66 beats/min, and respiratory rate was 16 breaths/min. On examination, he was alert, oriented, and without aphasia or dysarthria. Pupils were round and reactive to light; there was weak adduction of the left eye with dysconjugate nystagmus of the right eye during rightward gaze consistent with a left internuclear ophthalmoplegia. He had mild left arm and bilateral leg spasticity and lower extremity symmetrical hyperreflexia, poor tandem gait, negative Romberg sign, and normal limb coordination and sensory examination findings. Diagnoses considered at the time are shown in Table 61.1.

TESTING

Complete blood cell count and kidney function were normal. The erythrocyte sedimentation rate was 10 mm/h and C-reactive protein level was less than 3 mg/L. Head computed tomography without contrast showed no acute findings. Cerebrospinal fluid examination indicated mild lymphocytic pleocytosis with 9 cells/μL (reference range, 0-5/μL), protein value of 45 mg/dL (reference range, ≤35 mg/dL), and glucose level within normal limits. Cytologic analysis was negative for cancer. Extensive workup for infection was negative. Autoimmune serologic testing, including for antibodies to extractable nuclear antigen and cyclic citrullinated peptide, rheumatoid factor, antinuclear antibody, antineutrophil cytoplasmic antibody, and antiphospholipid panel, was negative. Brain magnetic resonance imaging (MRI) and magnetic resonance angiography (MRA) with contrast demonstrated a left caudate head infarction and leptomeningeal and perivascular enhancement involving bilateral temporal lobes, basal ganglia, and frontal lobes (Figure 61.1). Right middle cerebral artery wall enhancement was also noted. Conventional cerebral angiography showed diffuse dilatation and mural irregularity of the right middle cerebral artery M1 segment, as well as dilatation of the first 2 mm of the left anterior cerebral artery A1 segment. These findings were associated with vessel wall gadolinium enhancement on MRI, which raised concern for vasculitis.

Serum angiotensin-converting enzyme level (22 U/L) and calcium level (9.1 mg/dL) were normal. Computed tomography of the chest, abdomen, and pelvis showed no

Table 61.1 **DIFFERENTIAL DIAGNOSIS FOR INTERNUCLEAR OPHTHALMOPLEGIA (INO) IN THE CASE PATIENT**

POSSIBLE DIAGNOSES	COMMENT
Multiple sclerosis	Bilateral in most cases; associated with incomplete and slowed adduction; no prior episodes of demyelinating disease (eg, optic neuritis, inflammatory myelopathy)
Brainstem stroke (cerebrovascular disease, giant cell arteritis, primary central nervous system vasculitis)	Stroke and cerebrovascular disease is the most common cause of INO in middle-aged and older persons; INO is unilateral in most cases
Pseudo-INO of myasthenia gravis	No history of fatigable diplopia, dysphagia, dysarthria, ptosis, or generalized motor weakness
Pseudo-INO of Miller Fisher syndrome	Variant of Guillain-Barré syndrome (acute inflammatory demyelinating polyradiculoneuropathy); characterized by ophthalmoplegia, areflexia, and ataxia

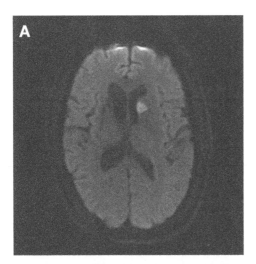

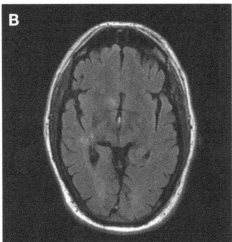

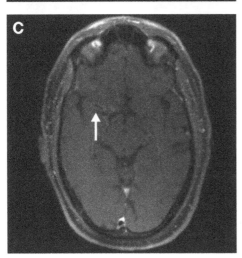

Figure 61.1 Brain Magnetic Resonance Imaging Findings for the Case Patient.
Axial sequences show (A) a left caudate infarct (diffusion-weighted imaging), (B) diffuse, nonspecific T2-signal abnormality (T2/fluid-attenuated inversion recovery), and (C) leptomeningeal and perivascular enhancement (right middle cerebral artery [arrow]; T1 post gadolinium).

evidence of malignancy or pulmonary findings suggestive of sarcoidosis. The patient was up to date on age-appropriate cancer screening. Transthoracic echocardiography indicated no abnormalities, and no dysrhythmias were recorded.

The patient was diagnosed with primary angiitis of the central nervous system (PACNS). The diagnosis was based on the presence of multiple ischemic infarcts, without cardioembolic source, abnormal brain MRI and MRA findings consistent with vasculitis, and the absence of systemic vasculitis, infection, and cancer.

MANAGEMENT

After diagnosis, the patient was started on intravenous methylprednisolone 1,000 mg for 3 consecutive days, followed by oral prednisone 60 mg daily and intravenous cyclophosphamide 0.75 g/m^2 once monthly for 6 months. Because of some new areas of enhancement on MRI, the patient was subsequently treated with rituximab, 1 g, 2 doses, 2 weeks apart, every 6 months. Clinical and radiologic remission was achieved, although the patient had permanent residual gait difficulties.

DISCUSSION

Central nervous system (CNS) vasculitis is an inflammatory process of the blood vessels in the brain, meninges, and spinal cord. It is called *PACNS* when the process is limited to the brain and, rarely, the spinal cord. In other circumstances, CNS vasculitis can be secondary to a systemic inflammatory syndrome or infectious process. Its incidence has been reported as 2.4 cases per 1 million person-years. The median age at onset is 50 years, and prevalence is equal in men and women.

The most common symptoms at presentation are headache, focal weakness, and altered cognition. Multiple strokes and transient ischemic attacks are present in more than half the patients with PACNS. Systemic symptoms such as fever, malaise, and weight loss are usually absent and if present should raise concern for a systemic process. If meninges are involved, PACNS presents as leptomeningitis.

Blood testing, including for acute phase proteins and autoantibodies, is generally unrevealing but assists in excluding other forms of autoimmune disease such as systemic vasculitis or systemic lupus erythematosus. Cerebrospinal fluid findings, however, are abnormal in 80% to 90% of patients with documented disease, generally showing an aseptic meningitis pattern with lymphocytic pleocytosis, increased protein concentration, and normal glucose values.

Neuroimaging findings are variable but include ischemic lesions in multiple vascular territories, blood vessel irregularities, arterial stenosis, tumorlike lesions, and leptomeningeal enhancement. On MRI, concentric vessel wall enhancement may be seen. Angiographic findings suggestive of vasculitis include alternating areas of narrowing and dilatation (beading) and areas of arterial occlusion in the absence of proximal atherosclerosis. Angiographic findings should be correlated clinically and with laboratory and MRI and MRA findings. Many patients are diagnosed on the basis of conventional cerebral angiography findings.

Meningeal and cerebral biopsy is commonly used to ensure the diagnosis and exclude infectious and neoplastic causes,

Table 61.2 | PRIMARY ANGIITIS OF THE CNS (PACNS) AND ITS MIMICKERS

DIAGNOSIS	DESCRIPTION
PACNS	Insidious onset; progressive headache and neurologic abnormalities; CSF with pleocytosis and increased protein concentration; angiography and MRI/MRA usually abnormal, demonstrating arterial irregularities with stenosis and enhancement; treatment with glucocorticoids and immunosuppressive medications
Intracranial atherosclerosis and cardioembolic strokes	More common than PACNS and can affect multiple vascular territories; age at presentation is generally older than 65 years; patients have multiple cardiovascular risk factors; usually noninflammatory CSF
Reversible cerebral vasoconstriction syndrome	Acute onset; characterized by a thunderclap headache in association with neurologic deficits and occasionally seizures; most frequent in women in the postpartum period or after exposure to vasoactive medications; multifocal segmental vasoconstriction is present on angiography or MRA, which spontaneously resolves over the following 3 months; usually noninflammatory CSF; treated with calcium channel blockers and discontinuation of vasoconstrictors
Cerebral amyloid angiopathy	Subacute onset; characterized by cognitive decline, headaches, and seizures; amyloid deposition leads to vessel fragility, which leads to intracerebral hemorrhages; associated vascular inflammation and response to immunosuppressive therapy; amyloid-β–related angiitis is considered by some to be a subset of PACNS
Susac syndrome	Microvascular disorder characterized by lesions in the corpus callosum, sensorineural hearing loss, and vision loss due to branch retinal artery occlusions

Abbreviations: CNS, central nervous system; CSF, cerebrospinal fluid; MRA, magnetic resonance angiography; MRI, magnetic resonance imaging.

with neuroimaging abnormalities identifying an appropriate neurosurgical target. Transmural vascular inflammation is the diagnostic standard for CNS vasculitis. The most common histopathologic pattern is granulomatous, followed by lymphocytic and necrotizing inflammation.

The diagnostic criteria proposed by Calabrese and Mallek include the presence of an acquired, otherwise unexplained, neuropsychiatric deficit; classic histopathologic or angiographic features of vasculitis; and the absence of systemic vasculitis. All criteria must be met for a diagnosis to be made.

When assessing a patient with possible PACNS, it is critical to rule out infections that can cause infectious angiitis; hematologic cancers, particularly lymphoma, which can cause leptomeningeal lesions and ischemic strokes; systemic autoimmune diseases; and other mimickers listed in Table 61.2.

Glucocorticoids alone or in association with cyclophosphamide have been the cornerstone of treatment in PACNS. Remission induction treatment should be initiated promptly to prevent further accrual of tissue damage due to vasculitis. Generally, patients are treated with pulse-dose glucocorticoids: 1,000 mg intravenous methylprednisolone daily for 3 days, followed by oral prednisone 1 mg/kg for 4 weeks, with a subsequent taper over 9 to 12 months depending on clinical progress. Cyclophosphamide can be given as intravenous monthly pulses or orally daily and is generally continued for 3 to 6 months. After remission is achieved, cyclophosphamide can be switched to azathioprine (1-2 mg/kg per day), mycophenolate mofetil (1-2 g/d), or methotrexate (20-25 mg/wk) for maintenance therapy. B-cell depletion with rituximab has

been reported to be of benefit in small case series, but further studies are required. All patients should receive prophylaxis against *Pneumocystis jirovecii* infection and prophylactic treatment for corticosteroid-induced bone loss.

MRI should be performed 4 to 6 weeks after starting treatment and subsequently every 3 to 4 months for the first year, or if a new neurologic deficit arises. In certain cases for which there are no abnormalities on MRI or MRA despite worsening clinical symptoms, a lumbar puncture or repeat angiography may be necessary. Long-term multidisciplinary follow-up by rheumatology, neurology, and physical therapy/rehabilitation specialists is essential.

KEY POINTS

- A high degree of suspicion is needed for diagnosis of PACNS. PACNS should be suspected in patients with multiterritory ischemic strokes, without a clear explanation and with inflammatory cerebrospinal fluid findings, chronic aseptic meningitis, and otherwise unexplained neurologic dysfunction.

- A thorough evaluation is required to rule out infection, cancer, systemic vasculitis, and other mimickers.

- Treatment should be initiated soon after diagnosis. Glucocorticoids and cyclophosphamide are the cornerstones of therapy.

- MRI and multidisciplinary follow-up are required.

SUBACUTE COGNITIVE DECLINE IN AN 86-YEAR-OLD WOMAN WITH PRIOR LOBAR INTRACEREBRAL HEMORRHAGE

Stephen W. English Jr, MD, MBA, and James P. Klaas, MD

CASE PRESENTATION

HISTORY AND EXAMINATION

An 86-year-old woman with a history of hypertension, hyperlipidemia, coronary artery disease, and hypothyroidism sought care for subacute, progressive cognitive decline. Five months earlier, she was hospitalized for a small, left temporal, lobar, intracerebral hemorrhage with associated receptive aphasia. Her language dysfunction gradually improved over weeks and she was discharged home after 3 days. Over the next several months, she had a precipitous cognitive decline; she stopped driving because of concerns from her family, and she was unable to recognize certain family members. She was prescribed memantine by her primary physician because of concern for dementia. One month before seeking care, she was found unconscious in her bathroom, which was believed to be an unwitnessed seizure. In the following month, she experienced further decline, particularly with sequencing common actions, including difficulty dressing, feeding, and taking medication.

On initial evaluation, neurologic examination indicated that she was inattentive, drowsy, and oriented to person but not place or time. She could follow some simple commands. She had mild dysarthria, but verbal output was markedly reduced. Cranial nerve examination was unremarkable. She did not track, but she blinked to threat bilaterally. Motor examination was limited by participation, but tone was normal and there was no obvious focal weakness. She exhibited brisk withdrawal response to pain in all 4 extremities.

TESTING

Brain magnetic resonance imaging (MRI) 1 month before the current evaluation showed a prior, small, left temporal hemorrhage and diffuse lobar microhemorrhages on gradient echo imaging, focal leptomeningeal gadolinium enhancement in the left temporal lobe, and multifocal T2 hyperintensity with mass effect, maximal in the left temporal lobe (Figure 62.1A-C). Magnetic resonance angiography showed no evidence of vasculitis. Electroencephalography

showed multifocal, independent epileptiform discharges. Cerebrospinal fluid (CSF) evaluation was acellular but showed an increased protein concentration (178 mg/dL; reference range, ≤35 mg/dL), no oligoclonal bands, and normal immunoglobulin G index. CSF cytologic evaluation was negative. Serum and CSF autoantibody evaluations were negative. She underwent open biopsy of the left temporal lobe, which indicated focal granulomatous inflammation causing vascular destruction, with β-amyloid plaques within the cortical and leptomeningeal vessels.

DIAGNOSIS

The findings were consistent with a diagnosis of amyloid-β-related angiitis (ABRA) in the setting of severe cerebral amyloid angiopathy.

MANAGEMENT

Because of concern for subclinical seizures and epileptiform discharges on electroencephalography, the patient was started on levetiracetam without substantial change in her mental status. After the biopsy findings demonstrated inflammatory changes consistent with ABRA, she was started on intravenous methylprednisolone 1,000 mg daily for 5 days, followed by transition to prednisone 60 mg daily. Cyclophosphamide was considered, but because of her age and substantial comorbid conditions, she remained on corticosteroids only, with gradual taper after 3 months. After 6 months of treatment, she had significant clinical and radiographic improvement. Follow-up MRI at that time showed interval improvement in the T2 hyperintensity and mass effect in the left temporal lobe (Figure 62.1D). She was again independent with her activities of daily living, and memantine was discontinued.

DISCUSSION

Cerebral amyloid angiopathy (CAA) encompasses a heterogeneous group of diseases characterized by amyloid-β peptide (Aβ) deposition in the media and adventitia of cortical and

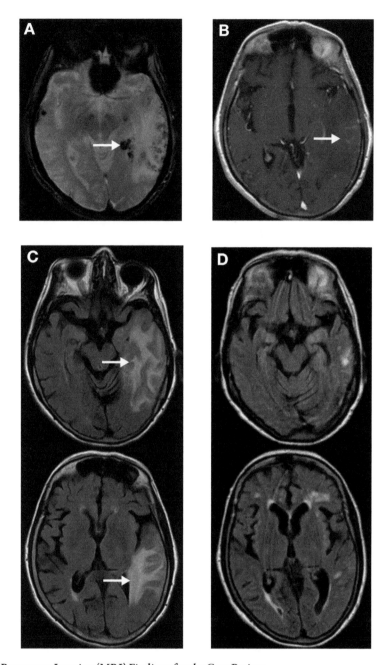

Figure 62.1 **Brain Magnetic Resonance Imaging (MRI) Findings for the Case Patient.**
A-C, MRI 1 month before our evaluation. A, Gradient echo sequence shows a prior, small, left temporal hemorrhage (arrow) and diffuse lobar microhemorrhages. B, T1 sequence with contrast shows focal leptomeningeal gadolinium enhancement in the left temporal lobe (arrow). C, T2/fluid-attenuated inversion recovery (FLAIR) sequences at 2 levels show subcortical white matter hyperintensity with mass effect
in the left temporal lobe (arrows). D, Repeated MRI at 2 levels (axial T2/FLAIR) after 6 months of corticosteroid treatment shows marked interval improvement of abnormal T2 white matter hyperintensity
and mass effect in the left temporal lobe.

leptomeningeal blood vessels. Aβ deposition can affect almost 30% of normal older persons but tends to be more severe and more frequent in patients with Alzheimer disease. The most common clinical manifestation of CAA is lobar intracere- bral hemorrhage, which can be multifocal and recurrent but can also result in cerebral ischemia and ischemic leukoen- cephalopathy. A subset of patients have associated vascular inflammation of the vessels that contain extensive Aβ depo- sition. Two pathologic subtypes exist: *CAA-related inflam- mation* (CAA-RI), which is characterized by a perivascular nondestructive inflammatory infiltrate, and *ABRA*, which

describes a vasculitic, transmural, granulomatous infiltrate of affected vessels. Mounting evidence suggests that these sub- types represent an underlying immune-mediated response against Aβ within the vessels. This evidence includes 1) clini- cal and radiographic response of these subtypes to immu- nosuppressive or immunomodulatory agents, 2) the clear pathologic colocalization of the vascular Aβ deposits and the inflammatory response, and 3) results of a clinical trial in which patients with Alzheimer disease had development of a similar inflammatory response after receiving Aβ-containing vaccinations.

The most common clinical manifestations of ABRA and CAA-RI include cognitive decline, headaches, seizures, and focal neurologic deficits, but substantial phenotypic overlap exists between these groups. MRI can be useful to distinguish CAA from the inflammatory subtypes. Patients with CAA are more likely to have lobar hemorrhage, but leptomeningeal enhancement and underlying, nonenhancing, infiltrative, T2 white matter abnormalities are more likely to be associated with ABRA or CAA-RI. CSF analysis is useful to exclude infectious and neoplastic processes, but nonspecific findings, including a mild to moderate lymphocytic pleocytosis and increased protein concentration, have been reported. Currently, a definitive diagnosis can only be made by biopsy, but efforts are under way to create noninvasive diagnostic criteria based on clinical and radiographic features.

Accurate diagnosis is imperative, however, because patients with ABRA or CAA-RI can have a positive response to immunosuppression, with improved morbidity and survival. Few studies exist that address specific treatment in ABRA or CAA-RI, but favorable evidence supports an initial trial of high-dose corticosteroids. After clinical and radiologic improvement, certain steroid-sparing immunosuppressive agents including pulsed cyclophosphamide, methotrexate, or mycophenolate mofetil can be considered. Cyclophosphamide has the most evidence showing prevention of relapse or recurrence, but its substantial adverse effect profile has limited its use in older persons.

KEY POINTS

- A subset of patients with CAA may have associated inflammation at the site of Aβ deposition within cerebral vessel walls.

- A diagnosis of ABRA should be considered in patients with a history of lobar hemorrhage or multiple cerebral microhemorrhages who have subacute cognitive decline, headaches, seizures, or progressive focal neurologic deficits.

- Brain biopsy is the diagnostic standard for CAA and its subtypes. MRI changes including leptomeningeal enhancement and asymmetric, nonenhancing, infiltrative, T2 white matter abnormalities can be suggestive of an inflammatory variant of CAA.

- Patients with ABRA may respond to aggressive immunosuppression, including either high-dose corticosteroids or pulsed cyclophosphamide.

A 75-YEAR-OLD MAN WITH 5 DAYS OF PROGRESSIVE GAIT DIFFICULTIES AND CONFUSION

Julie E. Hammack, MD

CASE PRESENTATION

HISTORY AND EXAMINATION

A 75-year-old man with a history of chronic obstructive pulmonary disease and ischemic cardiomyopathy was brought to the emergency department after a fall at home. He had a 5-day history of progressive gait disturbance, right-sided weakness, and confusion. He had reported floaters in the right eye for the past month. He was previously well with no history of trauma, fever, anorexia, or change in body weight.

On examination, he was drowsy but arousable. He scored 22 of 30 on the Mini-Mental State Examination. Language examination indicated mild mixed aphasia. Cranial nerve examination showed right lower facial droop but was otherwise normal, including visual fields to confrontation and ophthalmoscopy. He had mild pyramidal weakness in the right arm and leg. Deep tendon reflexes were brisker on the right than the left, and both plantar responses were flexor. His gait was apraxic with mild right circumduction. Sensory examination was normal. There was no meningismus. Noncontrast head computed tomography (CT) performed in the emergency department showed left hemisphere vasogenic edema with a linear area of hyperdensity in the subependymal region of the left lateral ventricle and a few cortical sulci (Figure 63.1A). Brain magnetic resonance imaging (MRI) (T1 with contrast) showed confluent areas of intense periventricular enhancement, some of which had a perivenular pattern (Figure 63.1B). The lesion showed restriction on diffusion-weighted imaging (Figure 63.1C). Diagnoses considered at the time are shown in Table 63.1.

TESTING

Cerebrospinal fluid (CSF) evaluation showed an increased protein concentration (80 mg/dL; reference range, ≤35 mg/dL), normal glucose level, no red blood cells, and 4 white blood cells/μL. Cytologic and flow cytometry evaluations were negative. CT of the chest, abdomen, and pelvis indicated no adenopathy or visceral lesions. Slitlamp examination of the

right eye showed clumps of cells in the vitreous. Vitrectomy was performed, and analysis showed atypical monoclonal B cells consistent with large B-cell lymphoma.

DIAGNOSIS

The patient was diagnosed with primary central nervous system lymphoma (PCNSL).

MANAGEMENT

The patient had an excellent initial clinical response to intravenous corticosteroids (dexamethasone) administered after vitrectomy. Subsequent staging showed no systemic lymphoma. He had hematology-oncology evaluations and was treated with chemotherapy (high-dose intravenous methotrexate, temozolomide, and rituximab) together with intravitreal rituximab for 1 year. He had an excellent clinical and radiographic response to treatment (Figure 63.2). He remained in complete remission until his death 6 years later (age 81 years) of pneumonia.

DISCUSSION

PCNSL accounts for approximately 4% of primary brain tumors and occurs more commonly in persons older than 60 years and those with compromised immune systems (eg, with AIDS, congenital immunodeficiency, and organ transplant). The tumor represents an extranodal form of non-Hodgkin lymphoma and is typically of the diffuse large B-cell type. In immunocompromised patients, PCNSL usually represents a lymphoproliferative process driven by Epstein-Barr virus. The incidence of PCNSL in immunocompetent patients older than 65 years has increased in the past decade for unknown reasons. Most patients do not have evidence of systemic lymphoma at the time of diagnosis; 40% have evidence of leptomeningeal involvement, and 15% to 20% have clinical evidence of ocular involvement (usually increased cells in the vitreous). CSF sampling (if clinically safe) and slitlamp examination of the eye is recommended in all patients with

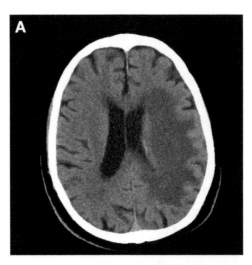

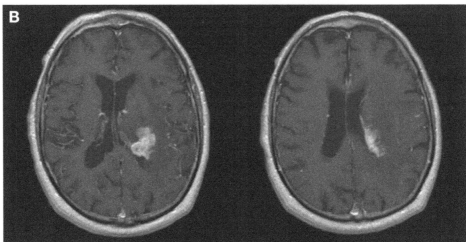

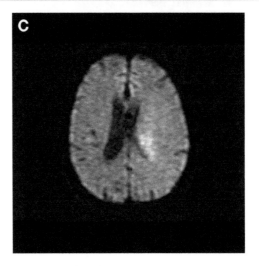

Figure 63.1 Imaging Findings for the Case Patient at Initial Evaluation.

A, Noncontrast computed tomography shows vasogenic edema and mass effect in the left cerebral hemisphere. B, T1-weighted magnetic resonance imaging with contrast at 2 different levels shows a homogeneously enhancing lesion in the periventricular white matter. C, Diffusion-weighted imaging shows restricted diffusion in the lesion, indicating hypercellularity.

suspected PCNSL. Isolation of monoclonal lymphocytes from the CSF or vitreous is diagnostic and can eliminate the need for brain biopsy.

Clinically, PCNSL usually presents with subacute, progressive, focal neurologic deficits. Cognitive changes are common. Headache and other symptoms of increased intracranial pressure occur in one-third of patients. Ocular symptoms (usually painless floaters) are present in only 4% of patients at presentation. Seizures are relatively rare, reflecting the subcortical location of most lesions.

Table 63.1 | DIFFERENTIAL DIAGNOSIS FOR THE CASE PATIENT

POSSIBLE DIAGNOSES	PERTINENT NEGATIVES	PERTINENT POSITIVES
Glioma	None	
Primary central nervous system lymphoma	None	Ocular symptoms
Tumefactive demyelination	Advanced age of patient No history of demyelination	
Granulomatous disease	None	
Cerebral abscess	Lack of radiographic necrosis No history of systemic infection No fever	
Subacute cerebral infarct	Subacute onset (temporal profile) Lesion crosses vascular territories	

On MRI, PCNSL appears as a homogeneously enhancing subcortical lesion or lesions. They are often periventricular. Immunocompromised patients with PCNSL often have lesions that show central necrosis on MRI and CT. Most of these lesions are supratentorial, although brainstem, cerebellar, and spinal cord lesions may occur. Leptomeningeal involvement is common (40%), although exclusive involvement of the leptomeninges is rare in PCNSL and occurs more commonly when systemic lymphoma spreads to the central nervous system. Involvement of bone marrow, lymph nodes, and viscera is exceedingly rare at the time of PCNSL presentation.

The differential diagnosis of PCNSL includes demyelinating disease and other inflammatory disorders including sarcoidosis. Subacute infarction may have a similar radiographic appearance to PCNSL, although the clinical history in stroke would have an acute onset as opposed to a subacute one in PCNSL. High-grade gliomas may have an identical clinical presentation and radiographic appearance to PCNSL. Metastatic tumors to the brain typically have central necrosis, unlike typical PCNSL.

Patients with indeterminate enhancing brain lesions should have a complete history and physical examination. CT of the chest, abdomen, and pelvis with contrast or positron emission tomography/CT of the body should be performed to investigate for adenopathy and visceral lesions (as may be present in the setting of granulomatous disease or metastatic neoplasm). CSF examination should be performed (if it is deemed to be clinically safe), including protein and glucose levels, blood cell count, oligoclonal bands, cytologic analysis, and flow cytometry. Even in the absence of ocular symptoms, the patient should have a complete eye examination including slitlamp evaluation. If a diagnosis cannot be made through these means, a biopsy of the brain lesion is required.

Corticosteroids, unless clinically essential, should be avoided before biopsy because they have a cytotoxic effect on lymphoma and may obscure the diagnosis. Surgical resection is not indicated for PCNSL. The lesions have a high risk of hemorrhage. Moreover, other therapies (chemotherapy and/or radiation) are typically effective, obviating the need for surgical resection.

Therapy for PCNSL is evolving. Currently, high-dose methotrexate-based chemotherapy combined with other agents including rituximab (an anti-CD20 antibody) is the current therapy of choice if the patient has adequate kidney function. Historically, whole-brain radiotherapy was the initial treatment of choice. However, it carries high risk of toxicity (leukoencephalopathy) and does not produce results superior

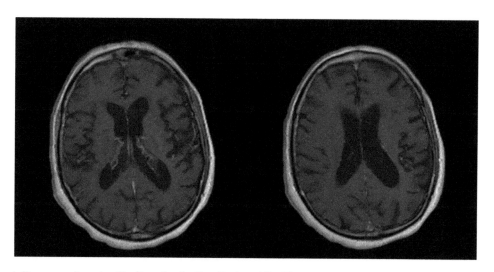

Figure 63.2 Magnetic Resonance Imaging Findings for the Case Patient After Treatment.
T1-weighted axial images with contrast at 2 different levels show response to treatment (near-resolution of enhancement, as compared with Figure 63.1B).

to chemotherapy (which shows less long-term neurotoxicity). Intrathecal chemotherapy usually is not required, even in patients with leptomeningeal involvement. Methotrexate has relatively good CSF penetration. Ocular involvement by PCNSL usually requires intraocular therapy (methotrexate or rituximab) or radiotherapy.

A high percentage of patients with PCNSL may achieve remission with medical therapy, sometimes for many years. Relapsed PCNSL usually behaves aggressively and can be treated with chemotherapy (sometimes with hematopoietic stem cell transplant) or whole-brain radiotherapy. Evaluation of novel therapies, including small molecule inhibitors and immunotherapy, is ongoing and as yet unproved.

Age and performance status are the most important factors influencing survival. In patients with good performance status, median survival of 3 to 4 years is common, and 5-year survival is approximately 30% in immunocompetent patients.

KEY POINTS

- PCNSL is an aggressive, relatively rare, extranodal non-Hodgkin lymphoma that presents with subacute progressive neurologic symptoms and may be mistaken clinically and radiographically for glioma, brain metastasis, or an inflammatory lesion (demyelinating or granulomatous disease).

- PCNSL is more common in older persons and in patients with conditions that suppress the immune system (HIV/AIDS, congenital immunodeficiency, and patients on immunosuppressant medications).

- Brain biopsy is usually required for diagnosis, although diagnostic tissue can sometimes be obtained from the CSF or vitreous tumor.

- Therapy typically involves chemotherapy with a methotrexate-based, multidrug regimen.

- Whole-brain radiotherapy is usually reserved for patients whose tumors do not respond to chemotherapy or recur despite chemotherapy.

- Although the disease is deemed incurable, remission is possible. Long-term survival may be achieved in patients with good performance status whose tumors are sensitive to chemotherapy.

NIGHT SWEATS AND PARAPARESIS

David N. Abarbanel, MD, and Ivan D. Carabenciov, MD

CASE PRESENTATION

HISTORY AND EXAMINATION

A 78-year-old man sought care for saddle anesthesia, left lower extremity numbness, and bilateral lower extremity weakness. The sensory loss occurred suddenly while sitting down in church, starting initially in the left perianal region and over the course of 3 hours extending down to involve the entirety of the left lower extremity. Symptoms were stable until 3 weeks later, when he had a few episodes of urinary incontinence. During the car ride to a medical evaluation, diffuse, severe, bilateral, lower extremity weakness developed. No arm symptoms were noted. The patient reported 6 months of intermittent night sweats that preceded the development of neurologic symptoms, but review of systems was otherwise normal.

Multidomain cognitive abnormalities were identified, and he scored 27 of 38 on the Kokmen short test of mental status. Strength testing indicated left lower extremity paralysis with diffuse, moderately severe weakness in the right lower extremity. Patellar and ankle jerk reflexes were absent, and plantar responses were flexor bilaterally. Sensory examination showed saddle anesthesia, as well as impaired vibratory sense and pain sensation in both lower limbs. Diagnoses considered at the time are shown in Table 64.1.

Table 64.1 | **DIFFERENTIAL DIAGNOSIS FOR THE CASE PATIENT**

POSSIBLE DIAGNOSES	PERTINENT INFORMATION
Demyelinating disease (myelin oligodendrocyte glycoprotein autoantibody)	Patient's age atypical; lack of prior inflammatory attacks; reduced reflexes atypical
Sarcoidosis	Sudden deterioration would be rare with this diagnosis
Vasculitis	Lower thoracic cord involvement atypical; sudden deterioration and cognitive symptoms would be supportive
Lymphoma	Intermittent night sweats, sudden deterioration, and cognitive symptoms would be supportive

TESTING

Serum studies were notable for pancytopenia and increased erythrocyte sedimentation rate and levels of ferritin and lactate dehydrogenase. Serum studies for aquaporin-4–immunoglobulin G and myelin oligodendrocyte glycoprotein–immunoglobulin G autoantibodies, peripheral blood smear, and monoclonal gammopathy screen were normal. Lumbar puncture showed a mildly increased protein concentration with normal blood cell count, glucose value, and cytologic and flow cytometry findings.

Magnetic resonance imaging obtained 4 weeks after initial symptom onset showed multifocal regions of increased T2 signal throughout the central nervous system (CNS) including the cerebrum, cerebellum, upper cervical cord, lower thoracic cord, and conus medullaris (Figure 64.1A). Gadolinium enhancement was present in the corpus callosum, cerebellum, and dorsal lower thoracic cord (Figure 64.1B).

One week later, ^{18}F-fludeoxyglucose (FDG)–positron emission tomography (PET)/computed tomography (CT) showed patchy FDG activity in the cerebral parenchyma, as well as 2 cutaneous, FDG-avid soft-tissue nodules (Figure 64.1C). Fine-needle aspiration of 1 of these nodules indicated diffuse large B-cell lymphoma (DLBCL), with no dysplastic abnormalities identified on subsequent bone marrow biopsy. Incisional biopsy of the second soft-tissue nodule showed foci of DLBCL adherent to the lumina of a few small arteries, consistent with a diagnosis of intravascular lymphoma.

DIAGNOSIS

The patient was diagnosed with intravascular large B-cell lymphoma (IVLBCL).

MANAGEMENT

At initial evaluation at an outside facility, 5 days of empiric intravenous corticosteroids were administered. After the biopsy findings of IVLBCL, he was started on intermediate-dose methotrexate followed by rituximab, cyclophosphamide, doxorubicin, vincristine, and prednisone (MR-CHOP) therapy. Unfortunately, neurologic improvement was minimal, and

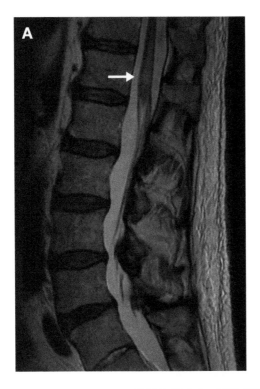
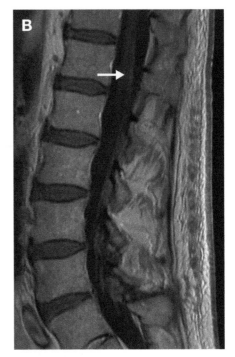
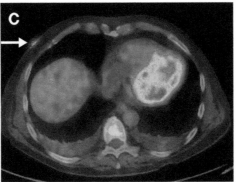

Figure 64.1 Imaging Findings for the Case Patient.

A, Sagittal, T2-weighted, lumbar spine magnetic resonance imaging (MRI) obtained 4 weeks after symptom onset shows an expansile, T2-hyperintense lesion involving the conus medullaris (arrow). B, Postcontrast, T1-weighted, lumbar spine MRI shows mild enhancement along the dorsal surface of the conus medullaris (arrow). C, ^{18}F-Fludeoxyglucose (FDG)–positron emission tomography/computed tomography obtained 5 weeks after symptom onset shows focal FDG activity overlying the right anterolateral chest wall (arrow).

he continued to experience severe, bilateral, lower extremity weakness and sensory loss. Two months after diagnosis of IVLBCL, he died of medical complications from chemotherapy.

DISCUSSION

Intravascular lymphoma is a rare lymphoma subtype that is typically of B-cell origin. The neoplastic cells preferentially grow within the lumen of blood vessels, potentially due to a lack of cellular machinery required for cellular extravasation and parenchymal invasion. IVLBCL typically occurs in patients older than 60 years. It can involve essentially any part of the nervous system, with highly variable neurologic manifestations depending on the site of involvement. Serum studies can show anemia, abnormal kidney or liver function, and increases in lactate dehydrogenase, ferritin, and inflammatory markers. Neuroimaging often identifies multifocal CNS involvement, but the imaging findings are usually nonspecific, overlapping with numerous inflammatory diseases.

Tissue biopsy is required for definitive diagnosis. PET/CT is a particularly useful test and is able to identify potential biopsy sites that are not apparent on conventional CT studies. If no biopsy sites are seen with PET/CT, random skin biopsies can be performed and have been shown to identify IVLBCL in some patients, even in the absence of skin lesions. Bone marrow biopsy also can be performed when lymphoma is being considered but often does not show diagnostic abnormalities. Malignant lymphocytes are rarely detected on cerebrospinal fluid analysis, even in cases of known CNS disease.

IVLBCL is an aggressive disease and is typically treated with combination chemotherapy. Prognosis has improved substantially since rituximab was added to the standard CHOP regimen. In cases with CNS involvement, high-dose methotrexate is added.

- Systemic clues, including B symptoms, increased serum lactate dehydrogenase levels, and hematologic abnormalities, are commonly present in patients with IVLBCL.

- Cerebrospinal fluid analysis, as well as imaging studies, can be nonspecific, and biopsy is needed for diagnosis.

- PET/CT can be a powerful diagnostic tool to assist in identifying optimal biopsy sites, particularly in areas that might be missed with traditional CT of the body.

A WOMAN WITH HEADACHES AND A TUMEFACTIVE BRAIN LESION

Andrew McKeon, MB, BCh, MD

CASE PRESENTATION

HISTORY AND EXAMINATION

A 65-year-old woman sought care for a 6-month history of confusion and emotional disturbance that was initially ascribed to stress. She then had development of headaches over several weeks, which prompted brain magnetic resonance imaging with contrast. Imaging showed a mass emanating bilaterally from the splenium of the corpus callosum with heterogeneous T1 postgadolinium enhancement (Figure 65.1A and 65.1B). Neurologic examination indicated left homonymous hemianopia, but she was otherwise normal. She had neither alexia nor other language deficit that may appear with a splenial corpus callosum lesion.

Her neurologic history and examination findings were not diagnosis specific. The main consideration in the differential diagnosis, on the basis of the radiologic appearance, was *butterfly glioma*, so called because of its appearance spreading out into both hemispheres (wings) from the corpus callosum (body). However, tumefactive demyelinating disease and lymphoma can also have a callosal localization and produce mass effect. Typical of a high-grade glioma, the enhancement pattern in this patient was heterogeneous (Figure 65.1B).

TESTING

A biopsy of the brain mass was performed.

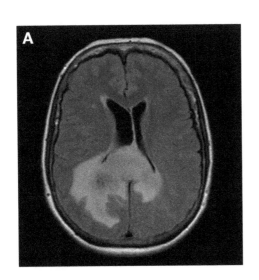
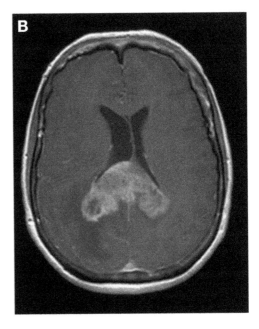

Figure 65.1 Axial Brain Magnetic Resonance Images.
T2/fluid-attenuated inversion recovery (A and C) and T1 postgadolinium (B, D, and E) images from the case patient (A and B) and example patients with tumefactive multiple sclerosis (C and D) and central nervous system (CNS) lymphoma (E). T2 signal appearance is similar for glioblastoma (A) and tumefactive demyelination (C), but the heterogeneous enhancement pattern of glioblastoma (B) is distinct from that of the ring enhancement pattern in tumefactive demyelination (D) and the homogeneous enhancement pattern of primary CNS lymphoma (E).
(E is from Chiavazza C, Pellerino A, Ferrio F, Cistaro A, Soffietti R, Ruda R. Primary CNS lymphomas: challenges in diagnosis and monitoring. Biomed Res Int. 2018 Jun 21;2018:3606970. Open access article distributed under the Creative Commons Attribution License [http://creativecommons.org/licenses/by/4.0/legalcode].)

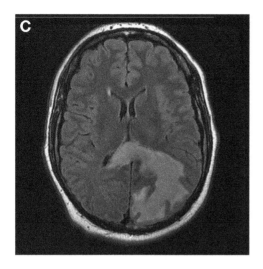

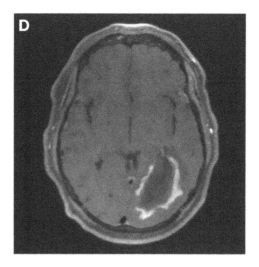

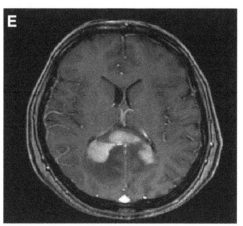

Figure 65.1 **Continued**

DIAGNOSIS

Histologic analysis of the biopsy specimen revealed glioblastoma multiforme.

MANAGEMENT

Corticosteroid treatment was prescribed, which relieved her headache. Radiation therapy and chemotherapy (temozolomide) were recommended. No further follow-up information was available.

DISCUSSION

In neurologic clinical practice, a large corpus callosum–based lesion is sometimes encountered. The localization of such lesions is not specific for any one diagnosis, but radiologic characteristics can aid clinical decision making. Although the radiologic appearance of a lesion spreading out into both hemispheres from the corpus callosum can indicate butterfly glioma, the differential diagnosis also includes tumefactive demyelinating disease and lymphoma, which can also have a callosal localization and produce mass effect. Occasionally, brain abscess may also localize to the corpus callosum. The

enhancement pattern in this patient was heterogeneous (Figure 65.1B). However, tumefactive demyelinating disease could also arise from the corpus callosum and could have had a similar appearance on T2 imaging, although ring enhancement (classically open ring) would be characteristic of multiple sclerosis lesions (Figure 65.1C and 65.1D, example images from a patient with tumefactive multiple sclerosis). Central nervous system lymphoma also could have had a similar appearance on T2 imaging, although the pattern of enhancement would be more homogeneous (Figure 65.1E, example images from a patient with central nervous system lymphoma). Case 7 includes a discussion pertaining to diagnosis and management of tumefactive demyelinating disease.

KEY POINTS

- Butterfly glioma and lymphoma may resemble tumefactive demyelinating disease on T2 imaging.

- The pattern of enhancement on T1 postgadolinium imaging should narrow the differential diagnosis, although biopsy is still required in suspected neoplasia (lymphoma or glioma) to confirm.

BEHAVIORAL CHANGE, SEIZURES, AND TEMPORAL LOBE LESION

Stuart J. McCarter, MD, and Andrew McKeon, MB, BCh, MD

CASE PRESENTATION

HISTORY AND EXAMINATION

A 56-year-old man with a history of type 2 diabetes, hypertension, hyperlipidemia, sleep apnea, alcohol use disorder in remission, renal cell carcinoma, and mucinous adenocarcinoma of the lung sought care at Mayo Clinic for evaluation of presumed limbic encephalitis.

Six months before evaluation at Mayo Clinic, he had development of anxiety, fatigue, and blurry vision. He was diagnosed with renal cell carcinoma, which was resected. Subsequently, worsening depression developed, which required self-admitted psychiatric hospitalization for suicidal ideation. After discharge he had subacute development of aphasia, inability to recognize family members, and delusions for which he was hospitalized at a local hospital. Brain magnetic resonance imaging (MRI) demonstrated a large, partly expansile, T2/fluid-attenuated inversion recovery (FLAIR)–hyperintense lesion involving the left hippocampus and parahippocampal gyrus, as well as temporal neocortex and white matter, which was interpreted as limbic encephalitis (Figure 66.1). Spinal fluid analysis showed 66 total nucleated cells/μL (reference range, ≤5/μL) with 93% lymphocytes, normal cytologic findings, protein concentration of 66 mg/dL (reference range, 15-40 mg/dL), and 15 erythrocytes/μL (reference range, <10 erythrocytes/μL). Cerebrospinal fluid (CSF) and serum paraneoplastic autoantibody evaluations were negative. Polymerase chain reaction testing of the CSF for herpes simplex virus was negative.

The patient then had a generalized tonic-clonic seizure and was started on levetiracetam. Positron emission tomography–computed tomography of the body showed a hypermetabolic lesion in the left lung that was resected and determined to be a stage IA mucinous adenocarcinoma of the lung. He was treated with 5 days of 1,000 mg intravenous methylprednisolone and intravenous immunoglobulin (IVIG) 1 g/kg every 2 weeks. His mental status reportedly improved, but it would worsen approximately 1 week after each dose of IVIG and improve again with the following treatment.

On evaluation at Mayo Clinic, he reported persistent difficulty with names, poor short-term memory, and insomnia but otherwise reported feeling well. At the time of his mucinous adenocarcinoma diagnosis, he had lost 22.7 kg (50 lb), which had since stabilized. His social history was negative for significant tobacco use, and he rarely used alcohol in the setting of his alcohol use disorder. There was no family history of autoimmunity.

TESTING

The Kokmen short test of mental status indicated mainly an amnestic profile without delirium, with a total score of 31 of 38. He lost 1 point for orientation, 1 point for attention, 1 point for general information, and all 4 points for delayed recall. The language examination was normal. He scored 4 of 20 on testing of famous faces, although he was able to accurately describe their personage. The remainder of his examination was unremarkable.

Given the patient's somewhat atypical neuroimaging findings for limbic encephalitis and lack of clear encephalopathy, the initial focus was confirming or ruling out the diagnosis of limbic encephalitis. Diagnoses considered at the time are shown in Table 66.1. He underwent repeated CSF analysis, which showed 3 total nucleated cells/μL with a protein concentration of 67 mg/dL. There were no oligoclonal bands. Serum autoantibody testing for encephalitis was negative, other than a low-titer glutamic acid decarboxylase 65-kDa isoform (GAD65) antibody value of 0.17 nmol/L (reference range, ≤0.02 nmol/L). Brain MRI 3 months after his initial MRI showed slight progression of the expansile, left temporal lobe, T2-hyperintense lesion, further involving the left parietal lobe white matter, temporal lobe neocortex, and splenium of the corpus callosum, without clear gadolinium enhancement (Figure 66.1).

Because he had had clinical improvement with IVIG, the patient was treated with 0.4 g/kg of IVIG per week for 6 weeks, with ongoing clinical improvement. Repeated MRI, however, demonstrated continued mild progression of the

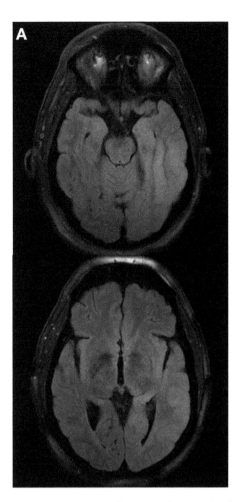
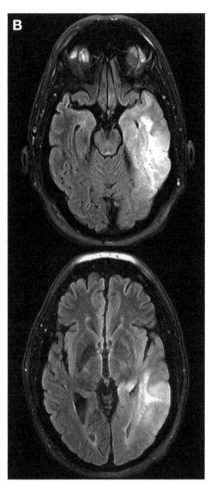
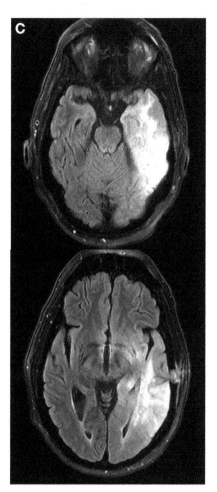

Figure 66.1 **Magnetic Resonance Imaging Findings for the Case Patient.**

Axial, T2-weighted, fluid-attenuated inversion recovery images at 2 levels demonstrate evolving size of the T2-hyperintense lesion in the left mesial temporal lobe, which extended into the neocortex of the temporal and parietal lobes despite immunotherapy. Images are at initial presentation (A), 3 months after symptom onset (B), and 5 months after symptom onset (C).

Table 66.1 | **DIFFERENTIAL DIAGNOSIS OF MESIAL TEMPORAL LOBE T2-HYPERINTENSE LESIONS**

POSSIBLE DIAGNOSIS	PERTINENT POSITIVES	PERTINENT NEGATIVES
Neoplasm	Focal masslike component	Clinical improvement with immunosuppression
	Minimal neuroimaging improvement with immunosuppression	Lack of contrast enhancement
		CSF pleocytosis
	Contiguous spread without involving the opposite hemisphere	
	History of primary neoplasm	
	Lack of fluctuating encephalopathy	
Autoimmune/inflammatory	Limbic involvement	More commonly bilateral
	Improvement immediately after immunosuppression	Lack of pathogenic autoantibody
	History of malignant process	Lack of fluctuating encephalopathy
	Seizures	
	Psychiatric disturbance	
	CSF with lymphocytic pleocytosis, with improvement after immunosuppression	
Infectious, particularly HSV	Mesial temporal lobe involvement	Absence of fever, headaches, or meningismus
	Sparing the basal ganglia	Lack of acute onset and rapid progression
	CSF with lymphocytic pleocytosis	Negative PCR for HSV
		Lack of encephalopathy
		Absence of pathognomonic antibody
Seizure	T2 hyperintensity involving the mesial temporal lobe	Involvement of extralimbic structures
	History of seizures	Progression of T2-hyperintense lesion without ongoing status epilepticus

Abbreviations: CSF, cerebrospinal fluid; HSV, herpes simplex virus; PCR, polymerase chain reaction.

left temporoparietal lobe lesion, with progressive involvement of the right posterior cingulate gyrus. Owing to ongoing disease progression, he underwent left temporal lobe biopsy. Results indicated anaplastic astrocytoma (World Health Organization [WHO] grade III), fibrillary type, isocitrate dehydrogenase 1 wild-type (associated with poorer prognosis).

DIAGNOSIS

A diagnosis of anaplastic astrocytoma (WHO grade III) was made.

MANAGEMENT

He was ultimately treated with 6 cycles of temozolomide and 33 fractions of radiotherapy, with radiographic improvement. However, he had development of medically refractory focal seizures with secondary generalization, considered most likely due to radiation necrosis. Serial follow-up of the left temporoparietal lesion showed radiographic stability. However, approximately 3 years after his initial diagnosis, the patient experienced significant functional decline, with brain MRI demonstrating multiple new, bihemispheric, T2-hyperintense lesions concerning for multifocal glioma. Further evaluation for evidence of metastatic disease was negative. Given his poor prognosis and functional status, the patient was transitioned to comfort care after discussion with his family.

DISCUSSION

The presentation of disease in this patient highlights the importance of neuroimaging interpretation in the context of clinical history. Although this case patient had some features that could suggest a paraneoplastic limbic encephalitis—including behavioral changes, seizure, systemic malignancy, and apparent clinical response to immunosuppression—several features were inconsistent with this diagnosis. First, although he had depression, he maintained insight and did not exhibit psychosis or encephalopathy; rather, he had focal neurologic deficits (anomia) attributable to left temporal lobe dysfunction without significant fluctuation. Second,

longitudinal imaging demonstrated progressive enlargement of the left temporal lobe mass, spreading beyond the limbic regions to contiguous structures without involvement of the contralateral mesial temporal lobe. This progression occurred despite immunotherapy, which also led to suspicion for primary central nervous system malignancy. Of note, IVIG therapy is a frequent cause of low (false) positive results in antibody diagnostic assays (such as GAD65 in this case). The increase in CSF white blood cell count was not entirely explained but was believed to be nonspecific. IVIG can also induce aseptic meningitis and thereby cause nonspecific increases in white blood cell count and protein concentration.

Anaplastic astrocytoma (WHO grade III) is an infiltrating cancer of astrocytic origin. Median survival is 2 to 3 years, with 23% of patients surviving 5 years. Prognosis is worse among those without sequence variations in isocitrate dehydrogenase 1. Treatment is largely limited to temozolomide chemotherapy, radiotherapy, and maximal safe surgical resection. Clinical symptoms are dependent on the location of the lesion. MRI typically demonstrates a poorly defined T2/FLAIR-hyperintense, T1-hypointense lesion. Gadolinium enhancement is variable and, when present, typically supports a higher-grade neoplasm. Importantly, infiltrating gliomas are one of a few causes of masses crossing the corpus callosum, as was observed in our patient. This does not occur in limbic encephalitis. Interestingly, our patient did have clinical improvement with corticosteroids, most likely an effect of decreasing peritumoral edema.

KEY POINTS

- A persistent, unilateral, mesial temporal lobe, T2/FLAIR-hyperintense lesion extending into neocortex on longitudinal imaging (particularly without involvement of the contralateral mesial temporal lobe) should raise concern for primary brain neoplasm.

- The absence of fluctuating cognition or mental status (delirium) argues against limbic encephalitis.

- The time course and progression of symptoms is vitally important to aid in the interpretation of neuroimaging.

A YOUNG WOMAN WITH VESSEL DISSECTION AND BRAINSTEM LESIONS

Burcu Zeydan, MD, and Orhun H. Kantarci, MD

CASE PRESENTATION

HISTORY AND EXAMINATION

A 21-year-old woman with baseline depression, 1-year history of recurrent, painful, oral and vaginal ulcers, and cellulitis had a new, severe, acute-onset, left posterior headache with left shoulder pain. Within a few days, she sought chiropractic manipulation treatment. Within 24 hours of a second manipulation, incoordination of her left leg developed, and she was admitted to the hospital. On neurologic examination, she had mild right oculomotor and abducens nerve weakness and marked left upper extremity and moderate left lower extremity upper motor neuron–type paresis.

Given the patient's history and because of the sudden onset of her neurologic symptoms, a cerebrovascular event was considered. However, owing to her young age and not having high-risk factors for stroke such as hypertension, hyperlipidemia, and smoking, uncommon causes of stroke were in the differential diagnosis. Diagnoses considered included non-atherosclerotic angiopathies (eg, fibromuscular dysplasia, vertebral arterial dissection), hypercoagulable states (eg, factor V Leiden, antiphospholipid syndrome, lymphoma), cardiac involvement (eg, patent foramen ovale), and inflammatory (eg, vasculitis, neuro-Behçet syndrome, neurosarcoidosis), infectious (eg, tuberculous meningitis), and genetic causes (eg, CADASIL syndrome [cerebral autosomal dominant arteriopathy with subcortical infarcts and leukoencephalopathy], MELAS syndrome [mitochondrial encephalomyopathy, lactic acidosis, and stroke-like episodes]).

TESTING

Initial brain magnetic resonance imaging (MRI) showed acute ischemia involving the right pons, right midbrain, right cerebral peduncle, and internal capsule, extending into the right diencephalic region. Neck computed tomography (CT) angiography (later confirmed by magnetic resonance angiography) identified a right vertebral artery dissection at the C3 level (Figure 67.1A-C). Follow-up conventional angiography

showed no evidence of medium- to small-vessel vasculitis. Electrocardiography showed no cardiac arrhythmia, and transesophageal echocardiography did not reveal a cardioembolic source of her ischemic event.

Cerebrospinal fluid analysis showed a marked neutrophilic pleocytosis with a reported "high" white blood cell count, but it was negative for infectious agents and malignant cells. Chest CT findings were normal. Serum testing for vasculitis and infectious etiologies was negative. *HLA-B51* testing was positive. Pathergy testing was not done, but the patient had had many previous needle sticks with no evidence of local skin reaction. Biopsies of her ulcers indicated nonspecific inflammation with no infectious sources.

Although the chiropractic manipulation may have facilitated the development of vertebral artery dissection, her severe headache preceding the manipulations, along with recurrent, painful, oral and genital ulcers (recurrent aphthous stomatitis), cerebrospinal fluid pleocytosis, and brainstem involvement after a vertebral artery dissection, raised concern for Behçet syndrome and eventually neurologic involvement of Behçet syndrome.

DIAGNOSIS

Recurrent corticosteroid-responsive oral ulcers plus recurrent genital ulcers and skin lesions (cellulitis) fulfill the criteria for Behçet syndrome, with possible neurologic involvement (*neuro-Behçet syndrome*). The patient was of Dominican descent; remote ancestry was unknown (Middle Eastern, Eastern Mediterranean, or Asian ancestry being pertinent). The positive *HLA-B51* testing was consistent with the diagnosis of Behçet syndrome.

MANAGEMENT

Treatment was initiated with low-dose aspirin and intravenous methylprednisolone, after which her neurologic status started to improve. Oral prednisone (slowly tapered after 6 months) and azathioprine were added for long-term treatment. With this treatment regimen, she remained

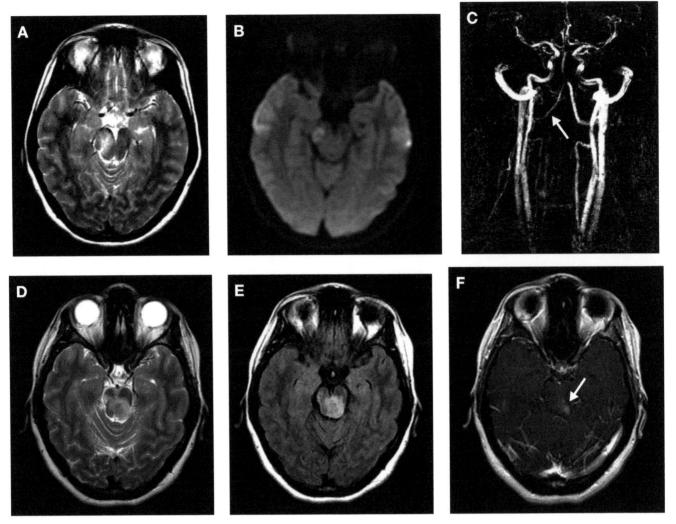

Figure 67.1 Imaging Findings for the Case Patient.
A and B, Axial brain magnetic resonance imaging (MRI) demonstrates acute stroke involving the right central pons, extending into the right midbrain, right cerebral peduncle, and posterior limb of the right internal capsule, with mild swelling of the brainstem on T2 (A) and diffusion-weighted imaging (B). C, Computed tomography angiography shows apparent dissection of the right vertebral artery (arrow), best localized to the level of C3, with the artery remaining patent throughout its course. D-F, During a relapse of symptoms after pregnancy and before reinitiation of immunosuppression, axial MRI shows new inflammatory T2 changes on T2 (D) and fluid-attenuated inversion recovery (E) images and subtle contrast enhancement (arrow) in the left pons and cerebellar peduncle on T1 postgadolinium imaging (F) extending along the posterior left aspect of the midbrain.

clinically stable for 4 years, except for fluctuating levels of oral ulcers during the switch between oral prednisone and azathioprine.

At age 25 years, she discontinued azathioprine because she planned pregnancy. During the pregnancy and lactation period, the patient had no new symptoms of Behçet syndrome, including no new oral or genital ulcers. At age 27 years, within 1 month of stopping breastfeeding, she started having recurrence of oral and genital ulcers, along with axillary ulcerative skin lesions. New-onset diplopia and left-sided weakness also developed before corticosteroid and azathioprine could be reinitiated. MRI of the brain showed a new left pontine and cerebellar peduncle lesion with subtle contrast enhancement (Figure 67.1D-F). Intravenous methylprednisolone 1,000 mg/d for 5 days was initiated, followed by reinitiation of oral prednisone and the azathioprine regimen for long-term maintenance immunotherapy. The prednisone was slowly tapered after 3 months. The patient has been stable

neurologically since then and reports having oral ulcers only during menstruation, which are responsive to intermittent use of oral corticosteroid washes.

The final diagnosis for this patient was relapsing neuro-Behçet syndrome because she had 2 recurrent neurologic episodes associated with 1) vertebral artery dissection and 2) brainstem involvement. If she were to have further relapses, the plan was to administer a tumor necrosis factor (TNF)-α inhibitor, but her condition has been stable.

DISCUSSION

The case of this patient highlights 3 aspects of Behçet syndrome: 1) diagnosis of systemic Behçet syndrome is made on clinical grounds only, but even if the diagnostic criteria are not fulfilled, once neuro-Behçet syndrome develops, treatment should be initiated to curtail significant morbidity; 2) although rare, arterial involvement in neuro-Behçet syndrome should be recognized; and 3) there are notable sex-dependent factors in the evolution of Behçet syndrome.

Behçet syndrome is a multisystem autoimmune disease with perivenular and intravenular inflammation and intravenular thrombosis. Recurrent, painful, corticosteroid-responsive, oral and/or genital aphthous ulcers are cardinal for establishing the diagnosis, but Behçet syndrome can start solely as a skin disease, uveitis, arthritis, venous sinus thrombosis, central nervous system parenchymal disease, or arterial aneurysms, or as combined involvement of several of these systems. Patients with Behçet syndrome are likely to have *HLA-B51* and/or pathergy test positivity, although the sensitivity and specificity of these tests are variable in an east-west gradient across the world.

Generally, within 5 years of systemic symptom onset, 5% to 15% of patients with Behçet syndrome have neurologic symptoms referred to collectively as neuro-Behçet syndrome. Imaging and cerebrospinal fluid evaluation aid in the diagnosis. Lesions associated with neuro-Behçet syndrome are clinically and radiologically associated with the brainstem and diencephalic region and cause substantial morbidity and mortality. Therefore, after neurologic involvement ensues, it should be treated promptly without awaiting the full systemic disease to develop. First-line agents are typically azathioprine and, in patients for whom first-line treatments fail, TNF-α inhibitors have been used successfully. Neurologic, pulmonary, and gastrointestinal tract involvement are associated with poor prognosis; thus, we currently recommend TNF-α inhibitors as first-line therapy when these systems are involved.

Whereas most patients with neuro-Behçet syndrome have symptoms resulting from either parenchymal involvement (70%-80%) or venous sinus thrombosis (15%-20%), central nervous system arterial involvement is relatively rare (8%). Most patients with arteriopathy (≈85%) have an ischemic stroke at initial presentation. General stroke risk factors of older age, male sex, hypertension, and smoking seem to be more frequent in patients with arterial involvement. Additional cerebrovascular involvement associated with Behçet syndrome includes carotid artery stenosis, vertebral artery dissection, and intracranial aneurysm.

Both in Behçet syndrome and in young patients with stroke, the frequency of aneurysm and dissection is higher than in the normal population. In patients with Behçet syndrome and cerebral arterial involvement, other systemic vessels of different types and sizes are also commonly involved (eg, deep vein thrombosis, thrombophlebitis, and pulmonary artery aneurysms). In our experience, the association of deep vein thrombosis and systemic arterial involvement such as pulmonary artery aneurysm is higher in patients with arterial neuro-Behçet syndrome involvement. Therefore, in a young patient with stroke, deep vein thrombosis, and pulmonary artery aneurysm, Behçet syndrome should be in the differential diagnosis because the treatment requires immunosuppression in addition to vascular risk modification.

Behçet syndrome often affects young people, with a peak age of 20s to 40s, which generally overlaps with the reproductive period. The prognosis of Behçet syndrome seems to be worse in men. Systemic complications (including ocular, vascular, and neurologic) and pathergy test positivity are more common in men, whereas genital ulcers and joint involvement are more common in women.

During pregnancy, our patient had no disease activity despite discontinuation of azathioprine and corticosteroids. However, she had rapid resurgence of systemic symptoms followed by another relapse after pregnancy, as soon as she discontinued breastfeeding and within 1 month of resumption of her menses. Even after resuming azathioprine with significant improvement of her symptoms, she continued to report that her mild symptoms (oral and genital ulcers) were confined only to the week of her menses. Some studies have indicated that patients with Behçet syndrome may have decreased ovarian reserve during reproductive ages. This may be influenced by the disease pathogenesis itself but also by age, disease severity, and treatments used. Overall, there also seems to be an association between hormonal changes and Behçet syndrome activity, which should be considered when counseling young women with Behçet syndrome on pregnancy planning.

KEY POINTS

- Neuro-Behçet syndrome is associated with substantial morbidity and mortality. Therefore, it should be treated promptly with an aggressive immunomodulation strategy.

- Arterial involvement in Behçet syndrome should be recognized because it contributes substantially to morbidity and mortality of the disease.

- Behçet syndrome is associated with sex differences in disease activity and prognosis that should be considered in individualized patient treatment strategies.

HEADACHE, UVEITIS, AND LEPTOMENINGEAL ENHANCEMENT

Orhun H. Kantarci, MD

CASE PRESENTATION

HISTORY AND EXAMINATION

A 35-year-old man of mixed Chinese, Japanese, French, German, and Filipino descent sought care for a severe, acute-onset, pounding, bifrontal headache, photopsias, and nausea for 1 day. Initially, bilateral red eyes developed, and within 24 hours he had central blurred vision problems in the left eye. He reported that objects had a yellow tint with the left eye and looked "wavy" supranasally. An emergent evaluation documented bilateral red eyes, and an initial diagnosis of bilateral panuveitis was given. Ophthalmologic examination including fluorescein angiography and optical coherence tomography showed bilateral findings of predominant panuveitis, exudative retinal detachments, posterior pole choroidal hyperfluorescence, and subretinal fluid adjacent to the optic nerves. Examination also indicated shallow elevation of membrane throughout the posterior pole of the right eye and temporal posterior pole of the left eye, thickened posterior fundus in both eyes, and no mass in either eye or orbit (Figure 68.1). By 48 hours after symptom onset, he started vomiting. He also was feeling feverish and off-balance. He reported no tinnitus or hearing loss (confirmed by examination), any change in color of his eyelashes or eyebrows, alopecia, poliosis, or cognitive difficulties. An initial workup for infectious processes was negative.

On the fourth day of symptoms, he was started on oral prednisone with an 80-mg first dose, followed by 60 mg daily. By the seventh day of symptoms he was first seen in the neurology clinic; his vision had fully improved and his red eyes had recovered. His headaches had improved about 75%, with a mild, dull headache remaining. He had brisk reflexes in all 4 extremities but no other focal neurologic findings. He had a family history of systemic lupus erythematosus and a personal history of mild, untreated hypertension, regions of hypopigmented skin patches, and oral but not genital ulcers.

Magnetic resonance imaging (MRI) of the brain showed leptomeningeal enhancement (Figure 68.2). Cerebrospinal fluid studies showed increased protein concentration (113 mg/dL; reference range, ≤35 mg/dL) and lymphocytic pleocytosis (1 erythrocyte/μL and 329 white blood cells/μL [reference range, ≤5 cells/μL] with 94% lymphocytes and 6% monocytes/macrophages).

Given the patient's history and owing to the sudden onset of meningitis and uveitis, a uveomeningeal syndrome (disorders that involve the uvea, retina, and meninges) was first considered. The differential diagnosis of uveomeningeal syndromes includes infectious causes (tuberculosis, syphilis, cat-scratch disease, toxoplasmosis, varicella-zoster, histoplasmosis, candidiasis, aspergillosis, *Cryptococcus neoformans* infection), autoimmune causes (Behçet syndrome, Vogt-Koyanagi-Harada syndrome [VKH], sarcoidosis, granulomatosis with polyangiitis, sympathetic ophthalmia due to penetrating eye trauma, acute posterior multifocal placoid pigment epitheliopathy, inflammatory bowel disease, collapsin-response mediator protein 5 [CRMP5] paraneoplastic ophthalmitis, amyloid-β-related angiitis), and neoplastic causes (primary ocular central nervous system lymphoma, metastases). Because a uveomeningeal syndrome represents an emergency as soon as major acute infectious causes are ruled out, corticosteroid treatment is appropriate to preserve vision.

TESTING

Cervical MRI obtained because of the finding of hyperreflexia was unrevealing for any pathologic process. Additional testing included studies for infectious disease possibilities, which were negative. Autoimmune marker tests, including for CRMP5–immunoglobulin G, were negative. The patient had no evidence of lymphoma on imaging and eye-specific evaluations. Chest computed tomography was negative for infectious processes and sarcoidosis.

DIAGNOSIS

Given the patient's ethnic background, including Chinese, Japanese, and Filipino origin, and typical findings of

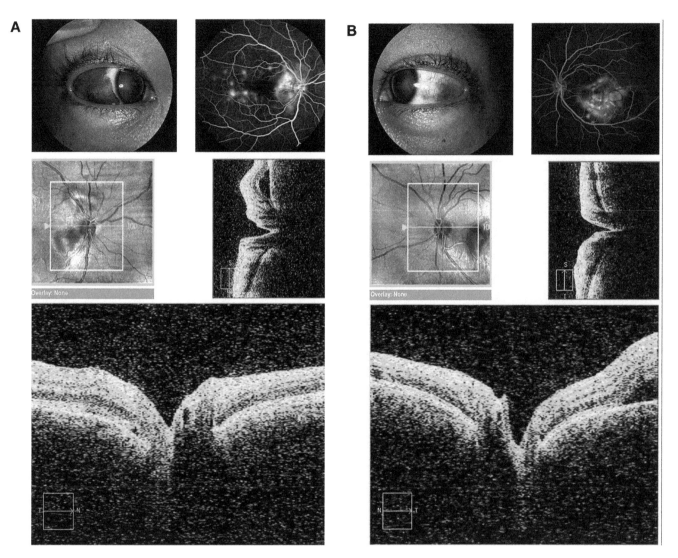

Figure 68.1 Ophthalmologic Examination Findings for the Case Patient.

A, Right eye with anterior uveitis. Fluorescein angiography (FA) shows posterior pole choroidal hyperfluorescence with no retinal leakage, along with subretinal fluid adjacent to nerve. Optical coherence tomography (OCT) shows retinal nerve fiber layer (RNFL) signal strength 9/10; average thickness, 158 μm. B, Left eye with anterior uveitis. FA shows diffuse choroidal fluorescence late within the posterior pole and large areas of subretinal fluid. OCT shows RNFL signal strength 8/10; average thickness, 110 μm.

uveomeningitis, he was diagnosed with probable VKH. There is no specific diagnostic test for this entity, and the diagnosis remains reliant on a combined interpretation of clinical and ancillary testing.

MANAGEMENT

The patient was kept on oral prednisone daily, and azathioprine was initiated, as well as prophylaxis against *Pneumocystis carinii* pneumonia and gastrointestinal tract hemorrhage. During the tapering phase of prednisone, liver function test abnormalities were found, so azathioprine was discontinued. He was maintained without difficulty on 10 mg prednisone daily. At 1-year follow-up, he had some mild skin flaking and weight gain from the corticosteroid therapy but no other symptoms, despite having discontinued azathioprine for 3 months. He continued to taper off prednisone to 5 mg and then by 1 mg per month until discontinued. Unfortunately, because of a recurrence of his uveitis, he resumed prednisone

therapy and was maintained on 5 mg/d for another year while training for a triathlon. He had development of bilateral hip pain; imaging showed bilateral aseptic hip necrosis. A decision was made to initiate tumor necrosis factor (TNF)-α inhibitors because of their known effects on uveitis and several other uveomeningeal syndromes. In the next 3 months, the patient was able to completely discontinue the corticosteroid with no recurrence of symptoms and continued with TNF-α inhibitor therapy alone until the last review 48 months into his symptom onset. He lost all the weight gained and recovered from the aseptic necrosis of the hip to be able to continue running. The final diagnosis was recurrent VKH.

DISCUSSION

VKH is an idiopathic inflammatory disease with panuveitis and neurologic involvement in the form of aseptic meningitis and/or hearing loss. Although the full spectrum of

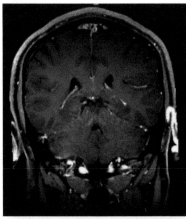

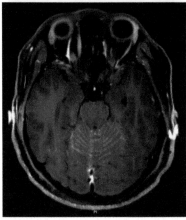

Figure 68.2 Magnetic Resonance Imaging Findings for the Case Patient.
Coronal (top) and axial (bottom) images with gadolinium contrast show leptomeningeal enhancement extending into the cerebellar hemispheres.

patients of Asian and Mexican ancestry. Melanin-associated antigen has been thought to be the target of autoimmunity, hence the spectrum of pigmentary changes in the retina to changes in the skin. VKH is also associated with a substantial interleukin (IL)-25 deficiency.

Although much is unknown about VKH, several key points have emerged over the years. 1) The differential diagnosis of uveomeningitis is relatively wide, with seemingly unrelated disorders ranging from infectious to autoimmune disorders being listed. It is therefore prudent to consider all possibilities in diagnoses and treatment. 2) Prompt treatment with corticosteroids substantially improves vision outcomes, so it should not be delayed. 3) There is no consensus treatment for long-term steroid-sparing immunomodulation. As illustrated in this case patient, however, recurrences can happen, so immunosuppression should be started early to facilitate corticosteroid taper. 4) If first-line immunomodulation such as azathioprine is not tolerated or fails, we recommend TNF-α inhibitor therapy.

The argument for use of TNF-α inhibitor therapy is anecdotal in VKH, but evidence from many other forms of uveitis, Behçet syndrome, sarcoidosis, and inflammatory bowel disease suggests that TNF-α inhibitor therapy can substantially alter morbidity and mortality. Interestingly, all the listed disorders can commonly cause uveitis, meningitis, and mucositis. A common pathway of autoimmunity responsive to TNF-α inhibition is most likely shared among these disorders. With the available and upcoming IL-1 and IL-6 therapies, many additional choices should be available for helping preserve vision in these patients. A well-organized international trial could help guide physicians in the future.

KEY POINTS

- VKH is a uveomeningeal syndrome characterized by a predominant uveitis and is more commonly associated with Asian ancestry.

- VKH and similar uveomeningeal syndromes seem to respond to TNF-α inhibition, which suggests a common immunopathogenesis.

- Prompt recognition and treatment of VKH is important for prevention of permanent ophthalmic injury.

the disorder may involve many skin changes and additional findings, most patients have incomplete disease because they are urgently treated with corticosteroids and the disorder is steroid responsive. The differential diagnosis includes many other causes of uveitis, but several predictive features have been identified: 1) exudative retinal detachment during the acute phase and 2) choroidal depigmentation or sunset glow fundus with chronic granulomatous anterior uveitis during the chronic-recurrent phase. The disease is extremely rare in those of European and African descent and more common in

WEAKNESS AND PUNCTATE ENHANCEMENT

W. Oliver Tobin, MB, BCh, BAO, PhD

CASE PRESENTATION

HISTORY AND EXAMINATION

A 40-year-old right-handed man sought care for a 3-year history of tingling in his cheeks and face, with progressive urinary urgency. He had a 1-year history of progressive binocular diplopia and ataxia that developed while playing football. On examination, he had decreased vibration sensation in his toes and a mild broad-based gait. The rest of the neurologic examination was normal.

TESTING

Complete blood cell count; erythrocyte sedimentation rate; liver enzyme, vitamin B$_{12}$, and folate levels; testing for Lyme disease and HIV; and antinuclear antigen, extractable nuclear antigen, serum immunoglobulins, antineutrophil cytoplasmic antibody, and antiphospholipid antibody were normal or negative. Magnetic resonance imaging (MRI) of the brain indicated mild fluid-attenuated inversion recovery (FLAIR) abnormality with punctate postgadolinium enhancement, primarily in the pons (Figure 69.1). Positron emission tomography/computed tomography of the body was normal. Spinal fluid analysis showed 2 white blood cells/µL (reference range, 0-5/µL) with 95% lymphocytes, protein value of 32 mg/dL (reference range, ≤35 mg/dL), 0 unique oligoclonal bands, and normal immunoglobulin G index (0.63; reference range, ≤0.85). Serologic testing for Whipple disease in serum and cerebrospinal fluid was negative. Pontine biopsy showed a polyclonal lymphocytic infiltrate, with a small polyclonal B-cell infiltrate. No granulomas or histiocytes were seen.

The patient was treated with a 5-day course of intravenous methylprednisolone. His symptoms markedly improved, and repeated brain MRI showed resolution of the enhancing lesions. Six months later he had progressive ataxia and

pseudobulbar affect. Repeated brain MRI showed a recurrence of the punctate enhancing lesions in the pons.

DIAGNOSIS

A diagnosis of chronic lymphocytic inflammation with pontine perivascular enhancement responsive to steroids (CLIPPERS) was made.

MANAGEMENT

The patient was treated with weekly intravenous methylprednisolone 1 g, oral methotrexate 15 mg/d, and folic acid supplementation. After 6 weeks, the methylprednisolone infusion interval was lengthened to 2 weeks for 12 weeks, then to 3 weeks for 12 weeks, and then to monthly infusions for 3 months, until finally discontinued. Serial MRI for 16 years after the original disease presentation showed no recurrence of enhancing brain lesions.

DISCUSSION

CLIPPERS is an inflammatory brainstem disorder of unknown cause. It presents with a progressive pontocerebellar dysfunction associated with punctate enhancing lesions centered on the pons and cerebellum. Published diagnostic criteria enable distinction of CLIPPERS from other causes of enhancing pontocerebellar lesions. Key clinical features include a subacute pontocerebellar dysfunction with improvement in symptoms in response to treatment with corticosteroids, absence of peripheral nervous system disease, and lack an alternative better explanation for the clinical presentation. MRI features are crucial to an accurate diagnosis. T2/FLAIR abnormalities are homogeneous and may be minimal in this disorder. The area of T2-signal abnormality does not significantly exceed the area of postgadolinium enhancement. Gadolinium-enhancing

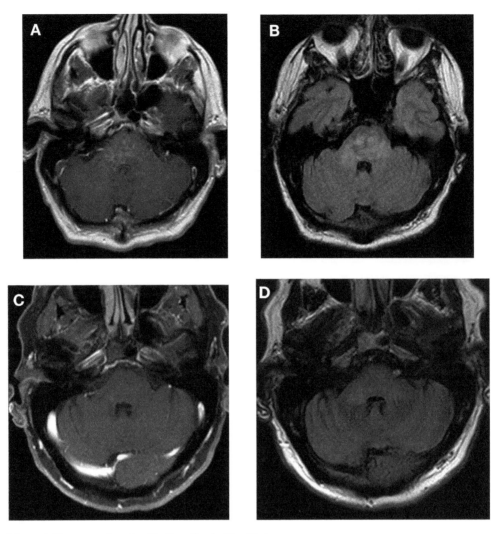

Figure 69.1 Brain Magnetic Resonance Imaging Findings for the Case Patient.

A and B, At initial evaluation, T1 postgadolinium (A) and fluid-attenuated inversion recovery (FLAIR) (B) imaging shows multiple punctate enhancing lesions, centered on the pons, with FLAIR abnormality that is similar in extent. C and D, Follow-up T1 postgadolinium (C) and FLAIR (D) imaging 12 years later, after treatment with corticosteroids and methotrexate, shows complete resolution of the enhancing lesions, with minimal residual FLAIR abnormality.

lesions are punctate, typically measuring less than 3 mm in diameter, without mass effect, and are centered on the pons or cerebellum, with variable involvement of the spinal cord and cerebral hemispheres. Enhancing lesions tend to respond exquisitely to treatment with corticosteroids. Neuropathologic evaluation shows lymphocytic perivascular inflammation with involvement of both white and gray matter. The lymphocytic infiltration is predominated by CD4+ lymphocytes, and myelin loss is minimal.

The differential diagnosis of enhancing brainstem lesions includes central nervous system (CNS) vasculitis, CNS lymphoma, intravascular lymphoma, lymphomatoid granulomatosis, neurosarcoidosis, CNS demyelinating disease, hemophagocytic lymphohistiocytosis, Behçet syndrome, chronic perivascular infections (tuberculosis, neurosyphilis, Whipple disease), autoimmune glial fibrillary acidic protein astrocytopathy, and histiocytic disorders. Patients

who do not clearly fulfill the proposed diagnostic criteria for CLIPPERS should be evaluated for alternative disorders before long-term immunotherapy is pursued. There is no definitive biomarker for CLIPPERS, so brain biopsy should be considered before pursuing long-term immunotherapy. The decision to pursue brain biopsy should be informed by the relative certainty of diagnosis and the expected operative risk, given the often eloquent location of these lesions. Red flags that should alert the provider to the possibility of an alternate diagnosis include a lack of substantial clinical or radiologic response to corticosteroids, lack of typical brainstem-predominant findings, progression to severe deficits within days, fever or marked B symptoms, early onset of seizures, depressed level of consciousness, and any other findings localizing outside the CNS. Suggested useful tests in the diagnostic evaluation of suspected CLIPPERS are shown in Table 69.1.

Table 69.1 | **SUGGESTED DIAGNOSTIC EVALUATION OF SUSPECTED CLIPPERS**

BLOOD TESTS	CSF TESTS	IMAGING
CBC	Blood cell count with differential	Brain MRI with contrast
ESR	Protein	Spine MRI with contrast
Proteins	Glucose	Intracranial vascular imaging
CRP	Oligoclonal bands	Whole-body PET/CT
ACE	IgG index	
Serum LDH	Cytologic analysis	
Cryoglobulins	Flow cytometry	
Monoclonal proteins	PCR for Whipple disease	
Antibodies	Paraneoplastic antibody screen	
ANA	GFAP-IgG	
ENA	VDRL test	
ANCA		
Anti-dsDNA		
RF		
Antiphospholipid antibodies		
Paraneoplastic antibody screen		
GFAP-IgG		
MOG-IgG		
Serum IgE		
Serologic/infectious disease testing		
Hepatitis B and C		
HIV		
Lyme disease		
Tuberculosis		
Syphilis		

Abbreviations: ACE, angiotensin-converting enzyme; ANA, antinuclear antibody; ANCA, antineutrophil cytoplasmic antibodies; anti-dsDNA, anti–double-stranded DNA; CBC, complete blood cell count; CLIPPERS, chronic lymphocytic inflammation with pontine perivascular enhancement responsive to steroids; CRP, C-reactive protein; CSF, cerebrospinal fluid; ENA, extractable nuclear antigen; ESR, erythrocyte sedimentation rate; GFAP, glial fibrillary acidic protein; Ig, immunoglobulin; LDH, lactate dehydrogenase; MOG, myelin oligodendrocyte glycoprotein; MRI, magnetic resonance imaging; PCR, polymerase chain reaction; PET/CT, positron emission tomography/computed tomography; RF, rheumatoid factor.

Modified from Zalewski NL, Tobin WO. CLIPPERS. Curr Neurol Neurosci Rep. 2017 Sep;17(9):65; used with permission.

KEY POINTS

• Patients who do not clearly fulfill the proposed diagnostic criteria for CLIPPERS should be evaluated for alternative disorders before long-term immunotherapy is pursued.

• MRI features are crucial to an accurate diagnosis of CLIPPERS. T2/FLAIR abnormalities are homogeneous and may be minimal in this disorder. The degree of T2-signal abnormality does not substantially exceed the area of postgadolinium enhancement. Gadolinium-enhancing lesions are punctate, typically smaller than 3 mm in diameter, without mass effect, and are centered on the pons or cerebellum, with variable involvement of the spinal cord and cerebral hemispheres. Enhancing lesions tend to respond exquisitely to treatment with corticosteroids.

BILATERAL PARESTHESIAS IN CROHN DISEASE

Amy C. Kunchok, MBBS, and Andrew McKeon, MB, BCh, MD

CASE PRESENTATION

HISTORY AND EXAMINATION

A 43-year-old woman sought care for bilateral lower limb numbness and paresthesias accompanied by a tight, bandlike sensation around her torso at the mid chest level. She had an episode 4 months earlier of bilateral arm paresthesias. The right arm paresthesias lasted several hours, but the left arm paresthesias persisted for 1 week. Urinary frequency had recently developed, but no incontinence. She had no associated limb weakness, facial numbness or weakness, or vision loss.

She had Crohn disease for 13 years, previously treated with mesalamine, azathioprine, and methotrexate. Adalimumab, a tumor necrosis factor (TNF)-α inhibitor (40 mg injection every other week) was commenced 10 years previously, with excellent efficacy. Two years before the current episode, a terminal ileal stricture developed requiring an ileocecectomy. Follow-up colonoscopy showed ulcers at the surgical site, and the adalimumab was increased to 80 mg every other week for 10 months, with ensuing remission. The dosage of adalimumab was then decreased to 40 mg every other week. She had no family history of neurologic disease,

autoimmunity, or cancer. She previously smoked 1 pack of cigarettes per day for 10 years, discontinuing 5 years before neurologic presentation.

On examination, the patient had normal cranial nerve findings, including visual acuity and Ishihara color testing. Ophthalmoscopy findings were normal. Her upper and lower limb examination was largely normal. Limb reflexes were diffusely but symmetrically brisk, and plantar reflexes were flexor. Sensory examination showed minimally reduced vibratory sense at the toes but normal at the ankles. Pinprick sensation was intact, and there was no sensory level. Her gait was normal. Romberg sign was positive. Cerebellar examination was normal. Diagnoses considered at the time are shown in Table 70.1.

TESTING

Electromyography and nerve conduction studies were normal. Magnetic resonance imaging (MRI) of the cervical spine showed multiple, short-segment, T2-hyperintense lesions (Figure 70.1A and 70.1B). C1 and C4-5 lesions demonstrated contrast enhancement (Figure 70.1C). MRI of the brain showed multiple ovoid areas of T2 hyperintensity involving the periventricular regions (Figure 70.1D and 70.1E).

Table 70.1 | **DIFFERENTIAL DIAGNOSIS FOR THE CASE PATIENT**

POSSIBLE DIAGNOSES	PERTINENT POSITIVES	PERTINENT NEGATIVES
Transverse myelopathy		
Inflammatory/demyelinating	Recurrent events	
	Association with Crohn disease and TNF-α inhibitors	
Infectious	Immunosuppressed	No systemic symptoms
Paraneoplastic	Autoimmune history, smoker	No systemic symptoms
Metabolic/nutritional	History of ileal surgery	Taking vitamin supplementation
Subacute sensory neuropathy		
Inflammatory/demyelinating	Association with Crohn disease and TNF-α inhibitors	Atypical history and signs, no systemic symptoms
Paraneoplastic	Immunosuppressed	Atypical history and signs, no systemic symptoms
Metabolic/nutritional	History of ileal surgery	Atypical history and signs, taking vitamin supplementation

Abbreviation: TNF, tumor necrosis factor.

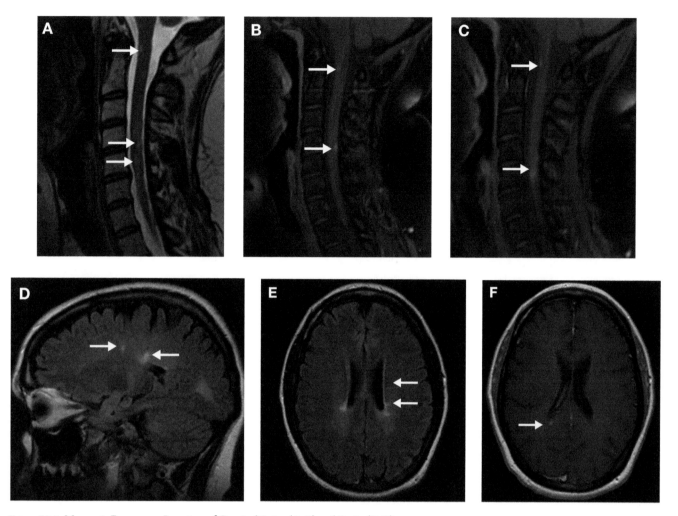

Figure 70.1 **Magnetic Resonance Imaging of Cervical Spine (A-C) and Brain (D-F).**
A, Sagittal, T2, fast-recovery, fast-spin echo sequence shows multiple foci of T2 hyperintensity (arrows). B and C, Sagittal, T1, postgadolinium, fluid-attenuated inversion recovery (FLAIR), fat-saturated sequence shows contrast enhancement at the C1 and C4-5 levels (arrows), typical of demyelinating disease. D and E, Sagittal (D) and axial (E) T2/FLAIR images show multiple ovoid areas of T2 hyperintensity involving the periventricular regions of the brain, including the corpus callosum (arrows). F, Axial, T1, postgadolinium image shows contrast-enhancing lesions adjacent to the posterior aspect of the right lateral ventricle (arrow).

Postcontrast images indicated 2 contrast-enhancing lesions adjacent to the posterior aspect of the right lateral ventricle (Figure 70.1F). MRI of the thoracic spine showed several T2-hyperintense lesions (posterior T2, right dorsolateral cord T7-8, central cord T11-12 and T12-L1) without contrast enhancement.

Serum studies, including biochemistry and inflammatory markers, were normal. Vitamin B_{12} level was low (171 ng/L; reference range, >180 ng/L; optimum value, >400 ng/L), but the methylmalonic acid level was normal. Cerebrospinal fluid (CSF) analysis revealed 1 nucleated cell/μL, protein concentration of 85 mg/dL (reference range, ≤35 mg/dL), and 17 CSF-exclusive oligoclonal bands (reference range, <4). Testing for JC polyoma virus was negative in the CSF by polymerase chain reaction, but serologic results were positive.

DIAGNOSIS

The patient was diagnosed with central nervous system (CNS) demyelination in association with Crohn disease and TNF-α inhibitor use.

MANAGEMENT

The patient discontinued adalimumab and started vedolizumab ($\alpha_4\beta_7$ integrin inhibitor) for her Crohn disease. Her vitamin B_{12} supplementation was increased and iron supplementation was commenced. The patient remained neurologically stable. MRI of the brain and cervical spine 3 months after the therapy changes showed 2 new periventricular lesions in the temporal lobes without contrast enhancement. MRI of the cervical spine was stable. Because of her seropositivity to JC polyoma virus and history of immunosuppression, natalizumab ($\alpha_4\beta_1$ and $\alpha_4\beta_7$ integrin inhibitor) was not recommended. After discussion regarding therapy choice from the remaining US Food and Drug Administration–approved treatments, with consideration of tolerance and potential adverse effects, the patient elected to start fingolimod.

DISCUSSION

Inflammatory bowel and connective tissue diseases are commonly treated with immunosuppressants including TNF-α inhibitors. TNF-α is a cytokine with a wide range of functions, including immune cell regulation, induction of the inflammatory response, inhibition of tumor growth, and induction of apoptosis.

TNF-α inhibitors are effective in the treatment of inflammatory bowel and connective tissue diseases via several proposed mechanisms, including reduction of other proinflammatory cytokine levels. Paradoxically, inflammatory conditions, including neurosarcoidosis, vasculitis, leptomeningitis, meningoencephalitis, and CNS demyelination, have been reported to occur during treatment with TNF-α inhibitors.

Inflammatory bowel and connective tissue diseases are also known to cluster with multiple sclerosis (MS) in some families, which suggests a possible genetic susceptibility to development of CNS inflammation in patients with inflammatory bowel disease and certain systemic autoimmune diseases. In addition, TNF-α inhibition may be a risk factor for development of CNS inflammatory disorders. Patients with MS treated with a TNF-α inhibitor (lenercept, a p55-TNF receptor fusion protein) had worsened frequency and severity of episodes, and 2 patients treated with infliximab had more gadolinium-enhancing lesions. It has been hypothesized that TNF-α inhibitors may cause dysregulation of apoptosis of autoreactive T cells.

Management of demyelinating and inflammatory CNS disorders occurring during treatment with TNF-α inhibitors must consider the benefit for the inflammatory bowel or connective tissue disease, along with the severity and risk of recurrence of the CNS disease. In general, our approach is to discontinue the TNF-α inhibitor in consultation with the gastroenterologist or rheumatologist and choose an alternative therapy. In the acute setting of a neurologic episode, use of acute immunosuppressive therapies may be indicated, such as methylprednisolone or plasma exchange. Additionally, commencement of a long-term disease-modifying MS therapy may be required in patients who fulfill MS diagnostic criteria. In patients with an isolated neurologic or radiologic event, close follow-up with MRI may suffice. Long-term neurologic follow-up is recommended to monitor disease course and potential recurrence.

KEY POINTS

- Demyelinating and other inflammatory CNS disorders can occur in patients with inflammatory bowel and connective tissue diseases treated with TNF-α inhibitors. Evaluation includes CSF testing and MRI of the neuraxis.

- Management points include:
  - Discontinuation of TNF-α inhibitors in consultation with a gastroenterologist or rheumatologist
  - Treatment directed at the CNS disease, including acute treatments (eg, corticosteroids) and MS-directed disease-modifying therapies
  - Long-term follow-up to monitor disease course

SEIZURES AND ENHANCING BRAIN LESIONS

Josephe Archie Honorat, MD, PhD, and Andrew McKeon, MB, BCh, MD

CASE PRESENTATION

HISTORY AND EXAMINATION

A 51-year-old man sought care for a 4-month history of generalized seizures, including 3 seizures over the previous month. The description of his seizures was consistent with generalized tonic-clonic seizures with focal onset (aura of seeing a ball of light or a feeling of reverberation). The patient had no history of head trauma or central nervous system infection and no family history of seizures. The patient reported having visual disturbances, described as blurred vision when looking down, for 2 years before the seizures. His medical and surgical history was unremarkable. Brain magnetic resonance imaging (MRI) showed left temporo-occipital, white matter, T2-signal intensity with gadolinium-enhancing lesions. His neurologic examination was normal, showing no cognitive impairment or focal motor or sensory deficit and normal reflexes. Diagnoses considered at the time are shown in Table 71.1.

TESTING

Electroencephalography findings were normal, as were extensive evaluations of serum and cerebrospinal fluid for systemic, metabolic, endocrine, autoimmune, and infectious causes.

Brain MRI showed patchy gadolinium enhancement with T2 hyperintensity in the left parietotemporal and occipital lobes (Figure 71.1). Spinal cord MRI findings were normal. Brain magnetic resonance angiography showed no evidence of vasculitis. Chest radiography was normal. Bilateral conjunctival biopsy showed no findings suggestive of sarcoidosis or neoplasia. Somatosensory and visual evoked potential testing was normal. Brain biopsy of the left temporal lobe showed white matter lesions with necrosis and chronic infiltration with macrophages and CD3-positive T lymphocytes and a predominant perivascular distribution. Focal, secondary vasculitis was present. There was no evidence of lymphoma. Testing for fungi, mycobacteria, and viral RNA was negative. A repeated brain biopsy of the parietal lobe after another inflammatory relapse showed pathologic findings identical to the first biopsy.

DIAGNOSIS

The patient was diagnosed with inflammatory encephalitis without additional defining features on biopsy.

MANAGEMENT

The patient received levetiracetam (1,500 mg twice daily [3,000 mg/d]) for seizure control, but the seizures remained

Table 71.1 DIFFERENTIAL DIAGNOSIS FOR THE CASE PATIENT

POSSIBLE DIAGNOSES	PERTINENT NEGATIVES
Infectious causes (eg, HIV, syphilis, cytomegalovirus, herpes simplex encephalitis)	Risk factors, fever, history of immunodeficiency
Primary CNS vasculitis	Headache with cognitive impairment and behavioral change; diagnostic angiography
Primary CNS lymphoma	Focal neurologic deficits, mental status and behavioral changes, symptoms of increased intracranial pressure; homogeneously enhancing single mass lesion on brain MRI; diffusion restriction on diffusion-weighted imaging
Acute disseminated encephalomyelitis	Encephalopathy, polyfocal neurologic deficits, rapid progression, younger age; deep gray matter involvement
Hashimoto encephalopathy	History of Hashimoto thyroiditis, cognitive impairment
Neurosarcoidosis	History of systemic sarcoidosis, meningeal symptoms and signs

Abbreviations: CNS, central nervous system; MRI, magnetic resonance imaging.

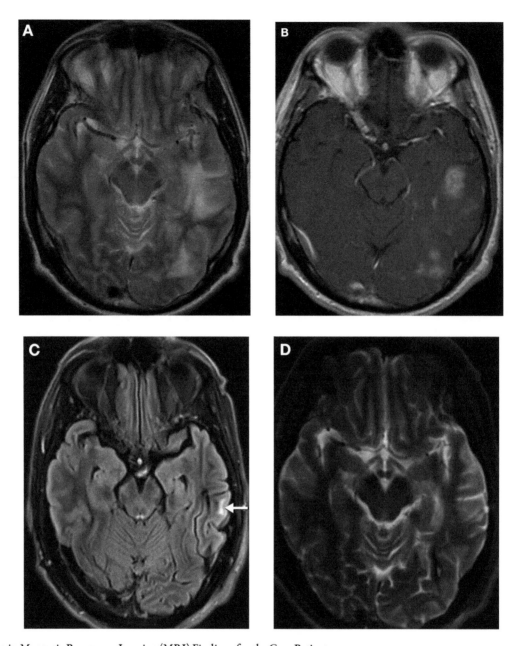

Figure 71.1 **Brain Magnetic Resonance Imaging (MRI) Findings for the Case Patient.**
A and B, Initial axial imaging showed a large hyperintense lesion in the left temporal and occipital lobes on T2-weighted sequences (A) and patchy enhancement of the same regions on T1 postgadolinium images (B). C and D, The patient's last follow-up brain MRI showed near-resolution of the lesion on axial, T2/fluid-attenuated inversion recovery imaging, with some mild residual gliotic change (C, arrow) but no enhancement on T1 postgadolinium imaging (D).

refractory. He then was treated with high doses of intravenous methylprednisolone (1,000 mg for 5 days) and then oral prednisone (80 mg/d). Simultaneously, mycophenolate mofetil was initiated (first 500 mg, then 1,000 mg twice daily [2,000 mg/d]). The patient was monitored every 3 months with complete blood cell counts and liver function tests. Three months later, the prednisone dose was slowly tapered, by 10 mg per month (from 80 mg/d to 10 mg/d), and then by 1 mg per month (from 10 mg/d to zero). During that process, the patient had no new seizures, and brain MRI showed no active inflammation (no new T2 lesions, no gadolinium-enhancing lesions).

After discontinuation of corticosteroids, the patient had a relapse with a generalized seizure, and brain MRI showed new gadolinium-enhancing lesions. Prednisone was resumed at 80 mg/d, with near-remission (the patient had persistent partial seizures, described as visual phenomena without dyscognitive features, as well as 1 generalized seizure per year, refractory to multiple antiseizure medications). He then reinitiated mycophenolate mofetil 1,000 mg twice daily (2,000 mg/d) and continued levetiracetam 1,500 mg twice daily (3,000 mg/d). With this regimen he remained clinically and radiologically stable, with only occasional visual phenomena that were possibly epileptic, although follow-up electroencephalography when he was symptomatic was normal.

DISCUSSION

Encephalitis of unknown origin represents approximately one-third of cases. This proportion is decreasing over time with the development of novel diagnostic technologies, such as sequencing techniques to identify causative infectious agents and advances in neural autoantibody diagnostics.

Patients with seronegative inflammatory encephalitis, without additional defining features on biopsy (such as noncaseating granulomas), should be treated after other well-defined inflammatory, autoimmune, infectious, and neoplastic causes have been reasonably excluded. Brain biopsy sometimes (but not always) has a vital role in helping to characterize those cases. Histologic evaluation combined with special staining may help to rule out a demyelinating, infectious, or neoplastic cause.

Because an inflammatory process was suggested by MRI and biopsy, the case patient was treated with immunosuppressive drugs, which led to substantial clinical and radiologic improvement and long-term remission. High-dose intravenous methylprednisolone is a reasonable first-line therapy in similar cases, followed by a prolonged course and taper of oral prednisone. Steroid-sparing maintenance immunosuppressive therapy can be achieved with mycophenolate mofetil or azathioprine, overlapping with the gradual tapering of corticosteroids. After 3 to 5 years without relapses, withdrawal of immunosuppressive therapy may be considered.

KEY POINTS

- Inflammatory encephalitides, not otherwise defined, are becoming less common because of advances in diagnostic technologies and should be distinguished from other detectable causes of encephalitis.

- Pathologic assessment with brain biopsy may be necessary.

- Immunotherapies, particularly high-dose corticosteroids, are a reasonable initial therapeutic approach.

A MAN WITH RECURRENT HEADACHE AND FOCAL NEUROLOGIC DEFICITS

Jaclyn R. Duvall, MD, and Jerry W. Swanson, MD, MHPE

CASE PRESENTATION

HISTORY AND EXAMINATION

A 42-year-old healthy man sought care for transient episodes of neurologic deficits followed by severe headache. The first episode began with left hand weakness, numbness, and dysarthria, followed approximately 1 hour later by a right temporal headache. His symptoms spontaneously resolved after 8 hours. He had a second episode 2 days later manifested by confusion and bilateral lower extremity numbness, again followed by severe headache with symptoms resolving within 12 hours. A total of 8 episodes occurred over 3 weeks, each lasting 8 to 24 hours, with spontaneous resolution each time. His most recent episode occurred during cerebral angiography. He and his wife reported that each episode seemed characteristic (although not completely stereotypical), generally preceded by left hand numbness followed by subsequent moderate to severe headache. Some episodes were additionally characterized by visual blurriness, intermittent involvement of the right hand, intermittent involvement of bilateral lower extremities, and difficulty with complex comprehension.

On examination, he was completely oriented but had difficulty performing higher-level tasks, including difficulty with calculation. He noted asymmetry in sensation in the left upper extremity but was unable to further elaborate. Neurologic examination was otherwise normal. The differential diagnosis considered at the time, for headache presenting with intermittent/fluctuating focal neurologic deficits, is shown in Table 72.1.

TESTING

Findings of brain magnetic resonance imaging (MRI) with and without gadolinium contrast were normal. Cerebrospinal fluid (CSF) evaluation showed opening pressure, 190 mm H_2O (reference range, 100-200 mm H_2O); white blood cells, 205/μL (reference range, ≤5/μL), 97% lymphocytes; protein, 95 mg/dL (reference range, ≤35 mg/dL); and glucose, 40 mg/dL (considered normal [60% of concurrently measured plasma glucose]). Electroencephalography (EEG) demonstrated right greater than left generalized slowing, with increased-voltage rhythmic delta wave activity, in the frontal regions predominantly. Conventional cerebral angiography findings were normal, but the test appeared to provoke the patient's previous episode. Computed tomography (CT) of the chest was normal. Extensive serum and CSF infectious and autoimmune evaluations were negative. Neurologic examination was normal after his most recent episode resolved, and no further episodes were reported.

DIAGNOSIS

This case highlights a typical presentation of transient headache and neurologic deficits with cerebrospinal fluid lymphocytosis (HaNDL syndrome). Diagnostic criteria according to the *International Classification of Headache Disorders*, 3rd edition, are shown in Box 72.1.

MANAGEMENT

Because the disorder was self-limited, treatment was aimed at symptomatic management of headache. In this case patient with a secure diagnosis of HaNDL syndrome (other processes had been excluded) and stereotypical episodes limited to 3 months after the initial presentation, additional testing was not indicated.

DISCUSSION

HaNDL syndrome is a rare, self-limited, benign condition with migrainelike headache episodes accompanied by transient neurologic deficits usually lasting more than 4 hours, with some deficits lasting more than 24 hours. This syndrome was first clearly characterized at Mayo Clinic in 1981 by Bartleson and colleagues. Previously used terms for this disorder include *migraine with cerebrospinal pleocytosis* and *pseudomigraine with temporary neurologic symptoms and lymphocytic pleocytosis*.

Table 72.1 | DIFFERENTIAL DIAGNOSIS FOR THE CASE PATIENT

POSSIBLE DIAGNOSES	COMMON PRESENTING SYMPTOMS/SIGNS	CLINICAL PEARLS
Migraine with aura	Progressive onset, spreads gradually over 5 minutes, lasting 5-60 minutes, aura accompanied or followed within 60 minutes by headache, although migrainous aura can occur in absence of headache	Stereotypical episodes, aura thought to be caused by cortical spreading depression Visual aura most common
	Auras: visual, sensory, motor (weakness may last longer than 60 minutes), speech or language, brainstem, retinal	
Ischemic stroke and transient ischemic attack	Sudden onset Pain is typically ipsilateral to ischemia	Incidence of headache with ischemic events varies from 15% to 65% between studies (average, 30%) More likely with posterior circulation ischemia Headache less common in lacunar infarction
Cerebral venous thrombosis	Seizure Headache generally diffuse and subacute	Headache is typically the most common and first presenting symptom
Carotid or vertebral artery dissection	Headache typically precedes ischemia Headache ipsilateral and severe	History of neck trauma may be present Oculosympathetic paresis may be present
HaNDL syndrome	Migrainelike headache episodes (typically 1-12 episodes over the illness duration of <3 mo) Accompanying hemiparesthesia, dysphasia, or hemiparesis lasting >4 h	Benign course, resolves spontaneously within 3 mo Associated with CSF lymphocytic pleocytosis (>15 white blood cells/μL) with negative studies for other causes
Reversible cerebral vasoconstriction syndrome	Thunderclap headache (66% of cases) Usually several episodes over several weeks Hemiplegia, ataxia, dysarthria, aphasia, numbness	Diffuse reversible cerebral vasoconstriction, cerebral catheter angiography is diagnostic standard and may need to be repeated Avoidance of vasoactive drugs is recommended
Posterior reversible encephalopathy syndrome	Seizure Altered mental status (encephalopathy) Visual disturbances Often with acute hypertension	Brain MRI shows T2/FLAIR white matter hyperintensities, most commonly in occipital and parietal lobes
Infectious	May have altered level of consciousness Inflammatory markers may be increased Abnormal serum/CSF studies	Neuroborreliosis, neurosyphilis, neurobrucellosis, mycoplasma, granulomatous, HIV meningitis, HSV meningitis, Mollaret meningitis
Inflammatory/vasculitis	Headache is most commonly reported symptom (60% of patients), usually subacute and insidious Cognitive impairment and stroke/TIA symptoms	PACNS, anti–NMDA receptor encephalitis, systemic vasculitis involving the brain (Behçet syndrome, polyarteritis nodosa, granulomatosis with polyangiitis, microscopic polyangiitis, Churg-Strauss syndrome), secondary vasculitis (SLE) May require angiography and/or cerebral biopsy for diagnosis confirmation

Abbreviations: CSF, cerebrospinal fluid; FLAIR, fluid-attenuated inversion recovery; HaNDL syndrome, transient headache and neurologic deficits with CSF lymphocytosis; HSV, herpes simplex virus; MRI, magnetic resonance imaging; NMDA, N-methyl-D-aspartate; PACNS, primary angiitis of the central nervous system; SLE, systemic lupus erythematosus; TIA, transient ischemic attack.

A range of neurologic deficits lasting 5 minutes to 3 days has been reported. Approximately 75% of patients experience repeated episodes that occur for weeks up to several months (range, 56-196 days). In the 2 largest reports, the mean durations of illness were 14 and 21 days. The most common neurologic manifestations include sensory symptoms (70%), followed by aphasia (66%) and motor deficits (42%). Visual symptoms are less common, reported in less than 20% of cases, and include decreased vision, homonymous hemianopsia, and photopsias. Additional rarer features include acute confusional state, papilledema, and sixth nerve palsy. Neurologic manifestations often vary from one episode to the next.

The headache associated with HaNDL syndrome is typically described as moderate to severe and throbbing in character and may be associated with photophobia, nausea, and vomiting. It may be unilateral or bilateral and usually lasts for several hours. Although headache may precede neurologic

deficits, it most often follows the onset of symptoms by 15 to 60 minutes.

HaNDL syndrome has been reported to occur in children as young as 5 years and in elderly persons but is most common in the third and fourth decades of life. No consistent sex or racial predominance has been identified. A minority of patients report prior history of migraine or family history of migraine. Preceding viral prodromal symptoms are reported in 20% to 40% of cases, including cough, rhinitis, generalized fatigue, and diarrhea.

The etiology of HaNDL syndrome is not well understood. Explanations proposed include rare migraine with aura variant, secondary to an infectious process, or an autoimmune mechanism. Isolated cases have been linked to echovirus 30, human herpesvirus 6, and human herpesvirus 7 infection. One study found antibodies to the CACNA1H subunit of the T-type voltage-gated calcium channel in 2

A. Episodes of migrainelike headache fulfilling criteria B and C

B. Both of the following:
   I. Accompanied or shortly preceded by the onset of at least 1 of the following transient neurologic deficits lasting >4 hours:
      a) Hemiparesthesia
      b) Dysphasia
      c) Hemiparesis
   II. Associated with CSF lymphocytic pleocytosis (>15 white blood cells/μL) with negative studies for other causes

C. Evidence of causation demonstrated by either or both of the following:
   I. Headache and transient neurologic deficits have developed or significantly worsened in temporal relation to the CSF lymphocytic pleocytosis or led to its discovery
   II. Headache and transient neurologic deficits have significantly improved in parallel with improvements in the CSF lymphocytic pleocytosis
   III. Not better accounted for by another ICHD-3 diagnosis

Abbreviations: CSF, cerebrospinal fluid; ICHD-3, *International Classification of Headache Disorders*, 3rd edition.

From Headache Classification Committee of the International Headache Society (IHS). The International Classification of Headache Disorders, 3rd edition (beta version). Cephalalgia. 2013 Jul;33(9):629-808; used with permission.

of 4 patients with HaNDL syndrome, compared with 0 of 30 healthy controls and 0 of 80 controls with other neurologic conditions. Linkage to the *CACNA1* gene has not been shown.

HaNDL syndrome is considered a diagnosis of exclusion. More-extensive testing for alternative diagnoses may be necessary if the diagnosis of HaNDL syndrome is not clear. CSF evaluation typically shows lymphocytic pleocytosis and can show other abnormalities such as increased opening pressure and protein concentration. Given the potential devastating nature of some of its mimickers, thorough evaluation should be completed if HaNDL syndrome is suspected. Findings on routine CT and MRI (with or without intravenous contrast) and angiography are expected to be normal. Given potential mimickers of HaNDL syndrome, MR angiography/CT angiography should be considered and are also expected to be normal. MR angiography/CT angiography are preferred to conventional vessel angiography, given the potential for the latter to potentially precipitate an episode. EEG and single-photon emission CT may show focally abnormal areas consistent with the focal neurologic deficits. Bacterial, viral, and fungal infections should be excluded by serum and CSF testing.

Treatment is aimed at symptomatic management of headache. Repeated episodes will invariably require emergent evaluation; however, patient education of this condition is paramount, with reassurance that HaNDL syndrome is self-limited.

KEY POINTS

- HaNDL syndrome is characterized by 1 or more episodes of headache with associated transient neurologic deficit and lymphocytic pleocytosis in the CSF. The most common transient neurologic symptoms are hemisensory deficit, hemiparesis, and aphasia.

- HaNDL syndrome is a self-limited, benign condition typically lasting hours and often recurring over the duration of the illness. It most commonly lasts 2 to 3 weeks but has been reported to recur for up to 3 months.

- Given the vast differential diagnosis of headache with transient neurologic deficit, diagnostic workup including MRI, EEG, cerebral angiography, and CSF evaluation is essential to rule out alternate diagnoses. HaNDL syndrome remains a diagnosis of exclusion.

- After a diagnosis of HaNDL syndrome has been established, treatment is aimed at symptomatic treatment of the headache. Subsequent episodes may warrant repeated investigation given the potential grim prognosis of a missed alternative diagnosis.

HEADACHE, RADICULAR PAIN, AND ENHANCING LESIONS

W. Oliver Tobin, MB, BCh, BAO, PhD

CASE PRESENTATION

HISTORY AND EXAMINATION

A 37-year-old right-handed woman sought care for a dull headache present for 6 months, which was followed by the development of radicular pain in the left leg radiating down the back of her leg into her foot, with associated left foot numbness. Magnetic resonance imaging (MRI) of the lumbar spine showed an enhancing lesion within the conus (Figure 73.1). She was referred for neurosurgical evaluation and underwent MRI of the entire neuraxis, which showed an enhancing lesion in the left cerebellum (Figure 73.1). She underwent a left cerebellar debulking surgical procedure. Postoperative diplopia developed for approximately 1 month and then subsequently resolved. She walked with a walker after surgery, with progressive deterioration in gait. Two months after surgery a postural tremor developed in the left arm and leg. She was referred for neurologic evaluation.

On examination, she had torsional nystagmus on left and right gaze. There was skew diplopia predominantly on left upgaze. Tone was decreased in the left arm with marked ataxia. She was hyporeflexic throughout; plantar responses were flexor. She had a left ankle contracture with weakness in the left leg in a pyramidal distribution, with foot dorsiflexion weakness, knee extension weakness, and hip flexion weakness on the left side. Sensory examination was normal. Her gait was ataxic.

TESTING

Pathologic evaluation of cerebellar tissue showed foamy histiocytes and xanthomatous cells that stained positive for CD68 (KP1). Staining for CD1a was negative. Tissue immunohistochemistry for the BRAF V600E sequence variation was negative. No hyponatremia was detected. Positron emission tomography/computed tomography (PET/CT) of the body from vertex to toes indicated hypermetabolism in the distal femur and proximal tibia (Figure 73.1).

DIAGNOSIS

Examination and imaging findings were consistent with a diagnosis of multifocal Erdheim-Chester disease.

MANAGEMENT

The patient was initially treated with pegylated interferon, with clinical and radiographic progression. She was subsequently treated with vemurafenib and dexamethasone, with continued radiologic progression. Treatment with radiotherapy and cladribine were also unsuccessful. At that point, next-generation sequencing of cerebellar tissue showed a BRAF V471F sequence variation. She was then treated with trametinib, which resulted in a decrease in size of the cerebellar lesion and growth stabilization of the conus lesion.

DISCUSSION

Histiocytic neoplasms are a heterogeneous group of multisystem disorders, primarily including Erdheim-Chester disease, Langerhans cell histiocytosis, and Rosai-Dorfman disease. Although initially thought to represent inflammatory processes, recent insights into their genomic architecture have shown that they are derived from macrophage-lineage neoplasms. Tissue-based genomics has demonstrated sequence variations in various components of the mitogen-activated protein kinase/extracellular signal–regulated kinase (MAPK/ERK) pathway, which has enabled potential treatment with targeted therapies in most patients. Although indolent neoplasms are often present, sometimes not requiring treatment, the presence of central nervous system (CNS) disease portends a poor prognosis and is typically associated with disability. CNS disease is most common in patients with Erdheim-Chester disease, with 40% of patients having CNS involvement (Table 73.1). Diabetes insipidus is a common early finding, with half of patients who have Erdheim-Chester disease–associated diabetes insipidus having normal brain MRI findings. Vemurafenib was the first drug to be approved for neoplasms with BRAF V600E and acts by B-Raf enzyme inhibition. Clinical trials are ongoing to assess

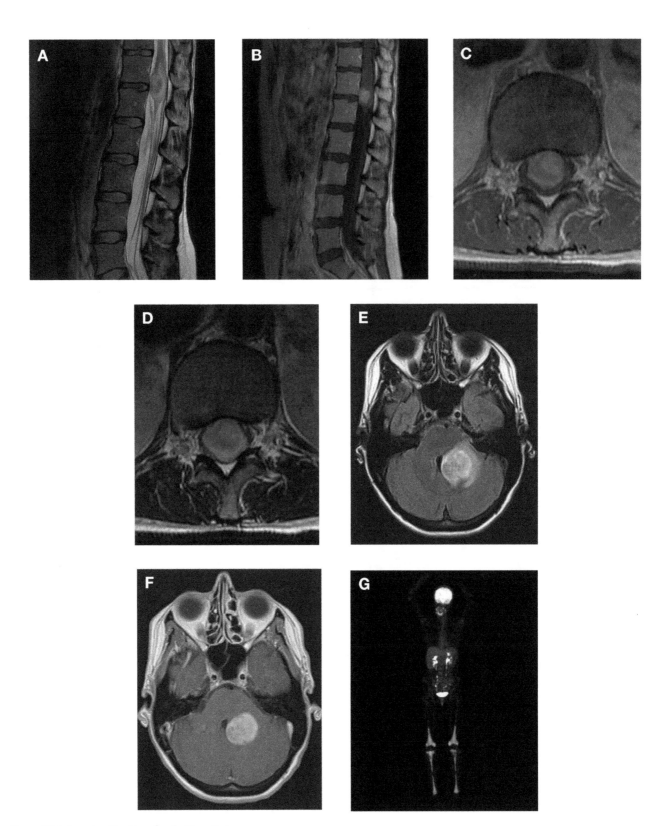

Figure 73.1 **Imaging Findings for the Case Patient.**
A-F, Magnetic resonance imaging of the spine (A-D) and brain (E-F) at initial evaluation shows a mass in the conus on T2-weighted imaging (A, sagittal; C and D, axial) with heterogeneous T1 postgadolinium enhancement (B, sagittal) and a left cerebellar peduncular mass on T2-weighted imaging (E, axial), also with T1 postgadolinium enhancement (F, axial). G, Positron emission tomography/computed tomography of the body from vertex to toes shows hypermetabolism in the distal femur and tibia.

Table 73.1 DIFFERENTIAL DIAGNOSIS OF HISTIOCYTIC DISORDERS

POSSIBLE DIAGNOSES	CLINICAL & RADIOLOGIC FEATURES
Erdheim-Chester disease	CNS involvement (40% of patients)
	Dural or pituitary stalk thickening
	Brainstem/cerebellar enhancing masses
	Cerebral white matter enhancement
	Clinical features of diabetes insipidus
Langerhans cell histiocytosis	CNS involvement (5% of patients)
	Globus pallidus/dentate nucleus T1 hyperintensity
	Brainstem/cerebellum T2 hyperintensity
	Dural lesion from intracranial extension of skull lesion
	Pituitary stalk thickening
Rosai-Dorfman disease	CNS involvement (10% of patients)
	Typically isolated dural lesions with extension into the parenchyma of the brain or spinal cord
	Rarely parenchymal lesions

Abbreviation: CNS, central nervous system.

the efficacy of other B-Raf inhibitors with better CNS penetration, in addition to agents targeting other sequence variations along the MAPK/ERK pathway, such as trametinib (a MEK1 and MEK2 inhibitor).

In the case patient, findings on PET/CT from vertex to toes were essentially diagnostic for Erdheim-Chester disease, with hypermetabolism in the distal femur and proximal tibia. Most standard PET/CT studies obtained for oncologic purposes are performed from orbits to mid thigh. This will not capture the long-bone disease seen in almost all patients with Erdheim-Chester disease. So-called hairy kidneys are a common finding on PET/CT, giving additional yield of PET/CT over that of bone scan.

Tissue-based BRAF immunohistochemistry did not demonstrate a BRAF V600E sequence variation. The patient did not have a clinical response to nontargeted therapies including corticosteroids, cladribine, radiotherapy, and pegylated interferon. Treatment with vemurafenib in the absence of BRAF V600E was also unsuccessful. Next-generation tissue-based sequencing identified an alternative target within the MAPK/ERK pathway, and initiation of trametinib resulted in sustained disease stability.

KEY POINTS

- PET/CT from vertex to toes is recommended to evaluate for bony lesions, in particular long-bone osteosclerosis at the metadiaphysis, which is pathognomonic for Erdheim-Chester disease. Soft-tissue hypermetabolic regions, such as hairy kidneys, are typically superior biopsy targets and are also identified on whole-body PET/CT.

- Testing for BRAF V600E by immunohistochemical analysis may have insufficient sensitivity to detect the variant protein in histiocytic neoplasms. Sensitivity is lower in decalcified bone tissue. Molecular testing methods are recommended to definitively exclude a sequence variation and to identify other potential treatment targets.

SEIZURES 3 MONTHS AFTER ENDARTERECTOMY

Andrew McKeon, MB, BCh, MD, and Robert D. Brown Jr, MD, MPH

CASE PRESENTATION

HISTORY AND EXAMINATION

A 57-year-old woman had development of acute-onset, right-sided weakness and sensory change (face, arm, and leg) when at a casino. She was brought to the emergency department, and her symptoms had essentially resolved upon her arrival. Brain magnetic resonance imaging (MRI) showed no acute stroke (Figure 74.1A), and a transient ischemic attack was diagnosed. She was transferred to an academic medical center. Investigations showed high-grade left internal carotid artery stenosis; the same day, a stent was placed via endovascular procedure by an interventional neuroradiologist.

The patient was discharged from the hospital and remained symptom free for the next 3 months. She then began to have episodic twitching in the upper and lower right side of her face, accompanied by a spasm-type feeling in her throat. With some episodes, she had a jacksonian march of muscle twitching from her hand into the right arm and then to her face. Other events triggered motor symptoms on the entire right side of the body. She had 2 episodes of loss of consciousness, surmised to be secondary generalized seizures. Headache and some occasional altered mental status were also noted. Despite anticonvulsant use, starting initially with levetiracetam (up to 1,500 mg twice daily [3,000 mg/d]), then with the addition of carbamazepine (400 mg twice daily [800 mg/d]) and divalproex sodium (2,500 mg/d in 2 divided doses), her seizures remained refractory. She also began to note persistent speech and language deficits, right-sided weakness, altered sensation in the right upper extremity, and fatigue. The differential diagnosis included cerebral infarction, brain abscess, central nervous system (CNS) sarcoidosis, focal CNS vasculitis, and neoplasia.

TESTING

MRI of the head showed an enhancing lesion with surrounding edema in the left frontal and parietal lobes at the cortex, also involving the nearby leptomeninges (Figure 74.1B). Electroencephalography showed potentially epileptogenic discharges over the left central head region. Brain biopsy was performed, which showed abundant CD68+ macrophages, granulomatous inflammation, and necrosis associated with foreign material. The associated lymphocytic infiltrates were predominantly composed of CD3+ T cells and only sparse CD20+ B cells. The foreign material seen was lamellated, amorphous, nonpolarizable, and nonrefractile, typical of hydrophilic polymers commonly used in intravascular medical devices.

DIAGNOSIS

The patient was diagnosed with seizures caused by multifocal, intracranial, foreign-body, granulomatous reaction to polymers that had embolized to brain parenchyma during the prior endovascular procedure.

MANAGEMENT

To suppress this inflammatory reaction, corticosteroids were initiated—intravenous methylprednisolone (IVMP) 1 g daily for 3 consecutive days, followed by an oral prednisone course, with a plan to gradually taper to zero over 2 months. Antiseizure medication was continued at the same doses. The patient's seizures remitted initially but relapsed upon corticosteroid dose reduction despite a very slow prednisone taper. She had further remissions from seizures and headache upon re-treating with prednisone starting at 60 mg/d on 3 occasions, but seizures would inevitably return at each subsequent taper to 10 mg/d of prednisone. In tandem with her clinical course, the amount of postgadolinium enhancement visible on MRI would fluctuate, becoming less prominent during high-dose prednisone treatment (Figure 74.1C) and recrudescing when prednisone was reduced to low doses (Figure 74.1D).

At that point, 18 months after the initial onset of seizures, the patient had cushingoid features, depression, and chronic insomnia. During the next year, 2 steroid-sparing strategies were employed sequentially in an attempt to bring about clinical and radiologic remission and freedom from corticosteroid treatment. Standard treatments for autoimmune

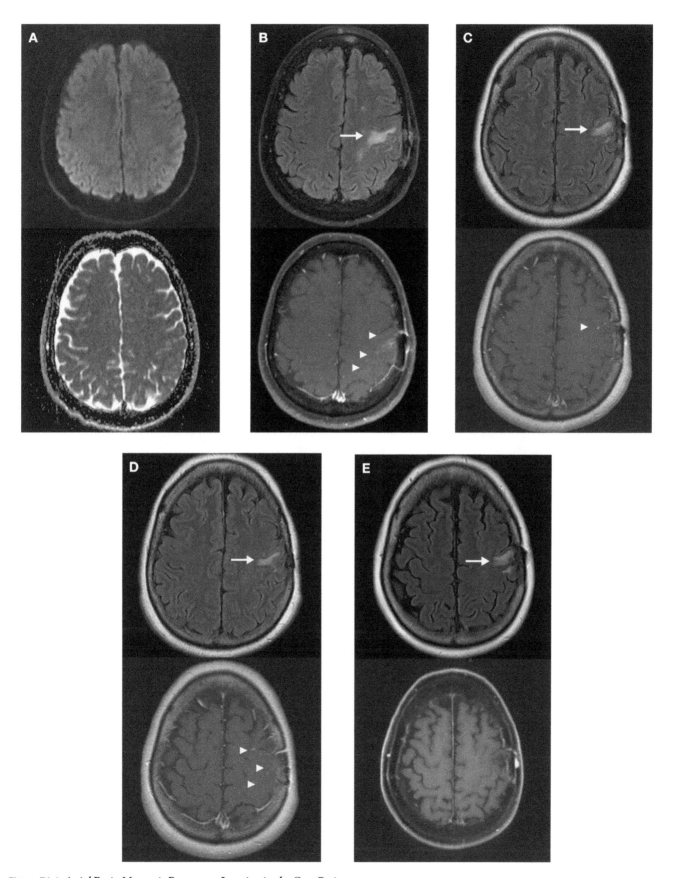

Figure 74.1 **Axial Brain Magnetic Resonance Imaging in the Case Patient.**
A, One day after initial presentation after the suspected cerebrovascular event, diffusion-weighted imaging (top) and apparent diffusion coefficient imaging (bottom) did not show acute stroke. B-E, T2/
fluid-attenuated inversion recovery (top) and T1 postgadolinium images (bottom), obtained at different time points during the patient's clinical course. The T2-signal abnormality due to postbiopsy gliosis
decreased and then stabilized in size over time (top, arrows). The degree of postgadolinium enhancement varied over time (bottom, arrowheads), from extensive before treatment (B), to decreased after corticosteroid treatment (C), to recrudescing after tapering to low-dose corticosteroid therapy, despite cyclophosphamide treatment (D), to finally remitted after tapering to low-dose corticosteroid therapy, combined with infliximab therapy (E).

encephalitis and CNS vasculitis (first, mycophenolate mofetil and, later, cyclophosphamide) were combined with prednisone 60 mg/d, with gradual reduction in prednisone dose over 6 months. On both occasions, despite the addition of those steroid-sparing immunosuppressants, the patient had breakthrough seizures and accompanying radiologic worsening with prednisone taper.

Because the pathologic process showed a granulomatous reaction and because more common granulomatous diseases (such as sarcoidosis) are known to remit with tumor necrosis factor α (TNFα) therapy, infliximab was started. A 5-mg/kg infusion was administered at weeks 0, 2, and 6, followed by an infusion every 8 weeks. In tandem, she started IVMP, 1 g weekly for 12 weeks, then every other week for 12 weeks, then every third week for 12 weeks, then every fourth week for 12 weeks, with a plan to stop altogether within 2 months. At one evaluation, 2 new, small areas of MRI enhancement were seen, without clinical correlate, which prompted an increase in the infliximab dose to 8 mg/kg every 8 weeks. The patient's condition remitted, which continued during her clinical course to the last follow-up, concomitant with the IVMP taper. At last follow-up, imaging showed near-resolution of the enhancement (Figure 74.1E). At this point, lifelong infliximab therapy is predicted to be required.

DISCUSSION

In patients who have received neurovascular medical device therapy and have subsequent development of seizures, focal neurologic deficit, headache, or encephalopathy, CNS inflammation triggered by retained foreign-body material should be considered as a potential cause. Radiologic clues include T2-signal change and enhancement in proximity to that medical device or, in this case patient, distal to the device (an arterial stent) but within the vascular territory of the artery stented.

This phenomenon is a previously reported outcome of carotid artery stenting. Symptoms may not be apparent immediately because the associated chronic inflammation, which causes the symptoms rather than the retained foreign-body material itself, takes time to evolve. Patients can have refractory neurologic syndromes as a consequence.

Biopsy of the lesion proved informative for securing the diagnosis and eliminating other differential diagnostic considerations and also aided treatment decision making. The most prominent inflammatory cell types noted were T lymphocytes and macrophage-enriched noncaseating granulomas. Although high doses of corticosteroid therapy serve as a catch-all therapy with rapid efficacy, it is inevitably accompanied by undesirable short-term and long-term adverse effects including insomnia, altered mood, obesity, hyperglycemia, hypertension, fluid retention, cushingoid appearance, osteoporosis, and cataracts, among others. Mycophenolate mofetil and cyclophosphamide were selected to target T lymphocytes but did not prove a successful surrogate for high-dose corticosteroids. TNFα promotes focused accumulation of immune cells at the site of infection, resulting in granulomas. Infliximab, which blocks TNFα receptors, prevents granuloma formation. We hypothesize that infliximab, by inhibiting T- and B-lymphocyte signaling and decreasing local adhesion molecule production, prevents organized chronic inflammation from occurring, thus eliminating postgadolinium contrast enhancement, and promotes remission from seizures. A potential downside of blocking this immunologic mechanism is opportunistic infection. In addition, some patients with autoimmune diseases, such as rheumatoid arthritis, have paradoxical development of CNS inflammation when treated with infliximab.

KEY POINTS

- Foreign-body polymer material embolization is an uncommon complication after carotid artery stenting.

- Presentation includes seizures, focal neurologic deficit, headache, and encephalopathy.

- Diagnosis can be made by demonstration of scattered T2 signal and punctate enhancement in the parenchyma vascularized by the stented vessel and targeted biopsy of one of those lesions, in a noneloquent region of brain, if possible.

- Treatment includes seizure management with standard antiepileptic therapies, although corticosteroids are generally needed to eliminate inflammation.

- Corticosteroid dependency may occur. Anti-TNFα therapy, such as infliximab, can be considered as a steroid-sparing agent.

75

PROGRESSIVE BILATERAL ARM PAIN, GAIT DISTURBANCE, CONSTIPATION, AND URINARY RETENTION

Ivan D. Carabenciov, MD, and Michael W. Ruff, MD

CASE PRESENTATION

HISTORY AND EXAMINATION

A previously healthy 48-year-old woman sought care for progressive right arm and hand pain with radial nerve–distribution sensory loss. As an athlete, she had a past history of multiple prior athletics-associated, musculoskeletal, upper cervical spine injuries. Her symptoms were initially attributed to a right C6 radiculopathy, and a targeted corticosteroid injection to the C6 nerve root resulted in transient improvement in her pain. Approximately 2 months after the injection, her pain returned and was refractory to further targeted injections. Over the next several months, the sensory loss spread to involve the entire right hand and subsequently the entire left hand. In addition, she had development of diffuse right hand weakness and a sense of imbalance that was particularly prominent while in the dark. In the 3 months before our evaluation, hypersensitivity and loss of temperature sensation developed from the neck down. Finally, she experienced progressive constipation and urinary retention.

On evaluation in our department, she had prominent right upper extremity weakness predominantly in the C8/T1 innervated musculature, with trace left interosseous muscle weakness. In addition, there was mild bilateral iliopsoas abductor weakness in the leg (right > left), which was more prominent with eyes closed. Biceps reflex was absent on the right, with reduced brachioradialis reflex on the right, absent brachioradialis reflex on the left, and slightly increased triceps reflexes bilaterally (left > right). Quadriceps and gastrocnemius reflexes were increased on the right. She had an extensor plantar response on the right and flexor plantar response on the left. She had moderately reduced joint position sense and vibratory sensation in the bilateral lower extremities (right > left). Diagnoses considered at the time are shown in Table 75.1.

TESTING

Magnetic resonance imaging (MRI) of the cervical spine showed an expanded cervical spinal cord from C3 through C7-T1 with diffuse T2-hyperintense changes and heterogeneous gadolinium enhancement most prominent at C5-6 (Figure 75.1). In combination with a congenitally small central canal, severe central canal narrowing was seen at C5-6 and moderate narrowing at C4-5. MRI of the brain and thoracic spine were normal, and MRI of the lumbar spine indicated only mild lumbar spondylosis.

On suspicion of a spinal cord neoplasm with a secondary compressive myelopathy, C3 through C7 laminectomy and posterior instrumented fusion from C2 through T1 was performed, with a biopsy obtained at the C5-6 level. Postoperatively, her gait and right upper extremity pain improved. The biopsy showed atypical glial cells. Neurofilament staining demonstrated an infiltrative pattern.

Table 75.1 | **DIFFERENTIAL DIAGNOSIS FOR THE CASE PATIENT**

POSSIBLE DIAGNOSES	PERTINENT INFORMATION
Compressive myelopathy	Previous cervical spine injuries; cervical spine localization of patient's symptoms; progressive decline
Demyelinating disease	Lack of prior inflammatory episodes; reduced upper extremity reflexes
Dural arteriovenous fistula	No report of "stepwise deterioration"; involves cervical spine without lower cord/conus involvement
Viral myelitis	No systemic symptoms; progressive symptoms over chronic time frame would be inconsistent with this diagnosis
Spinal cord glioma	Subacute time course would be consistent with this diagnosis

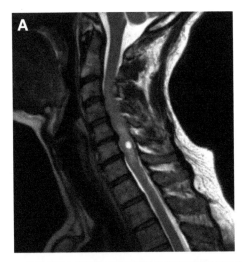

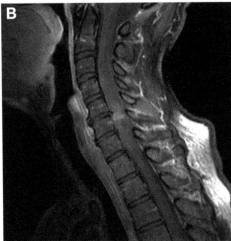

Figure 75.1 **Magnetic Resonance Imaging Findings for the Case Patient.**

A, T2-weighted sagittal image of the cervical spine shows an expansile T2-hyperintense lesion within the cervical spinal cord from C3 through T1, with a syrinx at the C6 segment. B, T1-weighted postcontrast image of the cervical spinal cord shows heterogeneous contrast enhancement slightly inferior to an area of severe canal narrowing at the C5-6 disk interspace.

Atypical cells were positive for glial fibrillary acidic protein, oligodendrocyte transcription factor 2, and a Lys27Met sequence variation of histone H3 (H3K27M), with overexpression of p53 on immunohistochemical staining. There was loss of H3 K27-trimethylation on the infiltrating cells, corresponding to the presence of H3K27M. The cells were negative for isocitrate dehydrogenase R132H and BRAF V600E sequence variations on immunohistochemistry.

DIAGNOSIS

These findings were diagnostic for diffuse midline glioma with H3K27M (World Health Organization grade IV).

MANAGEMENT

A total of 5,400 cGy of photon radiation was delivered in 30 fractions over 42 days. She was subsequently treated

with an oral histone deacetylase inhibitor, panobinostat, for 12 months. During this time, she had clinical response to treatment and reported improvement in balance and numbness. Follow-up MRI at 3 months showed a slight decrease in the size of the mass, and this response was sustained 1 year post radiotherapy.

DISCUSSION

Diffuse midline gliomas that contain H3K27M are incurable, often inoperable, midline brain tumors that are most commonly seen in the pediatric population. These tumors can also occur in adult patients and are considered high grade, even in the absence of features such as necrosis or microvascular proliferation. Substitution of this amino acid on histone H3 results in broad chromatin remodeling that ultimately impedes differentiation of the cell. Despite several advancements in understanding of the underlying genetic alterations, the prognosis in children with this neoplasm is poor, with a median survival of approximately 1 year from the time of diagnosis. H3K27M gliomas are a relatively newly recognized entity, and although this mutation is associated with an aggressive refractory course in children, where the sequence variation is found in the majority of diffuse intrinsic pontine gliomas, their behavior in adults may be more indolent.

Current standard treatment centers on fractionated radiation, administered to a total dose of 54 to 59 Gy in 30 fractions. Panobinostat is a general histone deacetylase inhibitor that has shown good in vitro efficacy against diffuse midline gliomas harboring H3K27M.

Distinct from this case, the most common spinal cord neoplasm in adults is ependymoma, which is characterized radiologically by a gadolinium-enhancing, centrally located, expansile tumor commonly associated with a syrinx and often with a hemosiderin "cap" indicating prior hemorrhage. Ependymoma was a diagnostic consideration in this case, particularly given the syrinx and the indolent disease course.

KEY POINTS

- Diffuse gliomas (eg, astrocytoma) are likely to be expansile, with imaging findings far more prominent than the clinical symptoms suggest, indicative of the chronicity of the lesion and infiltrative nature of the disease.

- Spinal cord tumors may be challenging to distinguish radiographically from inflammatory longitudinally extensive transverse myelitis. However, the clinical history can be exceedingly helpful to distinguish the 2 because inflammatory processes classically reach a nadir over a much briefer time course.

- Tumors with H3K27M can occur in adult patients and are considered high grade, even in the absence of features such as necrosis or microvascular proliferation.

76

A WOMAN WITH SUBACUTE NUMBNESS OF THE TRUNK, ARMS, AND LEGS

Eoin P. Flanagan, MB, BCh

CASE PRESENTATION

HISTORY AND EXAMINATION

A 39-year-old previously healthy woman had development of new-onset numbness in her left arm. This progressed over 2 to 3 weeks to involve the left axilla, trunk, lower extremities, and genital region. She had mild imbalance and left-sided weakness but remained ambulating without a gait aid. She had no bowel or bladder dysfunction. She had no preceding infection or vaccination and no shortness of breath, fevers, or chills. There was no accompanying nausea, vomiting, or hiccups. She did not have Lhermitte sign or repetitive tonic spasms.

Sagittal cervical spine magnetic resonance imaging (MRI) showed a longitudinally extensive T2 hyperintensity with gadolinium enhancement. Cerebrospinal fluid analysis showed an increased white blood cell count of 29/µL (reference range, 0-5/µL) but normal protein and glucose values and negative oligoclonal bands. Serum cell-based assays were negative for aquaporin-4 (AQP4)–immunoglobulin G (IgG) and myelin oligodendrocyte glycoprotein–IgG autoantibodies. She was diagnosed with idiopathic transverse myelitis and, subsequently, seronegative neuromyelitis optica spectrum disorder (NMOSD). She was treated initially with 1 g/d of intravenous methylprednisolone (IVMP) for 5 days, with transient improvement, but her symptoms recurred. Plasma exchange was recommended locally, but she sought a second opinion at Mayo Clinic.

Her neurologic examination at that time indicated a mild, face-sparing, upper motor neuron–pattern left hemiparesis and mildly decreased vibration sense in the left toe. There was no evidence of spasticity, and plantar responses were both flexor. Despite her subjective reports of sensory deficits, objective pinprick sensation was intact.

TESTING

Repeated MRI of the cervical spine showed the longitudinally extensive T2 lesion in a central location on axial

sequences (Figure 76.1A), with linear, dorsal, subpial gadolinium enhancement extending more than 2 vertebral segments (Figure 76.1B). The MRI findings were most suggestive of spinal cord neurosarcoidosis. Computed tomography (CT) of the chest showed bilateral hilar adenopathy. Serum levels of angiotensin-converting enzyme were normal. Transbronchial lung biopsy showed noncaseating granulomas.

DIAGNOSIS

Noncaseating granulomas were confirmatory of pulmonary sarcoidosis, which led to a diagnosis of spinal cord neurosarcoidosis.

MANAGEMENT

Treatment with 1 g/d IVMP for 5 days was repeated, followed by oral prednisone 1 mg/kg per day for 2 months. Her neurologic symptoms improved, and repeated MRI showed a marked decrease in T2 hyperintensity and gadolinium enhancement consistent with interval response to treatment. A slow prednisone taper over 9 months was initiated.

DISCUSSION

Spinal cord neurosarcoidosis often presents with an isolated myelopathy without symptoms of pulmonary sarcoidosis (eg, cough, dyspnea). The presentation can range from a subacute onset mimicking transverse myelitis (as in this case patient) to a more insidious progressive myelopathy over months to years. In those with a more insidious presentation, progression that occurs after the first month of neurologic symptoms helps distinguish this disease from an inflammatory myelopathy caused by relapsing-remitting multiple sclerosis, AQP4-IgG–seropositive NMOSD, or myelin oligodendrocyte glycoprotein–IgG myelitis that typically reaches nadir within 3 weeks. Early in the course, the clinical deficits are often less severe than with other disorders that are accompanied by longitudinally extensive spinal cord lesions (eg, AQP4-IgG–seropositive NMOSD) in which patients with

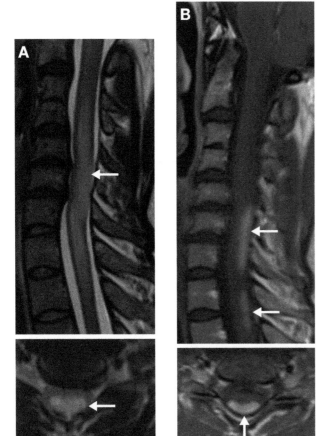

Figure 76.1 Spine Magnetic Resonance Imaging Findings for the Case Patient.

A, T2-weighted imaging shows a longitudinally extensive lesion on sagittal view (top, arrow) that is in a central location on axial view (bottom, arrow). B, T1 postgadolinium images show linear and dorsal, subpial enhancement extending more than 2 vertebral segments (top and bottom, arrows).

cord neurosarcoidosis and negative chest CT findings, ^{18}F-fludeoxyglucose–positron emission tomography should be performed. Moreover, it can help guide the optimal location for biopsy. Transbronchial lung biopsy via bronchoscopy or direct lymph node biopsy by mediastinoscopy may be used to obtain a tissue diagnosis by assessing for the characteristic noncaseating granulomas. Given the high risk of permanent disability, direct cord biopsy is generally not undertaken, and confirmation of sarcoidosis at an extraneurologic site is sufficient for a probable diagnosis of neurosarcoidosis. In patients with characteristic MRI features but without evidence of systemic sarcoidosis on imaging (sometimes owing to preceding corticosteroid use), an empiric corticosteroid treatment course with close imaging surveillance can be considered, with reassessment of the diagnosis in those without satisfactory treatment response.

The mainstay of treatment of spinal cord neurosarcoidosis is prolonged high-dose corticosteroids. A common dosing pattern is 1 g IVMP once daily for 5 days, followed by 1 mg/kg oral prednisone per day for at least 3 months, with a slow taper over the subsequent 9 to 12 months. Early relapse is common in those treated with short courses of IV corticosteroids alone or when oral corticosteroids are weaned too quickly, as occurred in the case patient. Steroid-sparing agents such as methotrexate, mycophenolate mofetil, or azathioprine are typically reserved for patients who have relapse during or after corticosteroid tapering. The tumor necrosis factor α inhibitor infliximab can be used as an acute treatment as a substitution for prednisone if the patient is intolerant of corticosteroids or they are contraindicated. After treatment for 1 to 2 years, the disease will often go into remission, and long-term immunotherapy beyond 2 years is often not necessary.

KEY POINTS

- Spinal cord neurosarcoidosis is frequently misdiagnosed as idiopathic transverse myelitis or seronegative NMOSD.

- Linear, dorsal, subpial enhancement extending for 2 or more vertebral segments on postgadolinium sagittal MRI is suggestive of spinal cord neurosarcoidosis.

- Chest CT is the initial diagnostic test for pulmonary sarcoidosis, but positron emission tomography/CT has greater sensitivity for diagnosis and is recommended if CT is negative and a high degree of clinical suspicion remains.

- Prolonged high-dose oral corticosteroids are required to achieve and maintain remission in spinal cord neurosarcoidosis.

severe motor weakness commonly become paraplegic or quadriplegic within a few weeks.

The T2-hyperintense lesion in spinal cord neurosarcoidosis is often indistinguishable from that of other causes, but the MRI gadolinium enhancement pattern may distinguish it. Specifically, the linear, dorsal, subpial enhancement extending inward from the posterior aspect of the cord, as seen in this case, is suggestive of spinal cord sarcoidosis. Occasionally, concurrent central canal enhancement is seen with a trident appearance on axial postgadolinium sequences.

The enlarged pulmonary hilar nodes can occasionally be visualized on thoracic spine MRI and give a clue to this diagnosis. Chest CT is often abnormal but may be less sensitive. In patients with a high clinical suspicion for spinal

A SEPTUAGENARIAN WITH PROGRESSIVE LOWER EXTREMITY WEAKNESS AND PAIN

Nicholas L. Zalewski, MD

CASE PRESENTATION

HISTORY AND EXAMINATION

A 75-year-old right-handed man was referred for evaluation of treatment-resistant transverse myelitis. His medical history included hypertension, coronary artery disease, benign prostatic hyperplasia, and chronic kidney disease. Eight years earlier, the patient noted development of radiating pain down the left lower extremity during long drives, which was relieved by lying down on his back. For the past 5 years, lower extremity weakness and pain would develop, on the left greater than right, when he walked more than half a block. He received epidural lumbar corticosteroid injections, given suspected symptomatic lumbar stenosis, which provided substantial pain relief, allowing him to sit and walk for longer periods. Nine months before the current evaluation, his symptoms became refractory, and he underwent surgical decompression with laminectomy at L3-L5. This provided substantial relief for the lower extremity pain.

Three months after the procedure, worsening weakness and numbness of the lower extremities developed, leading to many falls. Numbness was initially in his buttocks and feet and gradually progressed proximally from the feet over several months. He used a cane for 4 months and then a walker for 2 weeks because of progressive weakness and falls. He had difficulty voiding urine. He had nonspecific persistent pain in his calves, feet, and buttock region, worsening over months. One month before referral, magnetic resonance imaging (MRI) of the entire spine was performed, and he was told the findings were consistent with transverse myelitis. He began taking prednisone 40 mg daily; after 2 to 3 days he believed his symptoms were worsening rapidly and thus stopped the medication.

The patient's symptoms ultimately continued to worsen. He restarted the prednisone and sought a second opinion at Mayo Clinic because symptoms were worsening quickly again. Evaluation noted that his upper extremities were spared, he had no truncal sensory level, and he reported no prior neurologic or systemic symptoms. Neurologic examination showed severe paraparesis in an upper motor neuron pattern, normal resting tone, brisk lower extremity reflexes, mute plantar responses, and severe lower extremity multimodality sensory loss. Gait was consistent with severe paraparesis and sensory loss; he was able to cautiously walk a few steps with support.

Given the progressive myelopathy without contrast enhancement evolving over months, the idiopathic transverse myelitis diagnosis was discounted. Other diagnoses then considered are shown in Table 77.1.

TESTING

Review of outside MRI indicated multilevel lumbar stenosis before his surgery and possible, faint, T2-hyperintense cord signal extending into the conus (Figure 77.1). At the time his symptoms worsened, MRI of the thoracic spine showed longitudinally extensive T2 hyperintensity extending from the thoracic cord into the conus without contrast enhancement. MRI of the brain was unremarkable.

Evaluation in our department included cerebrospinal fluid analysis, which showed an increased protein concentration of 92 mg/dL (reference range, ≤35 mg/dL), 1 total nucleated cell/µL, normal immunoglobulin G (IgG) index, and no supernumerary oligoclonal bands; cytologic analysis and paraneoplastic autoantibody evaluation were negative. Serum aquaporin-4–IgG, myelin oligodendrocyte glycoprotein–IgG, and paraneoplastic autoantibody evaluation were negative. Serum serologic testing for HIV and syphilis were negative. Magnetic resonance angiography (MRA) of the spinal canal showed mild prominence of vascularity at T10-T12 but no clear spinal dural arteriovenous fistula (SDAVF). However, given the strong suspicion for SDAVF in an older man with progressive myelopathy worsening with corticosteroids, longitudinally extensive lesion extending into the conus, and no evidence

Table 77.1 DIFFERENTIAL DIAGNOSIS FOR THE CASE PATIENT

POSSIBLE DIAGNOSES	PERTINENT POSITIVES	PERTINENT NEGATIVES
Structural		
Arachnoiditis	Recent surgical procedure	No constricted site of cord/roots
	Progressive decline over months	No syrinx/dilated central canal
	T2 hyperintensity without enhancement	
Inflammatory		
Aquaporin-4–IgG–seropositive NMOSD	Longitudinally extensive T2 hyperintensity	Progressive decline over several months
	Older patient	No contrast enhancement
		Male
		Worsening with corticosteroids
Myelin oligodendrocyte glycoprotein–IgG myelitis	Longitudinally extensive T2 hyperintensity	Progressive decline over several months
	Extension into conus	Older age
	No clear contrast enhancement (or faint)	Worsening with corticosteroids
Sarcoidosis	Progression over months	No contrast enhancement
	Longitudinally extensive T2 hyperintensity	Worsening with corticosteroids
Glial fibrillary acidic protein–IgG myelitis	Prolonged time to nadir	No central canal enhancement
	Longitudinally extensive T2 hyperintensity	Lack of multifocal neurologic involvement/normal brain MRI
		Worsening with corticosteroids
Idiopathic transverse myelitis	Spinal cord T2 hyperintensity; complete cross-sectional cord signal	Nadir >21 d
		No evidence of truncal sensory level or inflammation
		No evaluation to rule out disease-associated causes of myelopathy
Paraneoplastic	Severe progression over months	Very rare in isolation, without other neurologic involvement
	No gadolinium enhancement	
	Older patient	No known cancer or systemic symptoms
Infectious		
Viral myelitis (eg, HIV), syphilis, Lyme disease, human T-lymphotropic virus	T2-hyperintense spinal cord lesion; poorly defined borders	No infectious symptoms, rash, etc
		Progressive decline over months
		No classic restricted clinical or radiographic pattern
Vascular		
Spinal dural arteriovenous fistula	Elderly man	No clear tortuous flow voids
	Progressive myelopathy	
	Longitudinally extensive lesion, extending into conus	
	Worsening with corticosteroids	
Neoplasm		
Spinal astrocytoma	Progressive myelopathy over many months	No focus of a mass component within lesion
	Longitudinally extensive T2 hyperintensity	No focus of contrast enhancement
Metabolic		
Vitamin B$_{12}$, copper, vitamin E deficiency	Progressive myelopathy over many months	Cross-sectional cord signal; no typical subacute combined degeneration pattern
		Severe multimodal decline within months; painful
		No risk factors

Abbreviations: IgG, immunoglobulin G; MRI, magnetic resonance imaging; NMOSD, neuromyelitis optica spectrum disorder.

of inflammation, spinal digital subtraction angiography (DSA) was performed.

DIAGNOSIS

The spinal DSA confirmed the diagnosis of left SDAVF at T11.

MANAGEMENT

A T11-12 laminectomy and ligation of the SDAVF was successfully performed without complication. The patient followed up with his local providers for rehabilitation.

DISCUSSION

SDAVF is the most common spinal arteriovenous malformation, arising from an acquired abnormal connection between a radicular artery and radiculomedullary vein. Progressive congestion and cord edema lead to neurologic deficits over time. Cases are commonly seen in older men with a history of back surgery or trauma. A delay in diagnosis of 1 to 3 years is common.

The vast majority of patients have a progressive thoracic myelopathy or conus syndrome affecting the lower extremities over the course of years. A peripheral process is often initially suspected because patients frequently lack clear upper motor neuron features and a truncal sensory level in many cases. Exertional- or Valsalva-induced worsening of deficits is commonly reported owing to transient worsening of venous hypertension. Dull low back pain is common, and radiation into the lower extremities can mimic a radiculopathy. Notably, substantial clinical worsening may occur with use of corticosteroids, which may be a strong clue to the underlying diagnosis.

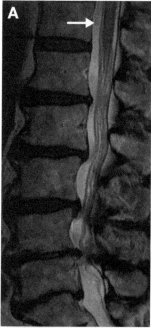
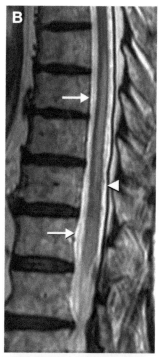
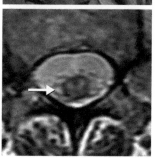
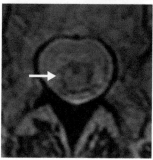

Figure 77.1 **Lumbar Spine Magnetic Resonance Imaging (MRI) Findings for the Case Patient.**

A, Initial images show multilevel central canal narrowing on sagittal views (top), with suspected faint T2-hyperintense signal extending into the conus on sagittal and axial (bottom) views (arrows). B, Several months after lumbar spine surgery, MRI shows longitudinally extensive T2-hyperintense signal extending from midthoracic cord into the conus (arrows), with faint, dorsal, tortuous flow void (arrowhead).

Spinal cord T2 hyperintensity is seen in more than 95% of patients; longitudinally extensive signal with edema is typical, and approximately 90% have extension to the conus. Tortuous vessel flow voids on sagittal views of T2-weighted imaging are seen in approximately 80%, but sensitivity is most likely higher with advanced sequences. Most cases of SDAVF show intraparenchymal gadolinium enhancement; enhancement is often nonspecifically hazy or patchy, but at times a unique pattern termed the *missing piece sign* can be seen, with an abrupt piece of contrast enhancement missing among holocord enhancement.

Findings of SDAVF, with flow in serpentine perimedullary veins, is detected on MRA of the spinal canal in approximately 80% to 95% and helps localize the fistula level to within 2 segments in approximately 95%. Conventional angiography remains the standard for detection and confirmation of SDAVF.

Surgical treatment through disconnection of the draining vein is highly effective (≈98%) and carries low morbidity at experienced centers. Endovascular occlusion of the draining vein using liquid embolic agents has demonstrated efficacy in approximately 70% to 80% of patients and can be performed at the time of initial angiography in select cases.

KEY POINTS

- Progressive myelopathy with T2-hyperintense signal extending into the conus should carry very high suspicion for SDAVF.

- Idiopathic transverse myelitis has specific diagnostic criteria, which most notably includes exclusion of other causes of myelopathy and nadir within 21 days.

- Not all SDAVFs have flow voids or abnormal MRA findings, thus a high index of suspicion is needed to appropriately pursue diagnostic DSA.

ACUTE QUADRIPARESIS IN A SMOKER

Nicholas L. Zalewski, MD

CASE PRESENTATION

HISTORY AND EXAMINATION

A 51-year-old woman was seen for evaluation of transverse myelitis. Pertinent medical history included hypertension, hyperlipidemia, and 50 pack-years of cigarette smoking. Two months earlier, she was shopping and suddenly had excruciating pain in her upper back. Two hours later, severe weakness of both hands developed abruptly. Over the next 8 hours, severe paraparesis and urinary retention developed, with inability to lift legs against gravity, and she reported a T1 sensory level.

In the local emergency department, her vital signs were normal. A cardiac evaluation and computed tomography angiography of the chest were obtained to rule out cardiac ischemia or aortic dissection, given her initial severe pain. Emergent magnetic resonance imaging (MRI) of the cervical and thoracic spine showed no compression and no abnormal signal in the spinal cord. Cerebrospinal fluid (CSF) analysis showed 2 total nucleated cells/μL, protein concentration of 76 mg/dL (reference range, ≤35 mg/dL), glucose value of 67 mg/dL, 0 supernumerary oligoclonal bands, and normal immunoglobulin G (IgG) index. With the increased CSF protein value and normal spinal cord imaging, Guillain-Barré syndrome was suspected, and intravenous immunoglobulin (IVIG) was initiated.

After 3 days of IVIG, there was no improvement. Repeated MRI showed a longitudinally extensive (≥3 vertebral segments) T2-hyperintense lesion from the lower cervical through the upper thoracic cord. The diagnosis was changed to transverse myelitis. MRI of the brain was normal. She had thorough serum and CSF evaluations for causes of an inflammatory or infectious myelopathy, including serum myelin oligodendrocyte glycoprotein–IgG and aquaporin-4–IgG autoantibodies, which were unremarkable. She received 5 days of intravenous (IV) methylprednisolone 1,000 mg; gradual improvement in strength was seen over months after intensive rehabilitation, with ability to walk with a cane. Her residual symptoms included lower extremity and hand weakness, neurogenic bladder, and severe neuropathic pain.

Her referring physicians considered her to have seronegative neuromyelitis optica spectrum disorder. On referral to our center, neurologic examination showed moderate upper motor neuron–pattern quadriparesis. She had brisk deep tendon reflexes, mild spasticity, and extensor plantar responses. Predominant pain and temperature sensory loss was found, with a T1 sensory level. Contact allodynia was noted on the trunk. On review of the previous MRI findings, a differential diagnosis was considered, shown in Table 78.1.

TESTING

Review of the outside MRI noted key imaging findings, including initially normal MRI within the first 12 hours of symptom presentation, and subsequent MRI on day 3 (Figure 78.1) showing anterior pencil-like hyperintensity on sagittal view and anterior U- or V-shaped pattern on axial view (termed *U/V pattern*), without associated gadolinium enhancement. Diffusion-weighted imaging was not obtained.

Given the rapid, severe deficits with pain, spinal cord infarction (SCI) was considered most likely, and the MRI findings were typical. Magnetic resonance angiography of the neck with T1-fat-saturated views was obtained and did not show dissection. Laboratory evaluation showed a low-density lipoprotein value of 124 mg/dL and hemoglobin A_{1c} of 6.2%.

DIAGNOSIS

The patient was diagnosed with probable spontaneous SCI on the basis of diagnostic criteria.

MANAGEMENT

The patient was counselled on smoking cessation, started on an aspirin and statin regimen, and followed up by a primary care provider for management of vascular risk factors. Residual neuropathic pain was treated with high doses of gabapentin. Importantly, unnecessary additional immunotherapy was avoided by establishing the correct diagnosis.

Table 78.1 | DIFFERENTIAL DIAGNOSIS FOR THE CASE PATIENT

POSSIBLE DIAGNOSES	HELPFUL FEATURES
Trauma	
Traumatic spinal cord injury	Trauma, motor vehicle accident
Severe spondylosis (with minor trauma worsening)	Severe spondylosis with canal narrowing and cord compression
	Minor fall/trauma, then decline
Inflammatory	
AQP4-IgG–seropositive NMOSD	Decline >24 hours (days)
	Previous episodes, typical brain lesions
	Serum AQP4-IgG, inflammatory CSF, MRI patchy/ring enhancement
MOG-IgG myelitis	Decline >24 hours (days)
	Previous episodes, typical brain lesions
	Serum MOG-IgG, inflammatory CSF
Sarcoidosis	Decline typically over weeks
	Thick dorsal subpial and/or trident gadolinium enhancement
	Inflammatory CSF (lymphocytic)
Multiple sclerosis	Decline >24 hours (days to weeks), mild episodes, sensory predominant
	Well-defined, short, ovoid lesions ≤2 vertebral body segments, typical brain lesions
	CSF oligoclonal bands, increased IgG index
Idiopathic transverse myelitis	Diagnosis of exclusion (criteria)
	Often recent infectious trigger
	Inflammatory CSF
Infectious	
VZV	Can be hyperacute (VZV vasculopathy)
	Recent shingles, immunocompromised
	Inflammatory CSF, VZV PCR-positive CSF
Acute flaccid myelitis	Predominantly in children
	Recent/current systemic infection, rapid decline, pure motor
	Inflammatory CSF, very long anterior gray matter on MRI
Viral myelitis (eg, cytomegalovirus, HIV)	Infectious symptoms, immunocompromised, risk factors
	Inflammatory CSF
Syphilis	Risk factors (eg, HIV seropositive)
	Can be hyperacute (syphilis vasculitis/aortitis)
Epidural abscess	Immunocompromised, intravenous drug use, fever, increased ESR/CRP
	MRI extra-axial mass (compressive)
Vascular	
Spinal dural arteriovenous fistula	Typical gradual decline with episodic worsening (≈5% acute)
	MRI lower thoracic/conus predominant, flow voids
Epidural hematoma	Anticoagulation, recent trauma
	MRI extra-axial mass (compressive)
Hematomyelia	Acute, or progressive myelopathy with acute decline (eg, AVM, cavernoma)
	Blood on MRI
Vasculitis	Systemic vasculitis history/findings
	Inflammatory CSF, multifocal central nervous system involvement
Ischemic stroke	In addition to the radiologic features described in the case patient, CT or MR angiography of neck and chest may show dissection
Toxic	
Heroin	Heroin reuse after abstinence
	Acute heroin intoxication with loss of consciousness
Nitrous oxide	Nitrous oxide exposure, dorsal column predominant
Neoplasm	
Metastatic epidural compression	History of cancer, back pain preceding
	MRI extra-axial mass (compressive)
Tumor hemorrhage	Progressive myelopathy with acute decline
	MRI spinal cord mass with blood products
	History of cancer, >24-hour decline
Spinal cord metastasis	MRI rim and flame signs

Abbreviations: AQP4, aquaporin-4; AVM, arteriovenous malformation; CRP, C-reactive protein; CSF, cerebrospinal fluid; CT, computed tomography; ESR, erythrocyte sedimentation rate; IgG, immunoglobulin G; MOG, myelin oligodendrocyte glycoprotein; MR, magnetic resonance; MRI, magnetic resonance imaging; NMOSD, neuromyelitis optica spectrum disorder; PCR, polymerase chain reaction; VZV, varicella-zoster virus.

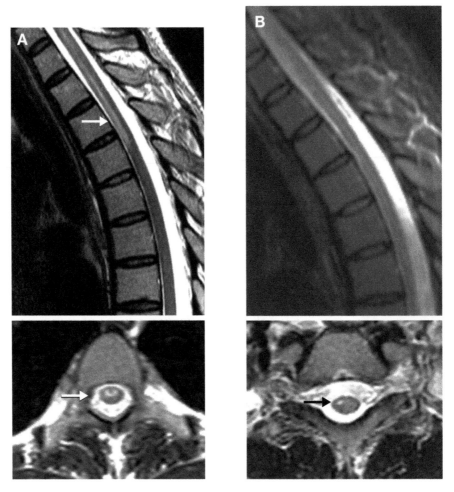

Figure 78.1 **Spinal Magnetic Resonance Imaging (MRI) Findings in a Patient With Acute Quadriparesis.**
A, MRI 3 days after symptom onset shows a longitudinally extensive, anterior, pencil-like hyperintensity from the lower cervical through the upper thoracic spinal cord on sagittal imaging (top, arrow) and an anterior U/V T2-hyperintense pattern on axial view (bottom, arrow). B, Subsequent MRI 2 months later was essentially normal on sagittal view (top), with small, anterior, horn cell, T2-hyperintense signal consistent with myelomalacia on axial view (bottom, arrow).

DISCUSSION

Spontaneous SCIs are an underrecognized cause of acute myelopathy. SCIs generally occur in older persons, with most cases associated with typical vascular risk factors, arterial dissection, and fibrocartilaginous embolism; historically, cases were often secondary to syphilis.

Diagnostic criteria for spontaneous SCI have been proposed and include the following components:

1) Clinical—onset of severe, nontraumatic, myelopathy deficits with nadir within 12 hours (or stuttering decline, with severe deficits within 12 hours)

2) MRI—a) no spinal cord compression, b) intramedullary T2-hyperintense lesion, and c) specific findings (diffusion restriction, adjacent arterial dissection/occlusion, vertebral body infarction)

3) CSF—noninflammatory

4) Alternative diagnosis is not more likely.

Level of confidence for spontaneous SCI is categorized as *definite* (components 1, 2 a-c, and 4), *probable* (components 1, 2 a-b, 3, and 4), or *possible* (components 1 and 4).

Notably, in this case patient, the severe deficits developed within hours, instead of seconds or minutes as with a typical stroke. It is unclear why patients with SCI commonly have a more prolonged decline to nadir than do those with cerebral ischemia, but this is important to recognize. About 60% to 70% of patients will report significant pain at or before onset, which may be caused by ischemia or the infarction mechanism (eg, dissection [aortic, vertebral artery] or fibrocartilaginous embolism). Although it is helpful if findings are restricted to a vascular territory (anterior or posterior spinal artery), SCI is often not neatly confined clinically or radiographically in a pure vascular territory. Truncal pain, sensory level, and bilateral symptoms acutely help localize deficits to the spinal cord, as opposed to other localizations that would raise alternative considerations.

Neuroimaging should be carefully reviewed in suspected SCI. Initially, spine MRI is often normal (hours), then typical T2 hyperintensity is seen (hours to day[s]), which may have associated gadolinium enhancement (linear craniocaudal strip, gray matter) and edema (days to weeks), and often resolves with residual cystic myelomalacia and/or regional spinal cord atrophy. Physicians should request diffusion-weighted imaging acutely and vascular imaging to look for adjacent dissection/occlusion. Adjacent vertebral bodies should be assessed for infarction. Spinal cord T2-hyperintensity patterns can vary widely depending on the location and size of infarct and the timing of imaging. Typical T2-hyperintense patterns in SCI include snake eyes, pencil-like hyperintensity, anterior U/V pattern, anteromedial spot, hologray, and holocord. CSF is generally unremarkable, often with an increased protein concentration, but some cases have mild inflammation.

Ideally, initial management includes rapid MRI to rule out alternative processes (eg, compressive myelopathy) and optimizing cord perfusion. Currently, data on treatment with IV tissue plasminogen activator or spinal drain with blood pressure augmentation are lacking. If an inflammatory myelopathy is believed possible, it is reasonable to treat with a short course of IV corticosteroids, but IVIG (prothrombotic) and plasma exchange (hypoperfusion) should be avoided if the index of suspicion for SCI is high.

A stroke investigation assessing the mechanism of infarction should be considered, but often a clear mechanism is not present. Despite severe acute deficits, many patients have substantial recovery. Aggressive rehabilitation, neurogenic bowel and bladder management, control of vascular risk factors, and treatment of residual neuropathic pain are all important.

KEY POINTS

- Severe, nontraumatic myelopathy developing in 12 hours or less is highly suspicious for SCI; acute pain is common but not universal.

- SCI T2-hyperintense patterns are diverse, but gadolinium enhancement is typically absent, or a linear craniocaudal strip might be seen subacutely; specific imaging findings should be sought.

- CSF in SCI is usually noninflammatory.

- Physicians should consider evaluation and management of SCI when suspected rather than treating as presumed transverse myelitis.

A 25-YEAR-OLD MAN WITH RECURRENT BACK PAIN AND RAPID-ONSET PARAPLEGIA

Nicholas L. Zalewski, MD

CASE PRESENTATION

HISTORY AND EXAMINATION

A 25-year-old man was transferred to Mayo Clinic for evaluation and management of severe transverse myelitis. He had no pertinent past medical history. His symptoms started approximately 6 months earlier with new, substantial low back pain for 2 days, followed by a 3-day history of lower extremity weakness. He could only ambulate with the help of a rolling chair and had to discontinue work because of the severity of the weakness, but his symptoms resolved spontaneously within a few days.

Six months later and approximately 10 days before transfer, acute low back pain developed lasting 2 days, followed by 3 days of progressive, symmetrical, bilateral, lower extremity weakness, sensory loss from the umbilicus to the toes, and bowel and bladder dysfunction. He was hospitalized locally.

Magnetic resonance imaging (MRI) of the spine and brain showed a lower thoracic spinal cord T2-hyperintense signal (Figure 79.1A). Cerebrospinal fluid (CSF) examination showed 17 total nucleated cells/μL (77% neutrophils), 459 erythrocytes/μL, protein concentration of 84 mg/dL (reference range, ≤35 mg/dL), and glucose value of 62 mg/dL. He was diagnosed with transverse myelitis, and a thorough serologic evaluation was undertaken to assess for a definable cause. The patient was started on a combination of intravenous methylprednisolone 1,000 mg daily and broad-spectrum antibiotics (vancomycin and cefepime) for 3 days to treat inflammatory transverse myelitis while also treating possible infection in the setting of neutrophilic pleocytosis seen on CSF examination. Given the rapid accumulation of severe deficits, a request was made for transfer to Mayo Clinic to consider escalation of treatment and further assessment.

The patient had no prior history of neurologic symptoms and had no fevers, chills, night sweats, new skin lesions, or weight loss. He reported no use of tobacco, alcohol, nutritional supplements, or illicit drugs. He had no family history of neurologic disease or other related medical issues.

On arrival to Mayo Clinic, he was hemodynamically stable and afebrile. Neurologic examination indicated flaccid, symmetrical paraplegia, T10 sensory level to all sensory modalities, decreased lower extremity reflexes, and mute plantar responses.

Review of serum laboratory testing from the outside facility included negative evaluations for aquaporin-4–immunoglobulin G (IgG), myelin oligodendrocyte glycoprotein–IgG, paraneoplastic autoantibody, connective tissue disease cascade, antineutrophil cytoplasmic antibody panel, antiphospholipid antibodies, anticardiolipin IgG and immunoglobulin M (IgM) antibodies, anti–beta-2 glycoprotein 1 IgG/IgM antibodies, and HIV and syphilis serologic testing. Specific testing of CSF included normal results for bacterial and fungal cultures, acid-fast bacillus stain and culture, VDRL test, and polymerase chain reaction testing for varicella-zoster virus, herpes simplex virus 1 and 2, and cytomegalovirus.

Review of outside thoracic spine MRI (Figure 79.1A) showed longitudinally extensive T2-hyperintense signal extending throughout the thoracic spinal cord, blood products in the low thoracic cord, and prominent T2-hypointense signal surrounding a focal masslike area along with surrounding T1-hyperintense signal. There was no additional gadolinium enhancement beyond the pregadolinium hyperintense T1 signal.

Given the significant focus of blood products, management shifted to a diagnostic approach assessing and treating spinal cord hemorrhage (hematomyelia). Diagnoses considered at the time are shown in Table 79.1.

Given the clinical and radiographic features, a cavernous malformation with recent hemorrhage was strongly suspected. However, given the extent of associated T2-hyperintense signal (consistent with severe associated

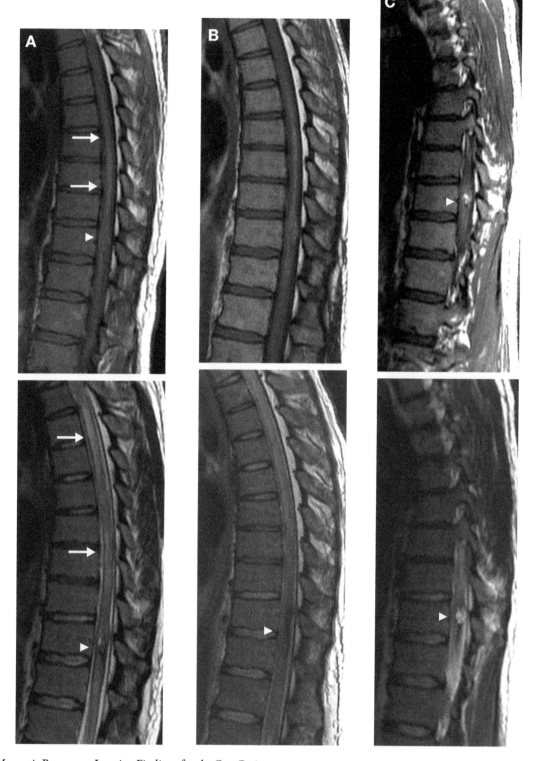

Figure 79.1 **Magnetic Resonance Imaging Findings for the Case Patient.**
A-C, T1-weighted (top row) and T2-weighted (bottom row) images show evolution of hematomyelia secondary to intramedullary spinal cavernous malformation (ISCM) from week 0 (A), week 1 (B), and week 4 (C). T1-hyperintense and dark T2-hypointense signal is demonstrated at the site of hemorrhage (arrowheads), associated with adjacent T1-hyperintense signal extending through the cord (arrows, upper row) and associated reactive T2-hyperintense edema (arrows, bottom row). With expected interval change after recent hemorrhage, a well-defined lobular mass with dark T2-hypointense rim (C) consistent with ISCM is best demonstrated approximately 4 weeks after hemorrhage onset.

Table 79.1 | DIFFERENTIAL DIAGNOSIS FOR THE CASE PATIENT

POSSIBLE DIAGNOSES	PERTINENT POSITIVES	PERTINENT NEGATIVES
Trauma	Most common cause of hematomyelia	No reported trauma
		Focal masslike component
Cavernous malformation	Common cause of hematomyelia	Extensive associated T2-hyperintense signal
	Young male patient	(edema) less common
	Heterogeneous lobular mass	
	Pain frequently precedes myelopathy deficits	
	Previous self-limited episode of pain with deficits	
	Heterogeneous T1- and T2-weighted signal, well-defined dark rim of T2 hypointensity	
Arteriovenous malformation	Common cause of hematomyelia	No flow voids identified on spinal cord magnetic resonance imaging
	Young patient	
	Previous self-limited episode of pain with deficits	
	Extensive associated T2-hyperintense signal (edema)	
Bleeding diatheses	Hematomyelia	No prior history of bleeding, no contributing medications or supplements
Neoplasm	Focal masslike component	No history of primary neoplasm
		No contrast enhancement
Miscellaneous (spinal cord aneurysm, intrasyringeal hemorrhage, vasculitis, radiation)	Hematomyelia	Rare
		Normal medical history and initial laboratory evaluation
Idiopathic	A common diagnosis of exclusion	Focal masslike component
		No history of hypertension as typical risk factor

Modified from Zalewski NL. Vascular myelopathies. Continuum (Minneap Minn). 2021 Feb 1;27(1):30-61; used with permission.

edema) and devastating presentation in this young patient, a thorough evaluation was required to rule out alternative causes of hematomyelia.

TESTING

Findings of repeated spinal cord MRI were consistent with evolution of a recent hemorrhage in the lower thoracic spinal cord (Figure 79.1B). Digital subtraction angiography (DSA) of the spinal canal showed normal findings, without evidence of arteriovenous malformation (AVM). Additional thorough evaluations for bleeding diatheses, drugs of abuse, thorough skin evaluation to exclude melanoma, and systemic imaging with computed tomography of the chest, abdomen, and pelvis and testicular ultrasonography were all normal.

DIAGNOSIS

Given the clinical timeline, the lobulated hemorrhagic appearance of the lesion with a surrounding T2-hypointense rim and heterogeneous T1 and T2 signal indicating recent hemorrhage, no pattern on imaging to suggest a neoplasm, with negative systemic evaluation and normal DSA, a diagnosis of hematomyelia due to intramedullary spinal cavernous malformation (ISCM) was made.

MANAGEMENT

No neurosurgical management was recommended given the complete cross-sectional spinal cord injury at the level of hemorrhage, with potential risk of surgery with resection of the ISCM. Short-interval follow-up imaging 3 weeks later (Figure 79.1C) showed expected evolution of the recent hemorrhage secondary to ISCM.

DISCUSSION

Hematomyelia may be caused by several potential mechanisms (Table 79.1). The most common nontraumatic causes are attributable to cavernous malformations and AVMs. Hematomyelia most commonly presents with acute back pain referable to the site of hemorrhage and myelopathy deficits with a range of severity (often severe).

Cavernous malformations are more common in the brain (0.5% general population) than the spinal cord. Overall, ISCMs account for approximately 5% to 12% of spinal vascular malformations. Most ISCM hemorrhages are spontaneous and sporadic, but some are secondary to prior radiation or familial inheritance. In addition to hematomyelia, progressive myelopathic symptoms may occur due to venous microhemorrhage leading to mass effect. Stepwise deterioration is often seen with recurrent hematomyelia (as in this case patient). This case showed typical MRI findings, especially with ongoing resolution of active hemorrhage, highlighting a lobular mass with heterogeneous T1- and T2-weighted signal intensity surrounded by a well-defined dark rim of T2 hypointensity due to hemosiderin deposition. ISCMs are not apparent on DSA, but DSA can be used to rule out important alternative considerations such as spinal AVM or hemangioblastoma. Surgical resection is aimed at avoiding deterioration by recurrent hemorrhage. Symptomatic improvement is possible, but most patients benefit from reduced risk of recurrent hemorrhage.

- Significant T2 hypointensity and T1 hyperintensity before gadolinium administration is consistent with hematomyelia rather than inflammatory myelopathies.

- ISCM and AVMs are the most common identifiable causes of nontraumatic hematomyelia.

- A thorough evaluation for bleeding diatheses and neoplasm should be undertaken, but no cause is found in many cases. Hypertension has been identified as a risk factor in idiopathic cases.

PROGRESSIVE MYELOPATHY AFTER NECK PAIN

Eoin P. Flanagan, MB, BCh

CASE PRESENTATION

HISTORY AND EXAMINATION

A 36-year-old woman with a background medical history of hypothyroidism, gout, fibromyalgia, depression, substance use disorder, and nephrolithiasis had development of neck pain. Three months later, she noted numbness in the left leg, which slowly worsened over the course of several months, spreading to involve the right leg and eventually forming a sensory level across the trunk at T8. At that time she also noted numbness in both hands. She had stiffness and weakness in both legs and had trouble emptying her bladder.

She sought care at a local facility, and cervical spine magnetic resonance imaging (MRI) showed a T2 hyperintensity extending 2 vertebral segments in sagittal view, with enhancement (Figure 80.1A and B). Cerebrospinal fluid analysis showed a normal white blood cell count, normal protein and glucose levels, and negative oligoclonal bands. She was initially diagnosed with idiopathic transverse myelitis and treated with 1 g of intravenous methylprednisolone once daily for 5 days. This treatment was associated with some transient clinical improvement, but after this her condition continued to worsen. She sought a second opinion at our center.

TESTING

Neurologic examination showed mild weakness restricted to the bilateral iliopsoas and hyperreflexia in the upper and lower extremities. Hoffmann and Babinski signs were positive bilaterally. There was moderate spasticity in both lower extremities and mild distal vibratory sensation loss, with a sensory level across the trunk at T8. Her gait examination indicated a spastic gait, and she had a mildly positive Romberg sign. On re-evaluation of her previous MRI, a transverse band or pancakelike enhancement pattern was noted (Figure 80.1B, top) at the center of a moderate to severely stenotic region of the cervical spine sparing gray matter on axial sequences (Figure 80.1B, bottom).

DIAGNOSIS

The MRI findings were highly suggestive of cervical spondylotic myelopathy.

MANAGEMENT

A neurosurgical referral was made, and the patient underwent anterior cervical discectomy with decompression and fusion from C4-C7. At her follow-up visit 4 months after surgery, the patient reported improvement in her strength and walking. Her neurologic examination showed normal lower extremity strength, resolution of spasticity, and negative Babinski sign bilaterally but persistent sensory deficits. MRI of the cervical spine at that time showed a decrease in the degree of T2 hyperintensity and enhancement, consistent with interval response to surgery (Figure 80.1C and D).

DISCUSSION

The presence of a progressive myelopathy over many months in this case patient argued against a diagnosis of transverse myelitis, which typically reaches nadir within 21 days. Furthermore, the cerebrospinal fluid was noninflammatory, which also favored cervical spondylosis over idiopathic transverse myelitis. However, the gadolinium enhancement pattern was the key diagnostic feature that strongly suggested cervical spondylotic myelopathy as the diagnosis and ultimately led to neurosurgical referral for decompression.

Cervical spondylosis is the most common nontraumatic cause of myelopathy. Given its frequency, it is important for neurologists and other clinicians to recognize less-common radiologic features that may accompany cervical spondylosis. Approximately 15% of patients will have associated parenchymal T2 hyperintensity (scar tissue, sometimes termed *myelomalacia*), which is generally well recognized by neurologists as a potential accompaniment of cervical spondylotic myelopathy. However, up to 7% of patients with cervical spondylotic myelopathy have accompanying gadolinium enhancement, which most likely results from focal breakdown of the blood–spinal cord barrier.

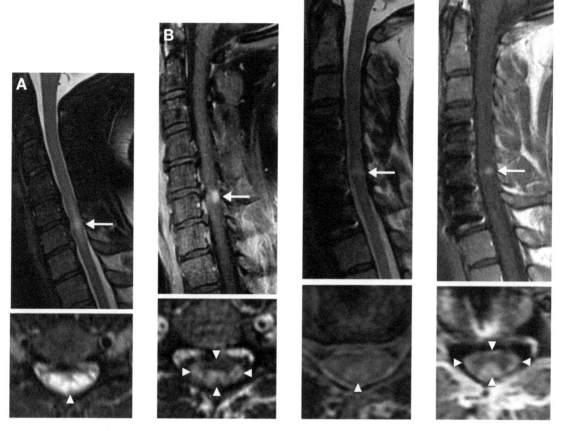

Figure 80.1 **Magnetic Resonance Imaging Findings for the Case Patient.**
A, At initial evaluation, T2-weighted imaging shows a T2-hyperintense lesion that extends 2 vertebral segments on sagittal view (top, arrow), is central on axial view (bottom, arrowhead), and is accompanied by moderate to severe stenosis in both views. B, On T1 postgadolinium imaging, a pancakelike band of enhancement is noted just below the site of maximal stenosis on sagittal images (top, arrow) that involves the white matter but spares the gray matter on axial images (bottom, arrowheads). C, Four months after decompressive surgery, the T2 hyperintensity has decreased, and stenosis is no longer evident on sagittal (top, arrow) and axial views (bottom, arrowhead). D, The degree of T1 postgadolinium enhancement has decreased and remains in a flat pancakelike transverse band pattern on sagittal view (top, arrow), sparing gray matter on axial view (bottom, arrowheads).

The presence of gadolinium enhancement often leads to confusion and misdiagnosis as transverse myelitis or neoplastic disease, with the potential for morbidity from inappropriate immunosuppression or unnecessary procedures (eg, spinal cord biopsy). The MRI gadolinium enhancement pattern is a strong clue to this disorder and helps distinguish it from other processes. There are 3 major characteristics of the enhancement pattern: 1) a flat transverse band on sagittal views that has been termed *pancakelike* given its flat appearance, with the width greater than or equal to the height; 2) location of the enhancement just below the site of maximal stenosis and at the center of the T2 hyperintensity; and 3) axial views showing enhancement circumferentially in the white matter, sparing gray matter.

The stenosis may appear moderate in the neutral position, which contributes to the diagnostic uncertainty, and in such situations MRI obtained in both maximal flexion and extension may reveal dynamic compression, particularly with the neck in extension. This transverse band of enhancement should be distinguished from transverse myelitis or neoplastic myelopathies in which the enhancement typically extends rostrocaudally throughout the T2 lesion. The enhancement

resolves slowly after surgery, often taking 1 to 2 years to resolve completely. Thus, the presence of persistent enhancement after surgical decompression should not rule out a diagnosis of cervical spondylosis in the absence of clinical or radiologic deterioration.

KEY POINTS

- Gadolinium enhancement occurs in 7% of patients with cervical spondylotic myelopathy and is often misdiagnosed as transverse myelitis or tumor.

- The presence of a transverse band or flat pancakelike appearance of gadolinium enhancement in which the width is greater than or equal to the height is suggestive of cervical spondylotic myelopathy.

- On axial views, a circumferential pattern of white matter enhancement sparing gray matter is typical.

- Gadolinium enhancement tends to resolve slowly after decompressive surgery and can take 1 to 2 years to disappear completely.

PROGRESSIVE IMBALANCE AND VISUAL IMPAIRMENT IN A PATIENT WITH DIABETES

Neeraj Kumar, MD

CASE PRESENTATION

HISTORY AND EXAMINATION

A 72-year-old man with hypothyroidism and type 2 diabetes (taking metformin) sought care for a 3-year history of slowly progressive, ascending lower limb paresthesias and imbalance. Three months earlier, he noted subacute onset of finger numbness and substantial worsening of imbalance with infrequent falls. He also had a 1-year history of progressive visual decline that persisted despite cataract surgery. Additional symptoms included intermittent light-headedness and confusion.

On examination, he required assistance for ambulation. He had an ataxic gait with a positive Romberg sign. Bilateral optic pallor was present. He had an upper motor neuron pattern of mild lower limb weakness. His lower limb reflexes were absent, and the plantar response was equivocal. Position perception was reduced at the toes. Vibration perception was reduced in the distal upper limbs and absent in the lower limbs. Diagnoses considered, for common causes of an insidiously progressive myelopathy or myeloneuropathy, are shown in Table 81.1.

Table 81.1 | **DIFFERENTIAL DIAGNOSIS FOR THE CASE PATIENT**

CAUSE OF MYELOPATHY	SPECIFIC DIAGNOSIS
Nutritional	
Deficiency	Vitamin B_{12}, copper, vitamin E, folate
Toxicity	Nitrous oxide (secondary vitamin B_{12} deficiency)
Infectious	HIV (often not due to HIV itself, vitamin B_{12} pathways implicated)
Geographic	
Nutritional	Lathyrism, konzo, fluorosis (compressive)
Infectious	Human T-lymphotropic virus
Toxic	
Toxins	Chemotherapy (methotrexate), heroin, organophosphates, solvents
Systemic	Liver disease
Vascular	Dural arteriovenous fistula
Neoplastic	Spinal cord tumor
Structural	Compression from degenerative arthritis

TESTING

Laboratory evaluations showed a decreased hemoglobin value (7.8 g/dL; reference range, 13.5-17.5 g/dL) and an increased mean corpuscular volume (138.6 fL; reference range, 81.2-95.1 fL). Macrocytic red blood cells were noted on a peripheral blood smear. Serum vitamin B_{12} level was less than 70 ng/L (reference range, 180-914 ng/L). Levels of plasma homocysteine and serum methylmalonic acid (MMA) were markedly increased to 375 μmol/L (reference range, <13 μmol/L) and 143 nmol/L (reference range, <0.4 nmol/L), respectively. Serum copper level was normal. Serum parietal cell antibodies were increased to 46 U (reference range, <20 U), and intrinsic factor antibodies were absent. Serum gastrin was markedly increased (2,477 pg/mL; reference range, <100 pg/mL).

DIAGNOSIS

The clinical presentation in this patient suggested a myeloneuropathy. His vitamin B_{12} level was undetectable and accompanied by a macrocytic anemia and increased MMA and homocysteine levels. Even though intrinsic factor antibodies were negative, the clinical picture was supportive of subacute combined degeneration (SACD) in the setting of pernicious anemia.

MANAGEMENT

The patient was started on vitamin B_{12} replacement, 1,000 μg/d subcutaneously for 5 days, then once a week for 4 weeks, and once a month thereafter. At 6-month follow-up he had striking improvement in gait and vision. The light-headedness and confusion were no longer present. His examination was remarkable only for mild impairment, with tandem gait and a slightly positive Romberg sign. The lower limb reflexes were reduced. Impaired position perception at the toes persisted, but vibration perception in the lower limbs improved. Laboratory investigations showed normalization of the hemoglobin, vitamin B_{12}, MMA, and homocysteine levels. The serum gastrin level had improved but was still increased at 742 pg/mL.

DISCUSSION

The term SACD was first used in 1900 to describe pathologic involvement of the dorsal and lateral columns in the spinal cord in patients with pernicious anemia. Nearly 5 decades later, vitamin B_{12} and folate were first synthesized, and the disorder was found to respond to supplementation of these vitamins.

The best-characterized neurologic manifestations of vitamin B_{12} deficiency include myelopathy and myeloneuropathy. Autonomic neuropathy, optic neuropathy, and neuropsychiatric manifestations have also been reported. Neurologic manifestations may occur without evidence of the characteristic hematologic derangement, megaloblastic anemia. Macrocytosis or hypersegmented neutrophils on peripheral blood smear may be clues.

If the cause of an insidiously progressive myelopathy or myeloneuropathy is unclear, neuroimaging and sometimes cerebrospinal fluid analysis are warranted. A compressive cause should be excluded. The presence of cerebrospinal fluid cellularity and evidence of enhancing lesions may suggest an infectious or inflammatory cause. The distinction of a vascular myelopathy (dural arteriovenous fistula, spinal cord infarction) from an infectious myelopathy can be particularly challenging. Often, patients with neurologic manifestations of vitamin B_{12} deficiency have a subacute symptom onset, hence the term *subacute combined degeneration*. Concomitant paresthesias in hands and feet are clues to a cervical myelopathy.

Gastrointestinal disorders other than pernicious anemia are often associated with multiple nutrient deficiency. Copper and vitamin E deficiency can also cause SACD, although neurologic manifestations of vitamin E deficiency often have a spinocerebellar component and mimic Friedreich ataxia. Because vitamin B_{12} replacement is routine after bariatric surgery, delayed neurologic manifestations such as myelopathy or myeloneuropathy after bariatric surgery are more commonly due to copper deficiency. Nitrous oxide (laughing gas) oxidizes the cobalt core of vitamin B_{12} and renders the vitamin B_{12} inactive. Thus, SACD due to nitrous oxide toxicity is a functional vitamin B_{12} deficiency. Nitrous oxide in the form of *whippets* is abused because of its euphoriant properties. It is also used as an anesthetic, particularly with dental procedures. It may precipitate *anesthesia paresthetica* in patients with borderline vitamin B_{12} levels. These borderline levels may be encountered in vegetarians because vitamin B_{12} is not found in plant foods. Vegetarians have subclinical or subtle vitamin B_{12} deficiency rather than overt clinically manifest disease, the significance of which is unclear. Vitamin B_{12} deficiency is particularly common in older persons due to atrophic gastritis–related hypochlorhydria. Other causes of vitamin B_{12} deficiency such as *Helicobacter pylori* infection and antacid therapy may coexist. Vitamin B_{12} deficiency reported with metformin use is also often subclinical. Patients with neurologic manifestations of vitamin B_{12} deficiency often have intrinsic factor–related malabsorption, as seen in pernicious anemia.

Although serum vitamin B_{12} measurement is a commonly used screening test, it lacks sensitivity and specificity for the diagnosis of vitamin B_{12} deficiency. Serum MMA and plasma homocysteine are useful ancillary tests but also have limitations. The specificity of MMA is superior to that of homocysteine; increases in homocysteine without corresponding MMA increase may be more suggestive of folate deficiency. Because vitamin B_{12} levels increase with parenteral vitamin B_{12} administration, vitamin B_{12} levels are of limited utility in assessing adequate replacement of vitamin B_{12} stores. Baseline MMA levels are useful to monitor adequacy of replacement.

It is important to determine the cause of vitamin B_{12} deficiency. Particularly important is to evaluate for pernicious anemia because its presence may warrant both surveillance for carcinoid or gastric cancer and management of coexisting autoimmune diseases such as thyroid disease and diabetes. Patients with pernicious anemia may have intrinsic factor antibodies; although their presence is specific (>90%) it has limited sensitivity (50%-70%). Gastric parietal cell antibodies may be present in pernicious anemia but are not specific; they are detected in 10% of the general population older than 70 years. Increased gastrin levels, a marker of hypochlorhydria, are commonly detected in older persons and are invariably increased in pernicious anemia. Absence of hypergastrinemia should cast doubt on the diagnosis of pernicious anemia.

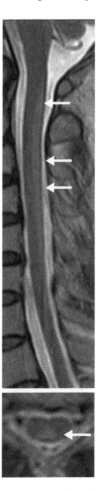

Figure 81.1 **Magnetic Resonance Imaging Findings for a Patient With Copper Deficiency Myelopathy.**
Sagittal (top) and axial (bottom) T2-weighted images show cervical spinal cord dorsal column hyperintensity (arrows).

Neurophysiologic studies may show slowed central conduction with or without a sensorimotor neuropathy. Magnetic resonance imaging abnormalities in vitamin B_{12} deficiency may include signal change in the posterior and lateral column, less commonly so in the subcortical white matter. This case patient had such classic findings that no imaging was required. Magnetic resonance imaging from another case encountered at Mayo Clinic, although with copper deficiency myelopathy, showed findings similar to those of pernicious anemia (Figure 81.1).

It has been suggested that if the dose of oral vitamin B_{12} is high enough, the amount of vitamin B_{12} absorbed may be enough to treat malabsorption-related vitamin B_{12} deficiency. This approach is not recommended in the setting of neurologic manifestations of vitamin B_{12} deficiency.

KEY POINTS

- Onset of hand paresthesias at the same time as foot paresthesias suggests a cervical myelopathy or myeloneuropathy.

- In patients with severe neurologic manifestations of vitamin B_{12} deficiency, intrinsic factor–related malabsorption is often responsible.

- A baseline MMA level should be measured before vitamin B_{12} therapy to monitor adequacy of vitamin B_{12} replacement.

- For the diagnosis of pernicious anemia, intrinsic factor antibodies are specific but not particularly sensitive.

- Multiple nutritional deficiencies can coexist, particularly in those with malabsorption.

PROGRESSIVE MYELOPATHY AFTER SPINE SURGERY

Andrew McKeon, MB, BCh, MD, and Nicholas L. Zalewski, MD

CASE PRESENTATION

HISTORY AND EXAMINATION

A 69-year-old man with a progressive myelopathy for 2 years was referred for evaluation of suspected transverse myelitis. His medical history included discectomies (L4-L5 and L5-S1) 28 years previously. Shortly before onset of the current symptoms, the patient had a severe episode of herpes simplex virus type 1 meningoencephalitis, with 1,039 total nucleated cells/μL (97% lymphocytic) and 139 red blood cells/μL detected in the cerebrospinal fluid (CSF), and he recovered over weeks with minimal residual cognitive deficits. Within a few months of recovery, he had development of insidiously progressive numbness and weakness of his hands. Cervical spine magnetic resonance imaging (MRI) showed 2 small, dural-based, gadolinium-enhancing lesions (Figure 82.1A). Biopsy of these lesions showed only normal neural tissue. Subsequently, the dura was stripped away surgically from the lower cervical region, in an effort to remove these lesions. During the next year, a sensory level developed at about the level of the nipples (T4), along with a squeezing sensation on his trunk below. Imbalance and bilateral lower extremity weakness and numbness then developed. MRI showed a longitudinally extensive cord signal abnormality, without gadolinium enhancement, worsening over 2 years (Figure 82.1B-D). An inflammatory cause was considered. Testing for serum aquaporin-4–immunoglobulin G (IgG) and myelin oligodendrocyte glycoprotein–IgG was negative, and positron emission tomography (PET)/computed tomography (CT) of the body showed no evidence of systemic sarcoidosis, neoplasm, or other hypermetabolic abnormality.

The patient received a prolonged course of empiric prednisone, 80 mg daily, with brief subjective improvement in strength, but then continued to worsen. Infliximab was added to treat possible neurosarcoidosis, despite the negative PET/CT findings. His progressive myelopathy and radiologic abnormalities continued to worsen. CSF evaluation showed 3 white blood cells/μL (reference range, ≤5/μL), with a markedly increased protein concentration of 186 mg/dL (reference range, ≤35 mg/dL). Spinal angiography did not indicate a dural arteriovenous fistula or other vascular abnormality. Spinal cord biopsy was performed, and pathologic analysis showed normal spinal cord parenchyma.

The patient was referred to Mayo Clinic, by which time he had neurogenic bladder and frequent lower extremity spasms and was walker dependent. He had a spastic quadriparesis, lower extremity hyperreflexia, and extensor plantar responses. He also had marked loss of vibratory sensation, with a severe sensory ataxia affecting the right greater than left lower extremity. Diagnoses considered at the time are shown in Table 82.1.

TESTING

The cause of the patient's initial subjective hand numbness and weakness was indeterminate but was not clearly attributable to the dural-based, contrast-enhancing lesions (most likely small neuromas). The onset of severely progressive symptoms after surgical removal of those lesions and the reported stripping of dura made it likely that the progressive cord edema was due to chronic adhesive arachnoiditis. His prior meningoencephalitis was a potential additional risk factor for arachnoiditis. CT myelography showed a markedly abnormal spinal canal with scalloping of the cord contour, with delayed flow of contrast above C6-C7, consistent with arachnoid adhesions causing obstruction of normal CSF flow (Figure 82.1E).

DIAGNOSIS

The patient was diagnosed with chronic adhesive arachnoiditis.

MANAGEMENT

A C4-C7 laminectomy and surgical lysis of the cord meningeal adhesions was performed, with subsequent intensive neurorehabilitation. Follow-up spinal cord MRI 6 months after surgery showed improvement of the T2-signal abnormality (Figure 82.1F) but persistent myelomalacia and spinal cord atrophy. Clinically, he had improvement in distal upper extremity and

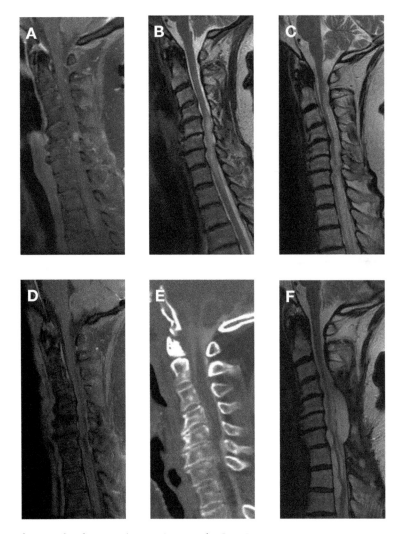

Figure 82.1 Sagittal Imaging of Cervical and Upper Thoracic Spine in the Case Patient.
A, T1-weighted magnetic resonance imaging (MRI) post gadolinium shows a dural-based lesion at the C5-C6 disc space; this was subsequently surgically removed, along with dura of dorsal cervical cord. B-D, Progressive lengthening of longitudinal MRI signal (B and C, T2-weighted) is non–contrast enhancing (D, T1-weighted). E, Computed tomography myelography shows pooling of cerebrospinal fluid within loculated collections resulting from meningeal adhesions. F, T2-weighted MRI shows regression of signal abnormality but with substantial residual spinal cord atrophy.

Table 82.1 DIFFERENTIAL DIAGNOSIS FOR THE CASE PATIENT

POSSIBLE DIAGNOSES	PERTINENT NEGATIVES
Longitudinally extensive transverse myelitis (typical of neuromyelitis optica spectrum disorders)	Progressive myelopathic course, lack of contrast enhancement on MRI, negative AQP4-IgG
Spinal dural arteriovenous fistula	Lack of dorsal venous flow voids, normal spinal angiography
Sarcoidosis	Lack of pial and subpial enhancement on MRI, normal CSF cell count, negative PET/CT
Glioma	Lack of mass effect on MRI, no contrast enhancement despite years of progression

Abbreviations: AQP4, aquaporin-4; CSF, cerebrospinal fluid; IgG, immunoglobulin G; MRI, magnetic resonance imaging; PET/CT, positron emission tomography/computed tomography.

bilateral lower extremity strength, with improved lower extremity sensation. Mild bowel and bladder dysfunction remained, and he required a walker for ambulation.

DISCUSSION

Adhesive arachnoiditis is an uncommon cause of progressive myelopathy resulting from an insult to the arachnoid meningeal layer, followed by inflammation and fibrosis. This process renders the arachnoid abnormally thick and adherent to the pia and dura mater. Abnormal adhesion of nerve roots or spinal cord to the dura produces neurologic impairment. Typical symptoms include back pain, paresthesias, lower limb weakness, and sensory loss. It is diagnosed clinically with supportive MRI and CT myelography findings.

During an 18-year period, 29 patients with myelopathy due to adhesive arachnoiditis were evaluated at Mayo Clinic.

The age range of these patients was 23 to 96 years, with 11 women and 18 men. Causative disorders (in descending order of frequency) were trauma, prior spinal surgery, nontraumatic subarachnoid hemorrhage, infection, myelography with iophendylate used as contrast medium, remote Guillain-Barré syndrome, and ankylosing spondylitis. Imaging findings included loculated CSF collections; nerve root clumping, enhancement, and displacement; spinal cord swelling with increased T2 signal; arachnoid septations; cord atrophy; syrinxes; and intrathecal calcifications. Ten patients underwent corrective surgical procedures, typically with clinical and radiologic stabilization but without marked improvement.

KEY POINTS

- Adhesive arachnoiditis should be considered in a patient with symptoms and signs of progressive myelopathy or myeloradiculopathy.

- Longitudinally extensive T2-signal abnormality of the spinal cord may be encountered and can mimic inflammatory disorders.

- Myelography can assist in diagnosis by demonstrating characteristic loculated collections of CSF.

- Surgical adhesiolysis may be considered on a case-by-case basis in an attempt to prevent progression of disability.

ALTERED MENTAL STATUS DURING THE COVID-19 PANDEMIC

Sara Mariotto, MD, Silvia Bozzetti, MD, Maria Elena De Rui, MD, Fulvia Mazzaferri, MD, PhD, Andrew McKeon, MB, BCh, MD, and Sergio Ferrari, MD

CASE PRESENTATION

HISTORY AND EXAMINATION

In March 2020, a 68-year-old man in Northern Italy with a history of pulmonary thromboembolism sought care at the emergency department for fever, cough, headache, and confusion. Because of severe respiratory failure, orotracheal intubation was required, and the patient was admitted to the intensive care unit, where bilateral deep vein thrombosis and hematemesis occurred. After 2 weeks, owing to respiratory improvement, the patient was weaned from ventilator support and sedation. However, persistent fluctuations in confusion, anxiety, agitation, and cognitive-motor slowing were noted. One week later, he was referred to the infectious diseases unit, where altered mental status persisted in the absence of fever, seizures, or episodes of impaired consciousness.

Neurologic examination was unremarkable except for confusion, short-term memory loss, anxiety, agitation, and cognitive-motor slowing. Meningeal signs were not observed.

The patient had subacute onset of encephalitic symptoms, which, along with the timing, suggested a possible metabolic, infectious, paraneoplastic, autoimmune, inflammatory, or neoplastic cause. The onset with fever and respiratory symptoms made the infectious origin (parainfectious or postinfectious) more probable. The concomitance of confusion and pneumonia suggested possible *Legionella pneumophila* infection or toxic-metabolic encephalopathy. In the context of the novel coronavirus disease 2019 (COVID-19) pandemic, which prominently affected Northern Italy in 2020, severe acute respiratory syndrome coronavirus 2 (SARS-CoV-2) infection was considered as a cause of pneumonia. The sudden occurrence of respiratory failure requiring invasive mechanical ventilation further supported this cause. A postinfectious autoimmune encephalitis is known to occasionally occur after other viral infections.

TESTING

Blood cultures, analyses for influenza A and B, and urine analyses yielded negative results. Chest radiography showed small, bilateral, ground-glass opacities. Brain magnetic resonance imaging (MRI) showed bilateral involvement of mesial temporal lobes and hippocampus on fluid-attenuated inversion recovery sequences, in the absence of contrast enhancement or restricted diffusion (Figure 83.1 A and B). Nasopharyngeal samples were positive for SARS-CoV-2 on reverse transcriptase–polymerase chain reaction testing. Cerebrospinal fluid (CSF) examination showed a slight increase in protein concentration (77 mg/dL; reference range, ≤35 mg/dL), 1 white blood cell/µL, and no evidence of central nervous system infection. In particular, SARS-CoV-2 RNA was not detected in the CSF, nor was herpes simplex virus type 1, 2, or 6, varicella-zoster virus, cytomegalovirus, enterovirus, or antigens for bacterial pathogens (*Escherichia coli, Haemophilus influenzae, Listeria monocytogenes, Neisseria meningitidis, Streptococcus pneumoniae,* and *Streptococcus agalactiae*). Serum and CSF analysis for antibodies to intracellular and surface antigens, including antibodies to glycine receptor, as well as antibodies to myelin oligodendrocyte glycoprotein were negative.

DIAGNOSIS

The patient was diagnosed with postinfectious inflammatory (limbic) encephalitis in the course of SARS-CoV-2 infection.

MANAGEMENT

The patient was treated with lopinavir/ritonavir and hydroxychloroquine. His recent thromboembolism prevented the administration of intravenous immunoglobulins, and high-dose corticosteroids were not administered because of the recent episode of hematemesis. Improvement in cognitive symptoms was noted 6 weeks after onset.

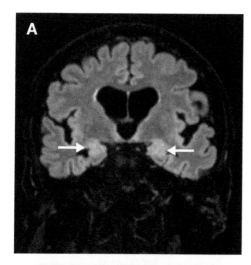

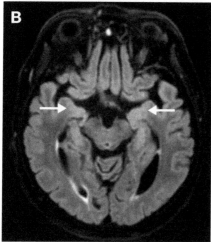

Figure 83.1 Brain Magnetic Resonance Imaging Findings for the Case Patient.
T2/fluid-attenuated inversion recovery sequences in coronal (A) and axial (B) views show hyperintensity of bilateral mesial temporal lobe regions (arrows).

DISCUSSION

At the time of this writing, May 2020, a few cases of encephalitis after COVID-19 had already been described. These have generally been characterized by fever, cognitive dysfunction, epileptic seizures, coma, and CSF inflammatory findings. It appears that a common MRI appearance in these patients is that of diffuse inflammatory encephalitis. In 1 of 4 cases, as in our case patient, MRI signs were restricted to mesial temporal lobe structures, consistent with limbic encephalitis. In 3 cases, SARS-CoV-2 RNA was detected in the nasopharyngeal

swab but not in CSF, and vice versa in the other patient. Improvement after corticosteroid treatment was reported in 1 case. Anosmia is an early symptom in many patients diagnosed with COVID-19, although no olfactory nerve invasion or neurologic significance has yet been demonstrated.

The cause or causes of COVID-19–related neurologic disorders remain to be elucidated. SARS-CoV-2 affects human host cells by interacting with high affinity with the angiotensin-converting enzyme 2 receptor, which is expressed in endothelial cells of the brain, glial cells, and neurons. Although SARS-CoV-2 virus has been demonstrated in CSF by genome sequencing, anecdotally most patients are negative for the virus in CSF by polymerase chain reaction. Some neurologic complications are akin to other clinically characterized, postviral, inflammatory neurologic disorders, including acute necrotizing hemorrhagic encephalopathy and Guillain-Barré syndrome. The occurrence of systemic and pulmonary cytokine storm in the course of COVID-19 also supports an inflammatory driver for neurologic complications. Some cases of stroke have also been reported, although the frequency of stroke does not appear to be increased in COVID-19 overall.

Agitation, corticospinal tract signs, and dysexecutive syndrome were recently described in patients with COVID-19, in some cases associated with enhancement in leptomeningeal spaces, bilateral frontotemporal hypoperfusion, and MRI features of ischemic stroke. Hypercoagulability (as a systemic consequence of infection) and vasculopathy are plausible mechanisms underlying brain ischemia. An increased frequency of a rare childhood vasculitis, Kawasaki syndrome, has been noted by some pediatricians among children who have had COVID-19.

KEY POINTS

- Encephalitis manifesting with headache, altered mental status, and short-term memory loss can occur in the course of SARS-CoV-2 infection.

- Patients can have MRI evidence of inflammatory encephalitides, including limbic encephalitis.

- Encephalitis can persist despite improvement of COVID-19–characteristic symptoms.

- The pathophysiologic process and biomarkers of encephalitis in the course of SARS-CoV-2 infection remain to be elucidated.

SECTION IV
QUESTIONS AND ANSWERS

Section I

CNS DEMYELINATING DISEASE QUESTIONS AND ANSWERS

MULTIPLE CHOICE
(CHOOSE THE BEST ANSWER)

I.1. Which statement is true regarding optic neuritis (ON) in multiple sclerosis?
   a. Corticosteroid-dependent ON is seen in 25%-50% of patients
   b. Only half of patients recover to 20/40 visual acuity or better
   c. Optic chiasm involvement is uncommon
   d. Half of patients have visible disc edema
   e. Eculizumab is the first-line agent for preventing relapse

I.2. A 23-year-old woman sought care for vision loss in both eyes for 7 days, followed by a decreased level of consciousness. Visual acuity was hand motion in both eyes, and prominent optic disc edema was present bilaterally. Neurologic examination showed hyperreflexia and bilateral positive Babinski sign. Magnetic resonance imaging showed multifocal white matter lesions in the subcortical frontal and parietal lobes. Bilateral optic nerve and optic nerve sheath enhancement was seen. What is the most likely diagnosis?
   a. Multiple sclerosis–associated optic neuritis (ON)
   b. Aquaporin-4–immunoglobulin G (IgG)–positive ON
   c. Glial fibrillary acidic protein-IgG–positive ON
   d. Collapsin-response mediator protein 5-IgG–positive ON
   e. Myelin oligodendrocyte glycoprotein-IgG–positive ON

I.3. Which of the following features is specific for idiopathic transverse myelitis (ITM)?
   a. Longitudinally extensive myelitis (>3 contiguous vertebral segments)
   b. Serum negative for immunoglobulin G antibodies to both aquaporin-4 and myelin oligodendrocyte glycoprotein
   c. Gadolinium enhancement
   d. Acute/subacute onset between 4 hours and 21 days, bilateral signs/symptoms of spinal cord dysfunction, clear sensory level of the trunk, and indirect evidence of spinal cord inflammation (gadolinium enhancement on magnetic resonance imaging or cerebrospinal fluid pleocytosis)
   e. None (there are no specific biomarkers for ITM)

I.4. What is the optimal initial treatment of idiopathic transverse myelitis?
   a. High-dose intravenous methylprednisolone (1,000 mg/d for 3-5 days)
   b. Plasma exchange
   c. Intravenous immunoglobulin
   d. Unknown
   e. Cyclophosphamide

I.5. McArdle sign (new or exaggerated finger extensor weakness detected upon neck flexion) is indicative of which cause of myelopathy?
   a. Compression
   b. Multiple sclerosis
   c. Vitamin B_{12} deficiency
   d. Paraneoplastic disorder
   e. Infarction

I.6. Which of the following *cannot* reliably distinguish glioma of the cervicomedullary junction from demyelinating disease (solitary sclerosis) in a patient with a slowly worsening myelopathy?
   a. T2-signal characteristics on magnetic resonance imaging (MRI)
   b. T1-signal characteristics on MRI after gadolinium administration
   c. Oligoclonal bands in cerebrospinal fluid
   d. Focal atrophy of the lesion
   e. Presence of McArdle sign

I.7. Which of the following clinical presentations is *atypical* of clinically isolated syndrome?
   a. Optic neuritis
   b. Facial numbness
   c. Partial myelitis
   d. Internuclear ophthalmoplegia
   e. Tonic spasms

I.8. In a patient with isolated optic neuritis, without brain magnetic resonance imaging abnormalities, what is the rate of conversion to multiple sclerosis over the following 15 years?
   a. 10%
   b. 25%
   c. 50%
   d. 75%
   e. 100%

I.9. A 48-year-old woman had a 2-year history of progressive right upper and lower extremity weakness in a pyramidal distribution with ipsilateral hyperreflexia and extensor plantar response. Sensory examination was intact and normal. She had never had symptoms of clinical relapse with improvement. Magnetic resonance imaging (MRI) of the brain showed a single area of abnormal T2 signal in the left temporal horn of the lateral ventricle. A nonenhancing, right-sided, hemicord

T2 lesion involving the lateral corticospinal tract was seen in the cervical spine at C2. The MRI findings were unchanged during the past 2 years. Cerebrospinal fluid (CSF) examination showed 4 unique CSF oligoclonal bands. Optical coherence tomography findings were normal. Which of the following is correct?

a. She has idiopathic inflammatory transverse myelitis

b. She has a clinically isolated syndrome of demyelination with a spinal cord onset

c. She has relapsing-remitting multiple sclerosis (MS)

d. She has progressive pauciclerotic MS with a critical demyelinating cervical spinal cord lesion

e. She has subacute combined degeneration of the spinal cord likely due to nutritional deficiency

I.10. Which of the following is consistent with the clinical and radiologic presentation of progressive pauciclerotic multiple sclerosis (MS)?

a. Progressive motor impairment can be anatomically linked to a "critical" demyelinating lesion

b. History is typically notable for many clinical relapses with resolution

c. Many brain magnetic resonance imaging (MRI) demyelinating lesions are present, often with gadolinium enhancement

d. Many spinal cord MRI demyelinating lesions are present, often with gadolinium enhancement

e. Disease-modifying therapy for MS is highly likely to be beneficial

I.11. In which of the following locations are progressive solitary sclerosis lesions typically found?

a. Spinal cord dorsal columns

b. Medullary pyramids or lateral columns

c. Central spinal cord

d. Dorsal brainstem

e. Dorsal root ganglion

I.12. Which of the following is a characteristic magnetic resonance imaging feature of lesions associated with progressive solitary sclerosis?

a. Persistent gadolinium enhancement over time

b. Progressive expansion over time

c. Development of focal atrophy over time

d. Longitudinally extensive T2 hyperintensity

e. Persistent diffusion-weighted abnormality

I.13. A 26-year-old woman seeks care for severe headache progressing over the past few weeks and sudden-onset, right-sided, upper motor neuron facial palsy, right arm paresis, and positive Babinski sign on the right. On magnetic resonance imaging (MRI), a large, 5-cm-diameter, left posterior frontal lesion is visualized, with associated edema, open ring enhancement, and peripheral restriction on diffusion-weighted imaging. The patient is given intravenous dexamethasone and improves markedly, with substantial decrease in lesion size on follow-up MRI 2 weeks later, although at this time 2 additional small (<2 cm) periventricular enhancing lesions are visualized. What should be the next step in the diagnostic plan for this patient?

a. Brain biopsy of the left frontal lesion

b. Testing of cerebrospinal fluid and serum for oligoclonal bands

c. Whole-body positron emission tomography

d. Radiotherapy

e. Observation

I.14. Which of the following may manifest as a tumefactive demyelinating lesion?

a. Acute disseminated encephalomyelitis

b. Prototypic multiple sclerosis

c. Neuromyelitis optica spectrum disorder

d. Baló concentric sclerosis

e. All of the above

I.15. Leukoaraiotic changes on brain magnetic resonance imaging refer to which of the following?

a. Demyelinating disease

b. Large-vessel strokes

c. Asymptomatic, age-related or microvascular disease–related changes

d. Susac syndrome

e. Amyotrophic lateral sclerosis

I.16. Which of the following statements about fibromyalgia is correct?

a. It is excluded if white matter changes are encountered on brain magnetic resonance imaging

b. It is a fictitious diagnosis

c. It is characterized by objective neurologic weakness

d. It is characterized by diffuse limb and axial pain

e. It is excluded if there are no tender points on examination

I.17. In demyelinating disease of the brain and spinal cord, what does radiologically isolated syndrome represent?

a. Multiple magnetic resonance imaging (MRI) lesions with occurrence of 1 typical clinical event

b. Multiple MRI lesions with multiple typical clinical events

c. Multiple MRI lesions without a typical clinical event

d. Solitary sclerosis

e. A false-positive result

I.18. Imaging findings in patients with acute disseminated encephalomyelitis are characterized by:

a. Rounded T2-hyperintense lesions predominantly in the corpus callosum

b. T2-hyperintense lesions perpendicular to the body of the lateral ventricles

c. Unilateral T1-hyperintense lesions with prominent contrast enhancement

d. Radial periventricular enhancement and long spinal cord lesions

e. Diffuse T2 hyperintensities in the subcortical white matter, thalami, and brainstem

I.19. The presence of antibodies to which of the following proteins is supportive of a diagnosis of acute disseminated encephalomyelitis?

a. GFAP (glial fibrillary acidic protein)

b. GAD65 (glutamic acid decarboxylase 65-kDa isoform)

c. MOG (myelin oligodendrocyte glycoprotein)

d. NMDAR (*N*-methyl-D-aspartate receptor)

e. GABA$_B$R (γ-aminobutyric acid$_B$ receptor)

I.20. Autoantibodies to which of the following proteins are associated with neuromyelitis optica spectrum disorders?

a. Glycine receptors

b. Glutamic acid decarboxylase 65-kDa isoform

c. Aquaporin-4

d. Glial fibrillary acidic protein

e. *N*-methyl-D-aspartate receptor

I.21. Which of the following is *not* a characteristic syndrome associated with neuromyelitis optica spectrum disorders?

a. Myelitis

b. Optic neuritis

c. Narcolepsy

d. Seizures

e. Intractable vomiting

I.22. Which of the following deficits in cognitive testing is most commonly found in patients with multiple sclerosis?

a. Anomia

b. Slow cognitive processing speed

c. Impaired cued recall

d. Receptive aphasia

e. Semantic memory deficits

I.23. Which of the following interventions are recommended for management of cognitive impairment associated with multiple sclerosis?

a. Cognitive rehabilitation, physical exercise, and management of contributing factors such as depression, sleep disruption, and polypharmacy

b. Acetylcholinesterase inhibitors

c. Memantine

d. *Ginkgo biloba*

e. Amantadine

I.24. When analyzing a cerebrospinal fluid (CSF) sample for a patient with central nervous system demyelinating disease, which of the following parameters most supports a diagnosis of multiple sclerosis?

a. CSF white blood cell count, 60 cells/μL

b. Immunoglobulin G index, 0.36

c. CSF synthesis rate, 12 mg/24 h

d. CSF kappa free light chains, 0.25 mg/dL

e. 3 Oligoclonal bands in CSF, 2 of which showed matching bands in serum

I.25. Which of the following is most predictive of motor disability in a patient with multiple sclerosis?

a. Magnetic resonance imaging finding of 2 gadolinium-enhancing paraventricular lesions

b. Immunoglobulin G index, 0.36

c. Symptomatic progression into irreversible clinical disability

d. Cerebrospinal fluid (CSF) kappa free light chains, 0.25 mg/dL

e. Eleven unique oligoclonal bands in CSF

I.26. Which of the following is more supportive of a diagnosis of pediatric aquaporin-4–immunoglobulin G (IgG)–positive neuromyelitis optica than of multiple sclerosis

or myelin oligodendrocyte glycoprotein-IgG–positive autoimmunity?

a. Optic neuritis

b. Myelitis

c. Encephalitis

d. A monophasic course

e. Permanent blindness

I.27. Which of the following treatments are US Food and Drug Administration approved for aquaporin-4–immunoglobulin G–positive neuromyelitis optica?

a. Rituximab, azathioprine, and mycophenolate mofetil

b. Eculizumab, inebilizumab, and satralizumab

c. Eculizumab, inebilizumab, and rituximab

d. Eculizumab, rituximab, and satralizumab

e. Eculizumab, inebilizumab, and mycophenolate mofetil

I.28. At what age do patients with late-onset multiple sclerosis have their first symptoms?

a. ≥30 years

b. ≥40 years

c. ≥50 years

d. ≥60 years

e. ≥70 years

I.29. At what age do patients with very late–onset multiple sclerosis have their first clinical symptoms?

a. ≥30 years

b. ≥40 years

c. ≥50 years

d. ≥60 years

e. ≥70 years

I.30. A 30-year-old woman with a history of fibromyalgia, diarrhea-predominant irritable bowel syndrome, and a new diagnosis of relapsing-remitting multiple sclerosis seeks medication counseling. She expresses a wish to avoid injections and use an oral medication. Which of the following disease-modifying therapies would be most suitable?

a. Teriflunomide

b. Fingolimod

c. Dimethyl fumarate

d. Cladribine

e. Low-dose naltrexone

I.31. A 26-year-old woman with a recent diagnosis of multiple sclerosis seeks medication counseling. She has plans to become pregnant in the following year but wishes to start disease-modifying therapy (DMT) before becoming pregnant. Which of the following DMTs is not associated with teratogenic effects?

a. Alemtuzumab

b. Fingolimod

c. Siponimod

d. Glatiramer acetate

e. Teriflunomide

I.32. A 45-year-old African American man seeks care for 4 clinical episodes of multiple sclerosis during the past year, including 2 spinal episodes and a significant radiologic burden of disease. He has not recovered well from his prior episodes. He has a history of smoking and obesity. Immunoglobulin G (IgG) antibodies to JC polyoma virus were detected in his serum. Testing for IgG antibodies to aquaporin-4 and myelin oligodendrocyte glycoprotein was negative. Which of the following disease-modifying therapies would be most appropriate?

a. Interferon beta-1a
b. Teriflunomide
c. Dimethyl fumarate
d. Natalizumab
e. Ocrelizumab

I.33. Which of the following is true regarding breakthrough disease activity (clinical or radiographic) in patients with multiple sclerosis (MS) on disease-modifying therapy?

a. Breakthrough disease activity is rare with current MS therapies
b. Breakthrough disease activity while on an MS therapy always mandates a change in therapy
c. Breakthrough disease activity is associated with worse long-term prognosis in MS, especially with new spinal lesions
d. Radiographic breakthrough disease activity on MS therapy is of no concern unless accompanied by clinical features
e. Evidence-based guidelines exist for what constitutes "acceptable" breakthrough disease activity on MS therapy

I.34. When assessing neurologic symptoms in patients with multiple sclerosis (MS) receiving disease-modifying therapy, which of the following is true?

a. New symptoms should always trigger repeated magnetic resonance imaging to objectively document new disease activity
b. New symptoms that last less than 24 hours should be treated with oral or intravenous corticosteroids
c. New symptoms should prompt initiation of another MS disease-modifying therapy
d. Worsening of previous symptoms should prompt investigation for possible causes of pseudorelapse
e. Worsening symptoms lasting more than 24 hours should be considered a new exacerbation of MS

I.35. Which of the following features, when present, is least associated with a risk of disability in patients with new-onset multiple sclerosis?

a. Male sex
b. African American ethnicity
c. Spinal cord lesions
d. Optic neuritis
e. Two gadolinium-enhancing T1-weighted lesions

I.36. In a patient who is positive for antibodies to JC polyoma virus and who has not been exposed to immunotherapy, what is the risk of progressive multifocal encephalopathy during the first 2 years of treatment with natalizumab?

a. 1/10
b. 1/100
c. 1/1,000
d. 1/10,000
e. No risk

I.37. Which drug's mechanism of action is binding to B cells expressing CD20 surface antigen, resulting in antibody-dependent cellular cytolysis and complement-mediated lysis?

a. Dimethyl fumarate
b. Natalizumab
c. Fingolimod
d. Alemtuzumab
e. Ocrelizumab

I.38. Dalfampridine should be avoided in a patient with a history of which symptoms?

a. Migraine headaches
b. Myocardial infarction
c. Spasticity
d. Seizures or epilepsy
e. Fatigue

I.39. A patient receiving natalizumab for multiple sclerosis sought care for 5 weeks of slowly progressive right hemiparesis involving his face and arm. Six months earlier he tested positive for antibodies to JC polyoma virus (JCV), with an index of 1.3. Magnetic resonance imaging of the brain shows a new, large, T2-hyperintense and T1-hypointense lesion in the left subcortical white matter without associated mass effect or enhancement. There is subtle restricted diffusion at the edges. Because of concern for progressive multifocal leukoencephalopathy, he undergoes lumbar puncture, which shows a mild lymphocytic pleocytosis and positive oligoclonal bands. JCV polymerase chain reaction (PCR) findings are negative. What is the best next step in management?

a. Start a course of daily high-dose intravenous methylprednisolone for 5 days
b. Discontinue natalizumab
c. Repeat cerebrospinal fluid JCV PCR
d. Switch therapy to ocrelizumab
e. Obtain brain biopsy

I.40. The same patient (as in the previous question) has a second cerebrospinal fluid evaluation, and JC polyoma virus polymerase chain reaction results are positive. Plasma exchange is initiated, but 1 week later his right hemiparesis worsens suddenly. Repeated magnetic resonance imaging shows speckled enhancement and edema associated with the previously described white matter lesion. What is the best next step in management?

a. Initiate 5 days of daily 0.4 g/kg intravenous immunoglobulin followed by a prednisone taper
b. Reinitiate natalizumab
c. Initiate 5 days of daily high-dose intravenous methylprednisolone followed by a prednisone taper
d. Observe
e. Obtain brain biopsy

I.41. Which of the following is best known to trigger or exacerbate a demyelinating process?

a. Head trauma
b. Stroke
c. Brain irradiation
d. Chemotherapy
e. Cancer surgery

SECTION I (CASES 1-21) ANSWERS

I.1. Answer c.

Approximately two-thirds of patients with multiple sclerosis–associated optic neuritis (MS-ON) have a normal optic nerve appearance at onset. Optic chiasm involvement is rare. Corticosteroid-dependent ON is seen in approximately 25% of myelin oligodendrocyte glycoprotein-immunoglobulin G–positive ON cases but not in MS-ON. Recovery to a visual acuity of 20/40 or better is seen in 92% of cases. Eculizumab can be a first-line agent for preventing relapse in neuromyelitis optica spectrum disorders, but it is not used for MS.

I.2. Answer e.

This patient has a classic presentation of myelin oligodendrocyte glycoprotein (MOG)–immunoglobulin G (IgG)–associated disorder. Elements suggestive of MOG-IgG–associated disorder include the bilateral optic neuritis (ON), prominent disc edema, perineural enhancement, and concomitant acute disseminated encephalomyelitis (ADEM). Glial fibrillary acidic protein-IgG and collapsin-response mediator protein 5-IgG are not associated with optic nerve enhancement. Multiple sclerosis–associated ON and aquaporin-4-IgG–positive ON do not tend to cause perineural enhancement of the optic nerve, ADEM, or significant optic disc edema.

I.3. Answer e.

Currently, there are no specific biomarkers for idiopathic transverse myelitis (ITM), which remains a diagnosis of exclusion. The diagnostic criteria listed in option d are characteristics of ITM but can be satisfied by other types of disease-associated transverse myelitis (eg, multiple sclerosis myelitis, aquaporin-4 [AQP4]–immunoglobulin G (IgG)– and myelin oligodendrocyte glycoprotein [MOG]-IgG–associated myelitis). Although AQP4-IgG and MOG-IgG frequently manifest with transverse myelitis, several other causes (eg, infectious, other inflammatory myelitis) must be excluded to make a diagnosis of ITM. The length of the myelitis lesion on spinal cord magnetic resonance imaging in ITM is variable, which reflects diverse underlying causes that are yet to be identified.

I.4. Answer d.

No randomized clinical trials have established the optimal treatment of idiopathic transverse myelitis. If infectious causes of myelitis have been reasonably excluded, an empiric therapeutic trial with high-dose corticosteroids is often used first, with plasma exchange or intravenous immunoglobulin used as second-line approaches for corticosteroid-refractory cases. Cyclophosphamide is reserved for severe demyelinating episodes that have not responded to the above-listed drugs.

I.5. Answer b.

McArdle sign alone is highly specific for multiple sclerosis involving the cervical cord or solitary sclerosis of the cervical cord. It has not been identified as a verified finding in any other kind of myelopathy.

I.6. Answer a.

Lesion characteristics on T2-weighted magnetic resonance imaging do not distinguish glioma and demyelinating disease. Gadolinium enhancement would be more consistent with a tumor in a patient with progressive myelopathy. Oligoclonal bands would be a strong clue to demyelinating disease. Focal lesion atrophy would be very suggestive of demyelination compared with tumor, which might show focal mass effect. McArdle sign is a new sign of exaggerated weakness of finger extensors with neck flexion that is specific for demyelinating disease.

I.7. Answer e.

Clinically isolated syndrome refers to an underlying pathologic process of multiple sclerosis. The presence of tonic spasms should raise concern for neuromyelitis optica. Testing for aquaporin-4–immunoglobulin G (IgG) and myelin oligodendrocyte glycoprotein-IgG antibodies should be performed in patients with this symptom.

I.8. Answer b.

Data from the Optic Neuritis Treatment Trial showed that patients with a single episode of optic neuritis without abnormalities on brain magnetic resonance imaging had a 25% chance of conversion to clinically definite multiple sclerosis over a 15-year period.

I.9. Answer d.

The progressive motor impairment associated with a critical demyelinating lesion in the cervical spinal cord, with highly restricted magnetic resonance imaging (MRI) lesion burden otherwise and typical cerebrospinal fluid abnormality, is characteristic of progressive paucisclerotic multiple sclerosis (MS). Idiopathic inflammatory transverse myelitis must reach a nadir within 20 days and is not associated with progressive impairment over years. Clinically isolated syndrome is a single episode–related demyelinating disease, often with improvement, without progressive motor impairment, and with no new MRI lesions or simultaneously gadolinium enhancing and nonenhancing lesions. Relapsing-remitting MS is defined by clinical stability between inflammatory episodes. Nutritional myelopathy such as subacute combined degeneration of the spinal cord is bilateral and symmetrical.

I.10. Answer a.

Progressive paucisclerotic multiple sclerosis (MS) is characterized by progressive motor impairment anatomically linked to a critical demyelinating lesion with highly restricted magnetic resonance imaging (MRI) lesion burden (no more than 5 lesions in the central nervous system). Many clinical relapses are uncommon in progressive paucisclerotic MS; most patients have motor progression from disease onset and a primary progressive disease course. Gadolinium-enhancing lesions and high MRI disease burden are both uncommon. Because markers of inflammation (relapses and number of MRI lesions) are minimal, current disease-modifying therapy for MS is unlikely to be beneficial.

I.11. Answer b.

Progressive solitary sclerosis lesions are typically associated with progressive motor impairment, and the accompanying lesions are located along eloquent corticospinal tract regions, particularly the pyramids of the medulla and lateral columns. Although multiple sclerosis (MS) demyelinating lesions are commonly located in the dorsal columns or dorsal brainstem, such lesions are not associated with progressive motor impairment that is characteristic of progressive solitary sclerosis. Central cord lesions are uncommon in MS and progressive solitary sclerosis, and these central nervous system diseases are not associated with dorsal root ganglion involvement.

I.12. Answer c.

The lesions in progressive solitary sclerosis develop focal atrophy over time. Progressive expansion over time or persistent enhancement would be more suspicious of a tumor or vascular malformation. Diffusion-weighted abnormalities may be seen in early multiple sclerosis (MS) lesions in the brain. Similar to other MS lesions, the lesions in progressive solitary sclerosis are not longitudinally extensive and generally extend over fewer than 3 vertebral segments on sagittal sequences.

I.13. Answer b.

The patient most likely has a tumefactive demyelinating lesion. At onset, the clinical and magnetic resonance imaging findings suggested a neoplasm. However, the decrease in lesion size after intravenous corticosteroids and subsequent appearance of additional periventricular lesions suggested demyelination, which made neoplasm less likely. Cerebrospinal fluid–specific oligoclonal bands would further support a demyelinating origin. Biopsy should be avoided whenever possible. Radiotherapy would only be an option if a neoplastic etiology was confirmed.

I.14. Answer e.

Tumefactive demyelinating lesions (TDLs) may be found in all of these conditions, including classic multiple sclerosis (MS), Baló concentric sclerosis, fulminant concentric Marburg variant MS, acute disseminated encephalomyelitis, and neuromyelitis optica spectrum disorders. They all must be considered carefully in the differential diagnosis for TDLs, because they require different therapeutic approaches.

I.15. Answer c.

Leukoaraiosis refers to multiple small areas of T2-signal change, mostly observed within cerebral hemispheric white matter as age-related change, or in patients with microvascular risk factors (without enhancement on T1 gadolinium imaging). Demyelinating disease (multiple sclerosis) lesions are ovoid and, in addition to residing in deep white matter, are distributed in key diagnostic sites (usually several of cerebral cortex, corpus callosum, brainstem, and cerebellum and spinal cord). Enhancement is commonly observed in new multiple sclerosis lesions. Large-vessel strokes follow large vascular territories. Susac syndrome lesions are prominent on magnetic resonance imaging in hemispheric deep white matter but are commonly observed in other sites, particularly corpus callosum. Before treatment, they are usually accompanied by parenchymal and leptomeningeal enhancement.

I.16. Answer d.

Fibromyalgia is a symptom-based diagnosis based on characteristic symptoms (usually diffuse limb and axial pain) and exclusion of other disorders. Leukoaraiosis (nonspecific age-related white matter changes, as distinct from inflammatory multiple sclerosis–related changes) are common in the general population and increase in frequency with age. Give-way weakness (subjective, poor effort) secondary to pain and deconditioning is a common examination finding. Tender points are characteristic but not required to make a diagnosis.

I.17. Answer c.

Radiologically isolated syndrome is defined as demonstration of magnetic resonance imaging (MRI) lesion dissemination in space by detection of 1 or more T2-hyperintense lesions involving at least 2 topographies (periventricular white matter, corticojuxtacortical, spinal cord, or infratentorial) without clinical evidence of multiple sclerosis or MRI abnormalities explained by any other disease process. Options a, b, and d are consistent with clinically active central nervous system demyelinating disease. The MRI findings are most likely indicative of subclinical demyelination rather than being a technical false-positive.

I.18. Answer e.

Imaging findings in acute disseminated encephalomyelitis are characterized by multifocal T2 hyperintensities that affect the deep and subcortical white matter diffusely and are usually bilateral and asymmetric. The basal ganglia, thalamus, and brainstem are often involved, and there is minimal contrast enhancement. Rounded callosal lesions are typical of Susac syndrome. Lesions perpendicular to the ventricles are typical of multiple sclerosis. T1 lesions are not hyperintense but hypointense, and prominent contrast enhancement is not typical. Radial periventricular lesions are typical of autoimmune glial fibrillary acidic protein astrocytopathy.

I.19. Answer c.

The presence of immunoglobulin G1 antibodies to myelin oligodendrocyte glycoprotein supports the diagnosis of acute disseminated encephalomyelitis; they are found in approximately 40% of patients. Transient seropositivity is associated with a monophasic disease course. Antibodies to the other proteins listed may be detected in other forms of autoimmune encephalitis.

I.20. Answer c.

Aquaporin-4 (AQP4), the dominant water channel in the central nervous system, is targeted by AQP4-immunoglobulin G antibody, which is a specific biomarker for neuromyelitis optica spectrum disorders. Glycine receptor and glutamic acid decarboxylase 65-kDa isoform are targets of autoimmune stiff-person spectrum disorders. Glial fibrillary acidic protein is targeted by an antibody associated with encephalopathy and a mild myelopathy; patients with this syndrome may have papillitis but not optic neuritis. N-methyl-D-aspartate receptor autoimmunity results in encephalopathy and movement disorders.

I.21. Answer d.

Seizures rarely occur in neuromyelitis optica spectrum disorders (NMOSDs). The most common syndromes are myelitis and optic neuritis, but syndromes affecting the area postrema in the dorsal medulla and certain hypothalamic syndromes, including vomiting and symptomatic narcolepsy, are also considered characteristic of NMOSDs.

I.22. Answer b.

All cognitive domains may be affected in multiple sclerosis, but the most common deficit is slow cognitive processing speed.

I.23. Answer a.

Cognitive rehabilitation, physical exercise, and management of contributing factors such as depression, sleep disruption, and polypharmacy are recommended for management of cognitive impairment in multiple sclerosis (MS). Acetylcholinesterase inhibitors, memantine, and *Ginkgo biloba* did not demonstrate significant benefit for patients with MS and cognitive impairment in clinical trials. Amantadine is used for the treatment of fatigue.

I.24. Answer d.

A cerebrospinal fluid (CSF) kappa free light chain value of 0.100 mg/dL or higher was shown to have similar sensitivity and specificity for the diagnosis of multiple sclerosis (MS) as the finding of 2 or more CSF-unique oligoclonal bands (OCB). Even though the CSF OCB were increased, paired serum samples are required to determine if these bands were CSF specific. In this situation, there is only 1 unique CSF band, which would mean a negative result. In MS, the CSF white blood cell count is usually normal and might be slightly increased (≤5 cells/μL) in less than one-third of patients. An increased CSF white blood cell count should prompt the exclusion of alternate disease processes such as infections or vasculitis. CSF immunoglobulin G index of 0.36 is within normal limits (<0.85), and normal CSF synthesis rate is ≤12 mg/24 h.

I.25. Answer c.

The single most adverse factor that influences prognosis in multiple sclerosis is the development of a progressive clinical course, or no recovery of neurologic function between episodes. Neither the number of oligoclonal bands nor immunoglobulin G index correlates with annualized relapse rate or the degree of clinical disability. Gadolinium-enhancing lesions do not correlate with the degree of disability. Enhancing lesions are found in conjunction with clinical relapses but also may be clinically silent. The type of disability depends on the functional location of the enhancing lesion. No association has been reported between cerebrospinal fluid kappa free light chain concentration and disability or disease severity.

I.26. Answer e.

Optic neuritis and myelitis can occur in multiple sclerosis, myelin oligodendrocyte glycoprotein (MOG)–immunoglobulin G (IgG) autoimmunity, or aquaporin-4 (AQP4)-IgG–positive neuromyelitis optica (NMO).

Encephalitis also can occur in pediatric MOG-IgG autoimmunity. Demyelinating disease, in general, can be monophasic or relapsing, but NMO is almost always relapsing. Poor recovery from episodes (eg, permanent blindness) is a hallmark of AQP4-IgG–positive NMO.

I.27. Answer b.

Eculizumab, inebilizumab, and satralizumab have been US Food and Drug Administration approved for relapse prevention of aquaporin-4–immunoglobulin G–positive neuromyelitis optica (as of 2019-2020). Azathioprine, mycophenolate mofetil, and rituximab are also commonly used to prevent neuromyelitis optica episodes but are off-label treatments.

I.28. Answer c.

Patients with late-onset multiple sclerosis have first symptoms at age 50 years or older.

I.29. Answer d.

Patients with very late–onset multiple sclerosis have first symptoms at age 60 years or older.

I.30. Answer b.

Teriflunomide and cladribine are contraindicated in patients who have the potential to become pregnant. Dimethyl fumarate causes abdominal cramping and can worsen irritable bowel syndrome. Low-dose naltrexone is not a disease-modifying therapy for relapsing-remitting multiple sclerosis. Of the options presented, fingolimod would have the lowest potential for adverse effects and would have reasonable efficacy for disease prevention.

I.31. Answer d.

Glatiramer acetate is not associated with risk of teratogenicity; therefore, it could be safely continued until conception and throughout pregnancy, if desired. Fingolimod, siponimod, teriflunomide, and alemtuzumab should be discontinued before conception. Teriflunomide requires an elimination protocol before conception.

I.32. Answer e.

This patient has multiple risk factors for disability accumulation in multiple sclerosis, including frequent episodes, spinal lesions, a high burden of radiologic disease, male sex, African descent, older age of disease onset, poor recovery from episodes, and tobacco use. Medication efficacy would be the priority for managing his disease. The presence of antibodies to JC polyoma virus in his serum is not an absolute contraindication to natalizumab, but the risk of progressive multifocal leukoencephalopathy would increase after 2 years of treatment with natalizumab. Therefore, ocrelizumab would be the most appropriate treatment recommendation in this patient with high disease activity. Interferon beta-1a, teriflunomide, and dimethyl fumarate are considered disease-modifying therapies for multiple sclerosis with modest efficacy compared with ocrelizumab.

I.33. Answer c.

Although there are no evidence-based consensus guidelines for how much, if any, breakthrough activity should be allowed while patients are on multiple sclerosis (MS) therapies, there is evidence that either clinical or radiographic disease activity during therapy predicts a worse long-term prognosis. NEDA (no evidence of disease activity) is a not a realistic goal for most current MS therapies but can help guide decision making as more effective therapies are developed. The decision to escalate therapy should be made with the patient after a thorough discussion of the risks and benefits of the proposed therapy and with consideration of the patient's risk tolerance, comorbid conditions, and other factors.

I.34. Answer d.

New or worsening symptoms in patients with multiple sclerosis (MS) receiving disease-modifying therapy must be evaluated objectively to determine whether symptoms are 1) consistent with the MS disease process and not better explained by another condition; 2) last at least 24 hours and are not better explained by fever, infection, or concurrent medical illness (ie, pseudorelapse); and 3) producing impairment or distress that warrant treatment for acute exacerbation (oral or intravenous corticosteroids or plasmapheresis).

I.35. Answer d.

Drug selection for disease-modifying therapy in patients with newly diagnosed multiple sclerosis is challenging, partly because of the paucity of head-to-head trials between disease-modifying therapy agents, and partly because of uncertainty regarding the efficacy of these medications for long-term prevention of disability. A strong argument can be made, however, for use of highly potent medications in patients with a high risk of disability. Poor recovery from the initial episode, male sex, African American ethnicity, brainstem and spinal cord lesions, and a large volume of T2 lesions and/or enhancing lesions at presentation or early in the course of treatment are associated with an increased risk of disability, and all should prompt consideration of highly active therapy in these patients. Optic neuritis as an initial clinical episode is associated with a lower subsequent risk of disability than episodes related to brainstem or spinal cord.

I.36. Answer c.

In patients with highly active multiple sclerosis, the use of natalizumab in the first 2 years of treatment is relatively safe, with a risk of progressive multifocal encephalopathy (PML) of less than 1/1,000, regardless of the JC polyoma virus antibody status. In patients who test negative for JC polyoma virus antibody, the risk of PML remains less than 1/1,000 for up to 6 years, regardless of other risk factors. In patients positive for JC polyoma virus antibody, the risk of PML increases after 2 years of treatment to 3/1,000, and after 4 years of treatment to 6/1,000. This risk is increased if patients have been previously exposed to immunosuppressant medications. Other US Food and Drug Administration–approved options for highly active disease-modifying therapy in patients with highly active multiple sclerosis include ocrelizumab, alemtuzumab, and oral cladribine.

I.37. Answer e.

Ocrelizumab selectively binds to B cells expressing CD20 surface antigen, which results in antibody-dependent cellular cytolysis and complement-mediated lysis. Dimethyl fumarate activates the nuclear factor (erythroid-derived 2)-like 2 transcriptional pathway involved in cellular response to oxidative stress. Natalizumab binds to $\alpha_4\beta_1$ integrin on lymphocytes, preventing ingress of those cells into the central nervous system. Fingolimod modulates sphingosine 1-phosphate receptor to block lymphocyte egression from lymph nodes. Alemtuzumab binds to CD52 cell surface antigen on T and B cells.

I.38. Answer d.

Dalfampridine is a US Food and Drug Administration–approved medication to improve walking speed in patients with multiple sclerosis. It is a broad-spectrum potassium channel blocker that can increase conduction of action potentials in demyelinated axons, as shown in animal studies. It is advised to avoid dalfampridine in those with a history of seizures or epilepsy or with a creatinine clearance less than 60 mL/min. The other suggested answers are not contraindications to the use of dalfampridine.

I.39. Answer b.

The JC polyoma virus (JCV) antibody index is increased, and the patient is at high risk for progressive multifocal leukoencephalopathy (PML). The subacute onset and imaging characteristics are concerning for PML. Natalizumab should be withdrawn immediately in this setting given the high index of suspicion, even though the JCV polymerase chain reaction (PCR) testing of the cerebrospinal fluid (CSF) was negative. Repeated PCR testing of the CSF for JCV should be performed in the coming weeks to help confirm the diagnosis. Imaging findings are not consistent with a multiple sclerosis exacerbation, and given the concern for PML, further immunosuppression with corticosteroid and ocrelizumab should be avoided. A brain biopsy may be reasonable if the diagnosis remains in doubt, but repeating the PCR for CSF JCV is less invasive and should be done first.

I.40. Answer c.

The paradoxical clinical worsening and associated enhancement on imaging after discontinuation of natalizumab is characteristic of immune reconstitution inflammatory syndrome (IRIS). Although data on efficacy are lacking, treatment with high-dose corticosteroids with or without a taper is generally recommended. Intravenous immunoglobulin is not recommended for the management of IRIS, and natalizumab should be avoided in this patient with progressive multifocal leukoencephalopathy. There is no concern about the underlying diagnosis, so a brain biopsy is not indicated. Observation could be considered, especially in mild cases. However, corticosteroids provide symptomatic relief and may improve outcome, although specific data supporting this are lacking.

I.41. Answer c.

Brain irradiation (but not the other disorders), including targeted techniques such as Gamma Knife radiosurgery, are known to sometimes trigger or worsen multiple sclerosis.

SECTION I (CASES 1-21) SUGGESTED READING

Bove RM, Healy B, Augustine A, Musallam A, Gholipour T, Chitnis T. Effect of gender on late-onset multiple sclerosis. Mult Scler. 2012;18(10):1472-9.

Bowen JD. Highly aggressive multiple sclerosis. Continuum (Minneap Minn). 2019 Jun;25(3):689–714.

Brownlee WJ, Altmann DR, Prados F, Miszkiel KA, Eshaghi A, Gandini Wheeler-Kingshott CAM, et al. Early imaging predictors of long-term outcomes in relapse-onset multiple sclerosis. Brain. 2019 Aug 1;142(8):2276–87.

Chen JJ, Flanagan EP, Jitprapaikulsan J, Lopez-Chiriboga ASS, Fryer JP, Leavitt JA, et al. Myelin oligodendrocyte glycoprotein antibody-positive optic neuritis: clinical characteristics, radiologic clues, and outcome. Am J Ophthalmol. 2018 Nov;195:8-15. Epub 2018 Jul 26.

Chitnis T. Pediatric central nervous system demyelinating diseases. Continuum (Minneap Minn). 2019 Jun;25(3):793–814.

Clauw DJ. Fibromyalgia and related conditions. Mayo Clin Proc. 2015 May;90(5):680–92.

De Stefano N, Giorgio A, Tintore M, Pia Amato M, Kappos L, Palace J, et al; MAGNIMS study group. Radiologically isolated syndrome or subclinical multiple sclerosis: MAGNIMS consensus recommendations. Mult Scler. 2018 Feb;24(2):214–21.

Freedman MS, Thompson EJ, Deisenhammer F, Giovannoni G, Grimsley G, Keir G, et al. Recommended standard of cerebrospinal fluid analysis in the diagnosis of multiple sclerosis: a consensus statement. Arch Neurol. 2005 Jun;62(6):865–70.

Giovannoni G, Turner B, Gnanapavan S, Offiah C, Schmierer K, Marta M. Is it time to target no evident disease activity (NEDA) in multiple sclerosis? Mult Scler Relat Disord. 2015 Jul;4(4):329-33. Epub 2015 May 8.

Goldenberg DL, Clauw DJ, Palmer RE, Clair AG. Opioid use in fibromyalgia: a cautionary tale. Mayo Clin Proc. 2016 May;91(5):640-8. Epub 2016 Mar 11.

Grebenciucova E, Berger JR. Immunosenescence: the role of aging in the predisposition to neuro-infectious complications arising from the treatment of multiple sclerosis. Curr Neurol Neurosci Rep. 2017;17(8):61.

Gurtner KM, Shosha E, Bryant SC, Andreguetto BD, Murray DL, Pittock SJ, et al. CSF free light chain identification of demyelinating disease: comparison with oligoclonal banding and other CSF indexes. Clin Chem Lab Med. 2018;56(7):1071–80.

Hardy TA, Reddel SW, Barnett MH, Palace J, Lucchinetti CF, Weinshenker BG. Atypical inflammatory demyelinating syndromes of the CNS. Lancet Neurol. 2016 Aug;15(9):967–81.

Hardy TA, Tobin WO, Lucchinetti CF. Exploring the overlap between multiple sclerosis, tumefactive demyelination and Balo's concentric sclerosis. Mult Scler. 2016 Jul;22(8):986-92. Epub 2016 Apr 1.

Hauser SL, Bar-Or A, Comi G, Giovannoni G, Hartung HP, Hemmer B, et al; OPERA I and OPERA II Clinical Investigators. Ocrelizumab versus interferon beta-1a in relapsing multiple sclerosis. N Engl J Med. 2017 Jan 19;376(3):221-34. Epub 2016 Dec 21.

Helis CA, McTyre E, Munley MT, Bourland JD, Lucas JT, Cramer CK, et al. Gamma knife radiosurgery for multiple sclerosis-associated trigeminal neuralgia. Neurosurgery. 2019 Nov 1;85(5):E933–9.

Jitprapaikulsan J, Chen JJ, Flanagan EP, Tobin WO, Fryer JP, Weinshenker BG, et al. Aquaporin-4 and myelin oligodendrocyte glycoprotein autoantibody status predict outcome of recurrent optic neuritis. Ophthalmology. 2018 Oct;125(10):1628-37. Epub 2018 Apr 30.

Kalb R, Beier M, Benedict RH, Charvet L, Costello K, Feinstein A, et al. Recommendations for cognitive screening and management in multiple sclerosis care. Mult Scler. 2018 Nov;24(13):1665-80. Epub 2018 Oct 10.

Kantarci OH. Phases and phenotypes of multiple sclerosis. Continuum (Minneap Minn). 2019 Jun;25(3):636–54.

Keegan BM, Kaufmann TJ, Weinshenker BG, Kantarci OH, Schmalstieg WF, Paz Soldan MM, et al. Progressive motor impairment from a critically located lesion in highly restricted CNS-demyelinating disease. Mult Scler. 2018 Oct;24(11):1445-52. Epub 2018 Jul 26.

Keegan BM, Kaufmann TJ, Weinshenker BG, Kantarci OH, Schmalstieg WF, Paz Soldan MM, et al. Progressive solitary sclerosis: gradual motor impairment from a single CNS demyelinating lesion. Neurology. 2016 Oct 18;87(16):1713-9. Epub 2016 Sep 16.

Kimbrough DJ, Fujihara K, Jacob A, Lana-Peixoto MA, Leite MI, Levy M, et al; GJCF-CC&BR. Treatment of neuromyelitis optica: review and recommendations. Mult Scler Relat Disord. 2012 Oct;1(4):180–7.

Kis B, Rumberg B, Berlit P. Clinical characteristics of patients with late-onset multiple sclerosis. J Neurol. 2008;255(5):697-702.

Koelman DL, Chahin S, Mar SS, Venkatesan A, Hoganson GM, Yeshokumar AK, et al. Acute disseminated encephalomyelitis in 228 patients: a retrospective, multicenter US study. Neurology. 2016 May 31;86(22):2085-93. Epub 2016 May 4.

Langer-Gould AM. Pregnancy and family planning in multiple sclerosis. Continuum (Minneap Minn). 2019 Jun;25(3):773–92.

Lopez-Chiriboga AS, Majed M, Fryer J, Dubey D, McKeon A, Flanagan EP, et al. Association of MOG-IgG serostatus with relapse after acute disseminated encephalomyelitis and proposed diagnostic criteria for MOG-IgG-associated disorders. JAMA Neurol. 2018 Nov 1;75(11):1355–63.

Lu G, Beadnall HN, Barton J, Hardy TA, Wang C, Barnett MH. The evolution of "no evidence of disease activity" in multiple sclerosis. Mult Scler Relat Disord. 2018 Feb;20:231-8. Epub 2017 Dec 25.

Lucchinetti CF, Gavrilova RH, Metz I, Parisi JE, Scheithauer BW, Weigand S, et al. Clinical and radiographic spectrum of pathologically confirmed tumefactive multiple sclerosis. Brain. 2008 Jul;131(Pt 7):1759-75. Epub 2008 Jun 5.

Luczynski P, Laule C, Hsiung GR, Moore GRW, Tremlett H. Coexistence of multiple sclerosis and Alzheimer's disease: a review. Mult Scler Relat Disord. 2019 Jan;27:232-8. Epub 2018 Oct 27.

McFarland HF. Examination of the role of magnetic resonance imaging in multiple sclerosis: a problem-oriented approach. Ann Indian Acad Neurol. 2009 Oct;12(4):254–63.

McKeon A, Lennon VA, Lotze T, Tenenbaum S, Ness JM, Rensel M, et al. CNS aquaporin-4 autoimmunity in children. Neurology. 2008 Jul 8;71(2):93-100. Epub 2008 May 28.

Metz LM. Clinically isolated syndrome and early relapsing multiple sclerosis. Continuum (Minneap Minn). 2019 Jun;25(3):670–88.

Miller RC, Lachance DH, Lucchinetti CF, Keegan BM, Gavrilova RH, Brown PD, et al. Multiple sclerosis, brain radiotherapy, and risk of neurotoxicity: the Mayo Clinic experience. Int J Radiat Oncol Biol Phys. 2006 Nov 15;66(4):1178-86. Epub 2006 Sep 11.

Montalban X, Hauser SL, Kappos L, Arnold DL, Bar-Or A, Comi G, et al; ORATORIO Clinical Investigators. Ocrelizumab versus placebo in primary progressive multiple sclerosis. N Engl J Med. 2017 Jan 19;376(3):209-20. Epub 2016 Dec 21.

Murphy CB, Hashimoto SA, Graeb D, Thiessen BA. Clinical exacerbation of multiple sclerosis following radiotherapy. Arch Neurol. 2003 Feb;60(2):273–5.

Price CC, Mitchell SM, Brumback B, Tanner JJ, Schmalfuss I, Lamar M, et al. MRI-leukoaraiosis thresholds and the phenotypic expression of dementia. Neurology. 2012 Aug 21;79(8):734-40. Epub 2012 Jul 25.

Rae-Grant A, Day GS, Marrie RA, Rabinstein A, Cree BAC, Gronseth GS, et al. Practice guideline recommendations summary: disease-modifying therapies for adults with multiple sclerosis: Report of the Guideline Development, Dissemination, and Implementation Subcommittee of the American Academy of Neurology [published correction appears in Neurology. 2019 Jan 8;92(2):112]. Neurology. 2018;90(17):777-88.

Reindl M, Di Pauli F, Rostasy K, Berger T. The spectrum of MOG autoantibody-associated demyelinating diseases. Nat Rev Neurol. 2013 Aug;9(8):455-61. Epub 2013 Jun 25.

Saadeh R, Pittock S, Bryant S, Murray D, Post M, Frinack J, et al. CSF kappa free light chains as a potential quantitative alternative to oligoclonal bands in multiple sclerosis. Neurology. 2019 Apr;92 (15 Supplement):S37.001.

Savoldi F, Nasr Z, Hu W, Schilaty ND, Delgado AM, Mandrekar J, et al. McArdle sign: a specific sign of multiple sclerosis. Mayo Clin Proc. 2019 Aug;94(8):1427-35. Epub 2019 Jul 11.

Schmalstieg WF, Keegan BM, Weinshenker BG. Solitary sclerosis: progressive myelopathy from solitary demyelinating lesion. Neurology. 2012 Feb 21;78(8):540-4. Epub 2012 Feb 8.

Schwab N, Schneider-Hohendorf T, Melzer N, Cutter G, Wiendl H. Natalizumab-associated PML: Challenges with incidence, resulting risk, and risk stratification. Neurology. 2017 Mar 21;88(12):1197-1205. Epub 2017 Feb 22.

Sechi E, Keegan BM, Kaufmann TJ, Kantarci OH, Weinshenker BG, Flanagan EP. Unilateral motor progression in MS: association with a critical corticospinal tract lesion. Neurology. 2019 Aug 13;93(7):e628-34. Epub 2019 Jul 9.

Sechi E, Shosha E, Williams JP, Pittock SJ, Weinshenker BG, Keegan BM, et al. Aquaporin-4 and MOG autoantibody discovery in idiopathic transverse myelitis epidemiology. Neurology. 2019 Jul 23;93(4):e414-20. Epub 2019 Jun 24.

Sumowski JF, Benedict R, Enzinger C, Filippi M, Geurts JJ, Hamalainen P, et al. Cognition in multiple sclerosis: state of the field and priorities for the future. Neurology. 2018 Feb 6;90(6):278-88. Epub 2018 Jan 17.

Thompson AJ, Banwell BL, Barkhof F, Carroll WM, Coetzee T, Comi G, et al. Diagnosis of multiple sclerosis: 2017 revisions of the McDonald criteria. Lancet Neurol. 2018 Feb;17(2):162-73. Epub 2017 Dec 21.

Thompson AJ, Baranzini SE, Geurts J, Hemmer B, Ciccarelli O. Multiple sclerosis. Lancet. 2018 Apr 21;391(10130):1622-36. Epub 2018 Mar 23.

Tobin WO. Management of multiple sclerosis symptoms and comorbidities. Continuum (Minneap Minn). 2019 Jun;25(3):753–72.

Weinshenker BG, Wingerchuk DM. Neuromyelitis spectrum disorders. Mayo Clin Proc. 2017 Apr;92(4):663–79.

Wijburg MT, Siepman D, van Eijk JJ, Killestein J, Wattjes MP. Concomitant granule cell neuronopathy in patients with natalizumab-associated PML. J Neurol. 2016 Apr;263(4):649-56. Epub 2016 Jan 25.

Wingerchuk DM, Banwell B, Bennett JL, Cabre P, Carroll W, Chitnis T, et al; International Panel for NMO Diagnosis. International consensus diagnostic criteria for neuromyelitis optica spectrum disorders. Neurology. 2015 Jul 14;85(2):177-89. Epub 2015 Jun 19.

Wingerchuk DM. Immune-mediated myelopathies. Continuum (Minneap Minn). 2018 Apr;24(2, Spinal Cord Disorders):497-522.

Section II

AUTOIMMUNE NEUROLOGIC DISORDERS QUESTIONS AND ANSWERS

SECTION II (CASES 22-52) QUESTIONS

MULTIPLE CHOICE (CHOOSE THE BEST ANSWER)

II.1. Which neoplasm is most likely to be detected in collapsin-response mediator protein 5–immunoglobulin G–associated optic neuropathy?
   a. Testicular germinoma
   b. Breast adenocarcinoma
   c. Small cell lung carcinoma
   d. Thymoma
   e. Testicular seminoma

II.2. What are the typical characteristics of collapsin-response mediator protein 5–immunoglobulin G–associated optic neuropathy?
   a. Optic disc edema, vitreous cells, and retinitis
   b. Retrobulbar optic neuritis and enhancement on magnetic resonance imaging
   c. Optic disc edema and headache
   d. Normal optic nerve appearance at onset
   e. Retinopathy only

II.3. An 80-year-old woman has subacute, bilateral, symmetric visual loss and photopsias; a diagnosis of autoimmune retinopathy is suspected. Which of the following is true?
   a. The fundus examination often demonstrates macular fibrosis and hemorrhage
   b. Normal findings of fluorescein angiography effectively eliminate the diagnosis of autoimmune retinopathy
   c. Electroretinography and optical coherence tomography often help to establish the diagnosis
   d. Serum retinal antibodies are sensitive and specific as diagnostic tests
   e. The diagnosis is unlikely without a prior history of cancer

II.4. Which of the following would *not* be included in appropriate management of autoimmune retinopathy?
   a. Corticosteroids
   b. Surveillance for neoplasm
   c. Plasma exchange
   d. Intravenous immunoglobulin
   e. Vitrectomy

II.5. What are the core clinical features of patients with limbic encephalitis?
   a. Behavioral changes, amnesia, seizures, and hallucinations
   b. Myoclonus, ataxia, and hyperekplexia

   c. Ophthalmoplegia, ataxia, and confusion
   d. Progressive gait apraxia, cognitive deficits, and urinary incontinence
   e. Progressive decline in visuospatial and praxis skills

II.6. Antibodies to which of the following are associated with faciobrachial dystonic seizures?
   a. Glial fibrillary acidic protein
   b. Leucine-rich, glioma-inactivated protein 1
   c. Glutamic acid decarboxylase 65-kDa isoform
   d. N-methyl-D-aspartate receptor
   e. γ-aminobutyric acid$_B$ receptor

II.7. Which is the most common initial manifestation of anti–N-methyl-D-aspartate receptor encephalitis?
   a. Flulike symptoms, nonspecific neurologic symptoms, and mood disturbance
   b. Dyskinesias
   c. Seizures
   d. Ataxia
   e. Abnormal behaviors

II.8. Which factors are predictive of good functional outcomes of anti–N-methyl-D-aspartate receptor encephalitis at long-term follow-up?
   a. No intensive care unit admission
   b. Early treatment initiation
   c. Lack of seizures at presentation
   d. a and b
   e. b and c

II.9. Which of the following statements is *incorrect* regarding a patient with suspected autoimmune encephalitis?
   a. Neural autoantibody testing should be performed in both serum and cerebrospinal fluid (CSF)
   b. The absence of a neural antibody detected in the serum or CSF excludes the diagnosis of autoimmune encephalitis
   c. Immunotherapy should be initiated when there is a high index of suspicion for autoimmune encephalitis, even before the neural autoantibody testing results are available
   d. Cancer screening should be performed
   e. Sometimes prolonged immunotherapy is necessary to evaluate treatment responses

II.10. Which of the following neural immunoglobulin G (IgG) autoantibodies has *not* been associated with autoimmune encephalitis?
   a. α-amino-3-hydroxy-5-methyl-4-isoxazolepropionic acid receptor–IgG
   b. N-methyl-D-aspartate receptor–IgG

c. Leucine-rich, glioma-inactivated protein 1–IgG
d. Acetylcholine receptor, muscle-type–IgG
e. Glutamic acid decarboxylase 65-kDa isoform–IgG

II.11. In a patient with subacute cognitive decline and the presence of thyroid peroxidase (TPO) antibodies, which of the following would support a diagnosis of SREAT (steroid-responsive encephalopathy associated with autoimmune thyroiditis)?
  a. Low thyrotropin level in serum
  b. Associated clinical features such as strokelike episodes, myoclonus or tremor, electroencephalography showing generalized slowing, inflammatory cerebrospinal fluid, and objective response to corticosteroids
  c. TPO antibodies alone
  d. Abnormal brain magnetic resonance imaging findings showing multiple bilateral strokes in different vascular territories
  e. Absence of objective response to treatment with corticosteroids

II.12. A 52-year-old woman sought care for cognitive difficulties for the past 8 weeks, episodes of left-sided weakness, and tremor. Magnetic resonance imaging findings were unremarkable. Cerebrospinal fluid showed increased protein concentration, and electroencephalography (EEG) showed mild diffuse slowing. Thyroid peroxidase (TPO) antibodies were increased. Testing for other infectious and autoimmune causes of encephalopathy in serum and cerebrospinal fluid was negative. Steroid-responsive encephalopathy associated with autoimmune thyroiditis is suspected. What are the next steps?
  a. Treatment trial with high-dose corticosteroids and follow-up measurement of TPO antibody titers to evaluate response to treatment
  b. Treatment with high-dose corticosteroids and long-term immunotherapy regardless of clinical response
  c. Neuropsychological testing, immunotherapy trial with high-dose corticosteroids, and repeated EEG and neuropsychological testing after treatment to evaluate clinical response objectively
  d. Treatment with rituximab because patients respond poorly to corticosteroid therapy
  e. Screening for cancer

II.13. Which of the following is *not* a typical clinical presentation of paraneoplastic autoimmune syndromes associated with neuronal antibodies to α-amino-3-hydroxy-5-methyl-4-isoxazolepropionic acid (AMPA) receptor?
  a. Behavioral change
  b. Short-term memory loss
  c. Confusion
  d. Neuropathy
  e. Seizures

II.14. Which investigation is not a reliable method to assess clinical outcomes in patients with autoimmune dementia at follow-up?

a. Electroencephalography
b. Positron emission tomography/computed tomography
c. Neuropsychological testing
d. Brain magnetic resonance imaging
e. Testing of antibody values

II.15. In which of the following clinical scenarios would autoimmune epilepsy associated with leucine-rich, glioma-inactivated protein 1–immunoglobulin G be suspected?
  a. A 75-year-old man with frequent, brief, tonic contractions of the face and arm occurring more than 50 times per day
  b. A 10-year-old boy with childhood-onset, highly stereotyped nocturnal events characterized by loud vocalization followed by stiffening and generalized shaking
  c. A 33-year-old woman with a history of neurocysticercosis with frequent episodes characterized by déjà vu and a rising butterfly sensation in her stomach followed by confusion
  d. A 27-year-old man with fever, headaches, neck stiffness, confusion, and generalized tonic-clonic seizures
  e. A 6-year-old boy with epilepsia partialis continua and brain imaging demonstrating hemicortical T2/fluid-attenuated inversion recovery hyperintensity and atrophy

II.16. Which of the following neurologic presentations is *not* associated with leucine-rich, glioma-inactivated protein 1–immunoglobulin G autoimmunity?
  a. Sensory and autonomic seizures presenting with piloerection and flushing
  b. Frequent paroxysmal episodes of dizziness lasting a few seconds, occurring multiple times per day without alteration of consciousness
  c. Neuropathic pain and dysautonomia
  d. Cramps, stiffness, fasciculations, depression, and amnesia
  e. Episodes of transient ataxia, dysarthria, and gait instability

II.17. A 45-year-old woman seeks care for new-onset headache, bilateral, painless, blurry vision, mild lower extremity weakness (fatigability), and sensory problems progressing over 1 month. She has optic disc edema, normal visual acuity, and subtle myelopathic signs. Brain magnetic resonance imaging (MRI) shows linear periventricular enhancement, and spine MRI shows a hazy T2 hyperintensity with some faint gadolinium central enhancement. Cerebrospinal fluid analysis shows marked lymphocytic pleocytosis (110 white blood cells/μL) with normal cytologic findings, increased protein concentration, and no oligoclonal bands. What is the most probable diagnosis?
  a. Aquaporin-4 autoimmunity
  b. Myelin oligodendrocyte glycoprotein autoimmunity
  c. Spinal cord tumor

d. Spinal cord infarct

e. Glial fibrillary acidic protein autoimmunity

II.18. Which of the following neural autoantibodies is most commonly encountered in children?

a. Glial fibrillary acidic protein–immunoglobulin G (IgG)

b. Antineuronal nuclear antibody type 2-IgG (anti-Ri)

c. Purkinje cell cytoplasmic autoantibody type 1-IgG (anti-Yo)

d. IgLON5-IgG

e. Collapsin-response mediator protein 5-IgG

II.19. A 58-year-old woman has development of subacute confusion and seizures 5 weeks after completing a 21-day course of acyclovir for herpes simplex virus (HSV) encephalitis. Upon dismissal from the hospital she had anterograde memory deficits but was fully alert and interactive. Over the past 2 weeks, she has become more somnolent, and her verbal output has decreased. Seizures are poorly controlled despite initiation of levetiracetam. She has been afebrile. Repeated imaging shows evolving gliosis of her left temporal pole and minimal residual enhancement. What is the best next step in management?

a. Restart acyclovir

b. Cerebrospinal fluid (CSF) analysis and HSV polymerase chain reaction testing

c. Initiate lamotrigine

d. CSF analysis for neural-based antibodies, including *N*-methyl-D-aspartate receptor antibodies

e. Consider epilepsy surgery

II.20. A 26-year-old man seeks care in January for confusion, seizures, and fever. Two days earlier, cough, myalgia, and fever developed. Magnetic resonance imaging of the brain shows scattered T2-hyperintense lesions with some associated enhancement. Cerebrospinal fluid (CSF) parameters are normal. Five days earlier, his sister had been diagnosed with influenza. Influenza-associated encephalopathy is suspected. What is the best testing to perform?

a. Polymerase chain reaction (PCR) of CSF for influenza

b. Serologic testing of CSF for influenza

c. PCR testing of nasopharyngeal sample for influenza

d. Testing of nasopharyngeal sample for influenza antigen

e. Testing for oligoclonal bands in CSF

II.21. What are the most common clinical manifestations of KLHL11 (kelch like family member 11) autoimmunity?

a. Seizures and encephalopathy

b. Vertigo, diplopia, and gait instability

c. Faciobrachial dystonic spells

d. Neuropsychiatric dysfunction

e. Meningoencephalomyelitis

II.22. What cancer is associated with KLHL11 (kelch like family member 11) autoimmunity?

a. Small cell lung cancer

b. Adenocarcinoma of the breast

c. Thymoma

d. Testicular germ cell tumor

e. Prostate adenocarcinoma

II.23. Which of the following sleep disorders is typically seen in IgLON family member 5 autoimmunity syndrome?

a. Restless legs syndrome

b. Excessive fragmentary myoclonus

c. Rapid eye movement sleep behavior disorder

d. Sleep walking

e. Cataplexy

II.24. To which of the following protein families does IgLON family member 5 belong?

a. Neuronal differentiation

b. Transglutaminase

c. Histidine decarboxylase

d. Myelin basic protein

e. Cell adhesion

II.25. Which of the following is a biomarker of autoimmune ataxia in female patients with occult ovarian or breast adenocarcinoma?

a. Metabotropic glutamate receptor 1–immunoglobulin G (IgG)

b. Purkinje cell cytoplasmic antibody type 1

c. Antineuronal nuclear antibody type 1

d. Glutamic acid decarboxylase 65-kDa isoform-IgG

e. Contactin-associated protein 2-IgG

II.26. An autoimmune ataxia–stiff-person syndrome overlap may be encountered in patients with which of the following antibodies?

a. Metabotropic glutamate receptor 1–immunoglobulin G (IgG)

b. Purkinje cell cytoplasmic antibody type 1

c. Antineuronal nuclear antibody type 1

d. Glutamic acid decarboxylase 65-kDa isoform-IgG

e. Contactin-associated protein 2-IgG

II.27. Which of the following is true regarding patients with chorea in the context of systemic lupus erythematosus?

a. They usually have occult small cell cancer

b. They do not improve with corticosteroid treatment

c. They usually have coexisting Purkinje cell cytoplasmic antibody type 1

d. They usually have a good prognosis

e. They are usually neuronal antibody positive

II.28. Which of the following is true regarding patients with chorea in the context of collapsin-response mediator protein 5–immunoglobulin G positivity?

a. They usually have small cell cancer

b. They usually improve with corticosteroid treatment

c. They usually have coexisting Purkinje cell cytoplasmic antibody type 1

d. They usually have a good prognosis

e. They are nonsmokers

II.29. Glycine receptor α1 subunit–immunoglobulin G antibody is a biomarker of which autoimmune syndrome?

a. Myelopathy

b. Ataxia
c. Stiff-person syndrome spectrum disorder
d. Peripheral neuropathy
e. Myasthenia gravis

II.30. Glutamic acid decarboxylase 65-kDa isoform–immunoglobulin G antibody is a biomarker of which autoimmune processes?
a. Ataxia, stiff-person syndrome (SPS), type 1 diabetes
b. Ataxia, SPS, psoriasis
c. Neuropathy, SPS, type 1 diabetes
d. Neuropathy, SPS, psoriasis
e. Neuropathy, SPS, ataxia

II.31. Symptoms observed in progressive encephalomyelitis with rigidity and myoclonus phenotypes include all of the following except:
a. Encephalopathy
b. Myoclonus
c. Diplopia
d. Faciobrachial dystonic spells
e. Exaggerated startle

II.32. Antibodies to which protein are associated with a favorable response to immunotherapy in stiff-person syndrome/progressive encephalomyelitis with rigidity and myoclonus phenotypes?
a. Glutamic acid decarboxylase 65-kDa isoform
b. Dipeptidyl-peptidase-like protein-6
c. Glycine receptor α1 subunit
d. N-methyl-D-aspartate receptor
e. Leucine-rich, glioma-inactivated protein 1

II.33. A 28-year-old woman with systemic lupus erythematosus reports a 2-week history of sudden onset of back pain, paresthesia, and weakness in her legs. She describes a tight, bandlike sensation of numbness and tingling from her mid back that descends into her buttocks and legs. Recently, she noticed an inability to completely void when urinating. She reports no fevers, headaches, eye pain, or visual deficits. On examination, she is alert and oriented and appropriately responds to questions. There is sensory loss to touch, pinprick, and temperature from the T12 dermatome extending into the saddle area and bilateral lower extremities. There is reduced anal sphincter tone. She has normal bulk and tone of her muscles but weakness of the bilateral hip flexors, hip extensors, and abductor and adductor muscles. There is no weakness of the upper extremity muscles. There is hyperreflexia of the patellar and Achilles tendons bilaterally. There is a positive Babinski sign bilaterally. Vibration and proprioception are intact. What is the most likely neurologic disorder?
a. Acute inflammatory demyelinating polyneuropathy
b. Transverse myelitis
c. Aseptic meningitis
d. Mononeuritis multiplex
e. Peripheral neuropathy

II.34. A 32-year-old woman with a history of systemic lupus erythematosus sought care for recurrent episodes of sudden, involuntary jerking of the left arm. She was diagnosed with an idiopathic, left lower extremity, deep venous thrombosis 2 years earlier and treated with 3 months of anticoagulation. Her examination revealed choreoathetoid movements of the left upper arm, hand, and wrist. There was no tremor, cogwheeling, or hemiballistic movement. Which antibody may be associated with the clinical presentation in this patient?
a. Aquaporin-4 antibody
b. Antiribosomal P antibody
c. Antiphospholipid antibody
d. Antinuclear antibody
e. N-methyl-D-aspartate receptor antibody

II.35. Which of the following features are characteristic of paraneoplastic myelopathy on spinal cord magnetic resonance imaging?
a. None (usually normal findings)
b. A longitudinally extensive, nonenhancing, tract-specific, T2 hyperintensity along the dorsal columns
c. Multiple, short, peripheral, T2-hyperintense lesions along the dorsal and lateral columns frequently associated with nodular or ring-like enhancement
d. A longitudinally extensive, tract-specific, T2 hyperintensity along the dorsal or lateral columns that enhances after gadolinium administration
e. A markedly edematous spinal cord T2-hyperintense lesion (either longitudinally extensive or not) with irregular intralesional enhancement after gadolinium, consistent with spinal cord neoplasm

II.36. What cancer type is most frequently associated with paraneoplastic myelopathies?
a. Teratoma
b. Spinal cord astrocytoma and ependymoma
c. Small cell lung and breast cancer
d. Prostate cancer
e. Melanoma

II.37. In which of the following patients should a diagnosis of Sjögren sensory ganglionopathy be suspected?
a. A 32-year-old woman with dryness of eyes and mouth, along with numbness and tingling involving her toes which progresses symmetrically up to the ankles
b. A 56-year-old woman with progressive distal weakness, gait instability, and tremors
c. A 72-year-old man with back pain radiating down the left lower extremity and left foot drop
d. A 56-year-old man with numbness and paresthesia involving left upper and right lower extremities and progressive gait instability
e. A 52-year-old woman with severe pain and paresthesia involving the dorsum of her left foot and left foot drop

II.38. Which of the following neuropathy phenotypes associated with Sjögren syndrome is least likely to respond to corticosteroids or intravenous immunoglobulin?
   a. Multiple mononeuropathy
   b. Cranial neuropathy
   d. Radiculoneuropathy
   d. Sensory ataxic neuropathy
   e. Painful sensory neuropathy without sensory ataxia

II.39. In which clinical scenario would a paraneoplastic myeloneuropathy associated with collapsin-response mediator protein 5 antibodies be suspected?
   a. A 45-year-old woman with sicca symptoms, subacute onset of painless numbness in all limbs, and progressive gait and limb ataxia
   b. A 75-year-old man with a 3-year history of numbness and tingling in both feet and hands, neck pain, and global hyperreflexia
   c. A 61-year-old man with 9 months of painful, asymmetric, ascending paresthesias and weakness in all limbs, severe gait ataxia, areflexia, extensor plantar reflex, and unintentional 9-kg (20-lb) weight loss
   d. A 23-year-old woman with a 2-week history of ascending paresthesias and weakness in all limbs, areflexia, and respiratory failure requiring mechanical ventilation
   e. A 37-year-old woman with kidney failure and acute onset of right wrist drop, followed 2 months later by left foot drop

II.40. Which statement is true regarding collapsin-response mediator protein 5 (CRMP5)-associated paraneoplastic syndromes?
   a. Small cell lung cancer and thymomas are the most common cancer associations
   b. There is no role for immunotherapies if oncologic treatment is initiated immediately after the diagnosis
   c. Ongoing cancer surveillance is not required if cancer is not found at the time of diagnosis because CRMP5 antibodies are not strongly associated with cancer
   d. Most patients have an excellent response to a combination of oncologic treatment and immunotherapies
   e. CRMP5-associated polyradiculoneuropathies are typically demyelinating

II.41. Which statement is true regarding antineuronal nuclear antibody type 1–immunoglobulin G (anti-Hu) autoimmune neuropathy?
   a. It is insidious in onset and exquisitely immunotherapy responsive
   b. It is almost always associated with cognitive decline
   c. It can present with a stiff-person–like syndrome
   d. It is most commonly associated with thymoma
   e. It is typically associated with severe pain

II.42. Paraneoplastic autoimmune neurologic presentations include:
   a. Subacute-onset radiculopathy, sensory neuronopathy, or length-dependent sensorimotor neuropathy

b. Progressive neuropathy over decades
   c. Carpal tunnel syndrome
   d. Tarsal tunnel syndrome
   e. Spinal stenosis

II.43. Chronic inflammatory demyelinating polyradiculoneuropathy is:
   a. An extremely rare inflammatory neuropathy
   b. An inflammatory axonal polyradiculoneuropathy
   c. A neuropathy commonly associated with malignancy
   d. Not treatable
   e. An inflammatory demyelinating polyradiculoneuropathy

II.44. In the evaluation of chronic inflammatory demyelinating polyradiculoneuropathy, what features should raise the possibility of an alternative diagnosis?
   a. Proximal and distal weakness; weight loss
   b. Increased cerebrospinal fluid protein levels; poor response to intravenous immunoglobulin
   c. Facial weakness; pain
   d. Severe autonomic dysfunction; dyspnea
   e. Symmetric weakness; demyelinating features on nerve conduction studies

II.45. Which statement is correct regarding contactin-associated protein 2 autoimmunity–associated pain?
   a. It is frequently immunotherapy responsive
   b. It is always associated with cognitive decline
   c. It is not associated with any cancer
   d. It does not respond to non-immunotherapies such as membrane-stabilizing medications
   e. It is linked with Morvan syndrome but not Isaacs syndrome

II.46. Which statement is true regarding the risk of cancer with contactin-associated protein 2–immunoglobulin G (IgG) autoimmunity?
   a. The risk is nonexistent
   b. It is most commonly associated with thymoma and is more common in persons with coexisting positivity for leucine-rich, glioma-inactivated protein 1-IgG autoantibody
   c. It is more common if patients have autoimmune pain
   d. It is strongly linked to hematologic cancers
   e. It is associated with poor prognosis

II.47. A 45-year-old woman is evaluated for subacute onset of nausea, vomiting, orthostatic hypotension, and urinary retention. She has severe dry mouth and dry eyes. Pupils are dilated and unreactive. An antibody directed against *which* of the following antigens is the most likely cause of this disorder?
   a. α1 subunit of nicotinic acetylcholine receptor
   b. α3 subunit of nicotinic acetylcholine receptor
   c. Muscarinic M3 receptor
   d. Auxiliary subunit of voltage-gated potassium channel
   e. L-type voltage-gated calcium channel

II.48. A 48-year-old man is evaluated for severe nausea, vomiting, and constipation. Abdominal radiography shows dilated intestinal loops indicating paralytic ileus, consistent with intestinal pseudo-obstruction. Which of the following paraneoplastic antibodies is classically associated with gastrointestinal tract dysmotility?

a. Antineuronal nuclear antibody type 1 (anti-Hu)
b. Anti-Ma2
c. Antiamphiphysin
d. Purkinje cell cytoplasmic antibody type 1 (anti-Yo)
e. Antineuronal nuclear antibody type 2 (anti-Ri)

II.49. Which of the following findings in a patient with gastrointestinal dysmotility would *not* warrant a consideration of immunotherapy?

a. Antineuronal nuclear antibody type 1 (anti-Hu) seropositivity
b. Dipeptidyl-peptidase-like protein-6–immunoglobulin G (IgG) seropositivity
c. Ganglionic (alpha 3) acetylcholine receptor-IgG seropositivity
d. History of dysautonomia and systemic lupus erythematosus
e. Hypermobile joints

II.50. Which of the following neural antibodies is most likely to be associated with autoimmune gastrointestinal dysmotility and small cell carcinoma?

a. Antineuronal nuclear antibody type 1 (anti-Hu)
b. Dipeptidyl-peptidase-like protein-6–immunoglobulin G (IgG)
c. *N*-methyl-D-aspartate receptor-IgG
d. Leucine-rich, glioma-inactivated protein 1-IgG
e. Contactin-associated protein 2-IgG

II.51. Which of the following autoimmune myasthenia gravis antibody profiles is associated with a high risk of thymoma?

a. Muscle-specific tyrosine kinase antibody
b. Acetylcholine receptor (AChR) antibodies (binding, modulating) and striational antibodies
c. Low-density lipoprotein receptor-related protein 4 antibody
d. Seronegative
e. AChR binding antibody positive, with modulating and striational antibodies negative

II.52. Which of the following long-term steroid-sparing treatments is commonly favored in muscle-specific tyrosine kinase–immunoglobulin G myasthenia gravis?

a. Pyridostigmine
b. Mycophenolate mofetil
c. Rituximab
d. Azathioprine
e. Cyclosporine A

II.53. What is the most common cancer detected in patients with Lambert-Eaton myasthenic syndrome?

a. Ovarian adenocarcinoma
b. Seminoma
c. Breast adenocarcinoma
d. Small cell lung carcinoma
e. Prostate adenocarcinoma

II.54. Lambert-Eaton myasthenic syndrome is associated most frequently with autoantibodies specific for:

a. Voltage-gated calcium channels
b. Neuronal acetylcholine receptors
c. Voltage-gated potassium channels
d. Muscle acetylcholine receptors
e. Muscle striational proteins

II.55. In a patient with subacute progressive proximal weakness and markedly increased creatine kinase level, which of the following findings would support a diagnosis of necrotizing autoimmune myopathy?

a. Positive anti–3-hydroxy-3-methylglutaryl–coenzyme A reductase antibodies
b. Positive anti–transcription intermediary factor 1-γ antibodies
c. Muscle biopsy showing rimmed vacuoles and sarcoplasmic congophilic deposits
d. Muscle biopsy showing prominent inflammatory exudate in the perimysium and atrophy of perifascicular myofibers
e. Weakness resolving after discontinuation of statins

II.56. Which of the following statements is correct regarding cancer and necrotizing autoimmune myopathy (NAM)?

a. NAM is not a paraneoplastic disorder, so cancer screening is not necessary
b. Seronegative and signal recognition particle (SRP) antibody–positive patients with NAM have higher incidence of cancer than the general population
c. Seronegative and 3-hydroxy-3-methylglutaryl-coenzyme A reductase (HMGCR) antibody–positive patients with NAM have a higher incidence of cancer than the general population
d. Seropositive (HMGCR or SRP antibodies) patients with NAM have a higher incidence of cancer than the general population
e. All patients with NAM, regardless of antibody status, have a higher incidence of cancer than the general population

II.57. A muscle biopsy from a 60-year-old man with muscle weakness shows atrophic, necrotic, and regenerating fibers in the perifascicular regions. What is the patient's most likely diagnosis?

a. Necrotizing autoimmune myopathy
b. Dermatomyositis
c. Inclusion body myositis
d. Polymyositis
e. Muscular dystrophy

II.58. Which of the following neuromuscular diseases is the most likely cause of weakness in a patient with dysphagia, difficulty climbing stairs, and positive nuclear matrix protein 2 autoantibodies?

a. Dermatomyositis
b. Inclusion body myositis
c. Necrotizing autoimmune myopathy

d. Myasthenia gravis

e. Lambert-Eaton myasthenic syndrome

II.59. Neurologic complications of immune checkpoint inhibitors (ICIs) can arise with the use of which ICI category?

a. Cytotoxic T-lymphocyte-associated protein 4 inhibitors alone

b. Programmed cell death protein 1 inhibitors alone

c. Programmed cell death ligand 1 inhibitors alone

d. Any category of ICI

e. None of the ICIs

II.60. A patient with melanoma is treated with combination immune checkpoint inhibitors (ICIs). After his third ICI cycle, he has development of double vision and nonfatigable neck and proximal upper and lower extremity weakness. Electromyography shows no neuromuscular junction defect. What are the next steps in this patient's care?

a. Edrophonium (Tensilon) test

b. Creatine kinase testing, cardiology workup, ICI discontinuation, and corticosteroid treatment

c. ICI discontinuation and watchful waiting

d. Quadriceps biopsy, and if there are no signs of inflammation, resume ICI treatment

e. Continue ICI treatment because this is a paraneoplastic manifestation and treating the cancer will improve the symptoms

II.61. High-titer striational antibodies are most strongly associated with which of the following?

a. Congenital myasthenic syndrome

b. Lambert-Eaton myasthenic syndrome

c. Necrotizing autoimmune myopathy

d. Thymoma without evidence of myasthenia gravis

e. Thymoma with evidence of myasthenia gravis

II.62. Testing for striational antibodies in the incorrect clinical context will result in which of the following?

a. Low clinical specificity

b. Low clinical sensitivity

c. Low positive predictive value

d. Low negative predictive value

e. High negative predictive value

SECTION II (CASES 22-52) ANSWERS

II.1. Answer c.

Detection of immunoglobulin G (IgG) antibodies to collapsin-response mediator protein 5 (CRMP5) supports a paraneoplastic cause. Small cell lung carcinoma is most frequently detected in those positive for CRMP5-IgG. Thymoma is also associated with CRMP5-IgG but less commonly so. Antibodies to Ma2 and kelch-like protein 11 are associated with testicular germinoma and seminoma, respectively. IgG antibodies to antineuronal nuclear antibody type 2 and Purkinje cell cytoplasmic antibody type 1 (Ri and Yo antibodies) and amphiphysin most commonly accompany breast adenocarcinoma.

II.2. Answer a.

Collapsin-response mediator protein 5–immunoglobulin G–associated optic neuropathy has optic nerve involvement typically seen as optic disc edema but without optic nerve enhancement on magnetic resonance imaging (MRI). The optic disc edema rarely presents in isolation and usually coexists with vitritis and retinitis. Paraneoplastic retinopathy in isolation is associated with antirecoverin antibody. The clinical features of vision loss, retrobulbar optic neuritis (absence of optic disc edema), pain with eye movements, and optic nerve enhancement on MRI are fitting with a diagnosis of optic neuritis. Bilateral optic disc edema and headache may be symptoms of increased intracranial pressure secondary to a compressive mass lesion or pseudotumor cerebri syndromes.

II.3. Answer c.

Electroretinography and optical coherence tomography can be helpful in diagnosing autoimmune retinopathy. The fundus examination is often normal or close to normal in appearance, and angiography is not helpful. Commercially available tests for serum retinal antibodies, with the exception of antirecoverin, have low clinical specificity. Autoimmune retinopathy can be nonparaneoplastic.

II.4. Answer e.

There is no class I evidence to support the treatment of these rare retinopathies. Trials of immunotherapy are generally undertaken. Screening for neoplasm may be antibody specific in patients with antirecoverin antibody (small cell carcinoma), and those patients may need surveillance every 3 to 6 months for up to 3 years if carcinoma remains undetected. In general, for other cases, comprehensive screening for cancer is done once. Vitrectomy has no role in the management of autoimmune retinopathy.

II.5. Answer a.

Limbic encephalitis is an inflammatory process that affects the limbic cortex, hippocampus, amygdala, hypothalamus, and cingulate gyrus. It presents with cognitive dysfunction, behavioral changes, visual and auditory hallucinations, prominent amnesia, and seizures. Myoclonus, ataxia, and hyperekplexia are more commonly encountered in patients with glutamic acid decarboxylase 65-kDa isoform autoimmunity. Ophthalmoplegia, ataxia, and confusion is the typical triad associated with Wernicke encephalopathy. Gait apraxia, cognitive deficits, and urinary incontinence are features of normal-pressure hydrocephalus. Declines in visuospatial and praxis skills are manifestations of neurodegenerative disorders.

II.6. Answer b.

Although seizures can be a manifestation of other antibody-mediated disorders, faciobrachial dystonic seizures (FBDS) only occur in patients with immunoglobulin G antibodies to leucine-rich, glioma-inactivated protein 1. FBDS are characterized by brief, frequent, dystonic movements that mostly affect the arm and ipsilateral hemiface. Response to antiepileptic drug therapy is limited, but immunotherapy can result in seizure freedom.

II.7. Answer a.

Anti–N-methyl-D-aspartate receptor encephalitis may have a prodrome of nonspecific viral-like and neurologic symptoms (headache, paresthesias), followed by altered mood, behavioral change (particularly in children), and cognitive impairment. Later in the disease course, seizures, dyskinesias, and ataxia will often manifest but are not the first symptoms noted.

II.8. Answer d.

The 2 factors that have been most strongly associated with improved 1-year functional outcomes of anti–N-methyl-D-aspartate receptor encephalitis on multivariate analysis are lack of intensive care unit admission at onset and early treatment initiation. Independently, however, lack of seizures at presentation is associated with good functional outcomes.

II.9. Answer b.

There are seronegative forms of autoimmune encephalitis. For that reason, if autoimmune encephalitis is suspected on the basis of the clinical presentation, cerebrospinal fluid (CSF) results, and imaging, even with negative neural autoantibody testing in both serum and CSF, cancer screening should be performed and an immunotherapy trial started.

II.10. Answer d.

All of the above autoantibodies have been associated with autoimmune encephalitis except for the muscle-type acetylcholine receptor immunoglobulin G, which is a biomarker of myasthenia gravis. In patients with thymoma and autoimmune encephalitis, muscle-type acetylcholine receptor antibody can be present even without evidence of myasthenia gravis and is a biomarker of the underlying thymoma.

II.11. Answer b.

Features required to diagnose SREAT (steroid-responsive encephalopathy associated with autoimmune thyroiditis) include 1) subacute and fluctuating encephalopathy, with 1 or more of strokelike episodes, seizures, myoclonus, and tremor; 2) detection of thyroid autoantibodies (which reflect a predisposition to an autoimmune neurologic disorder, but do not imply a pathogenic role for those antibodies); and 3) an objective neurologic response to immunotherapy. Encephalopathic-appearing electroencephalography findings and inflammatory cerebrospinal fluid support the diagnosis. Thyrotropin level is typically normal in patients with SREAT. Thyroid peroxidase antibodies alone are not enough to make a diagnosis of SREAT. The abnormal brain magnetic resonance imaging findings are suggestive of an alternative cause, such as central nervous system vasculitis. SREAT usually responds to treatment with corticosteroids.

II.12. **Answer c.**

Neuropsychological testing is helpful to evaluate the cognitive deficits before treatment and document objective improvements after immunotherapy. The patient had abnormal electroencephalography (EEG) findings, so repeated EEG after treatment would also assist in objective measurement of improvement. Thyroid peroxidase antibody titer has no value for monitoring response to immunotherapy. Long-term immunotherapy would not be appropriate if there is no response to the initial immunotherapy trial. SREAT (steroid-responsive encephalopathy associated with autoimmune thyroiditis) usually has a good response to corticosteroid therapy. SREAT is not typically associated with underlying neoplasm.

II.13. **Answer d.**

Autoimmune and paraneoplastic syndromes associated with α-amino-3-hydroxy-5-methyl-4-isoxazolepropionic acid (AMPA) receptor immunoglobulin G neuronal antibody typically present with fulminant limbic encephalitis (severe short-term memory loss, confusion, seizures, and psychiatric symptoms). However, the spectrum can include more subtle presentations of confusion and cognitive impairment that can mimic neurodegenerative diseases. Neuropathy is not a recognized manifestation of AMPA receptor autoimmunity.

II.14. **Answer e.**

It is important to identify an appropriate objective measure at the baseline clinical assessment of a patient with an autoimmune or paraneoplastic syndrome. This measure should be a reliable correlate with the patient's symptoms and be able to be repeated at regular intervals to determine a clinical response to immunotherapy. Common methods used in patients with autoimmune or paraneoplastic syndromes include electroencephalography, neuropsychological testing, positron emission tomography/computed tomography, and brain magnetic resonance imaging. Antibody values are not a reliable measure of neurologic outcome and can remain positive despite successful treatment and clinical improvement.

II.15. **Answer a.**

Faciobrachial dystonic seizure is a characteristic phenotype described among adult patients with leucine-rich, glioma-inactivated protein 1–immunoglobulin G–associated autoimmune epilepsy. These are brief focal motor seizures and occur multiple times a day. They are stereotypically characterized by dystonic contraction of the face and arm. Case description b is more suggestive of frontal lobe epilepsy. Case descriptions c and d are suggestive of seizures secondary to neurocysticercosis and infectious meningoencephalitis, respectively. The clinical presentation in description e is suggestive of Rasmussen encephalitis.

II.16. **Answer e.**

Neurologic presentations in options a through d have been described in association with leucine-rich, glioma-inactivated protein 1–immunoglobulin G (LGI1-IgG) antibodies. Seizure and memory deficits are the most common presentations of LGI1-IgG autoimmunity. Peripheral nervous system presentations such as neuromyotonia or neuropathic pain syndromes have also been described. *Paroxysmal dizzy spells* are brief and frequent episodes of dizziness (likely seizures) that may precede encephalopathy by 2 to 12 months. Episodic gait ataxia and dysarthria, however, is a phenotype associated with contactin-associated protein 2 autoimmunity but not with LGI1 autoimmunity.

II.17. **Answer e.**

The patient has subtle myelopathic signs and no clear evidence of optic neuritis, which makes aquaporin-4 and myelin oligodendrocyte glycoprotein autoimmunity less likely. The associated meningeal signs and symptoms, as well as the subacute onset of her symptoms, make spinal cord tumors or infarcts unlikely. The symptoms, examination, imaging, and testing described are characteristic of glial fibrillary acidic protein autoimmunity.

II.18. **Answer a.**

Glial fibrillary acidic protein–immunoglobulin G (IgG) autoimmunity can be encountered in children. Other neural autoantibodies commonly encountered in the pediatric population are specific for N-methyl-D-aspartate receptors, myelin oligodendrocyte glycoprotein, aquaporin-4, and γ-aminobutyric acid$_A$ receptor. The other neural autoantibodies (antineuronal nuclear antibody type 2-IgG, Purkinje cell cytoplasmic autoantibody type 1, IgLON5-IgG, and collapsin-response mediator protein 5-IgG) are encountered almost exclusively in adults.

II.19. **Answer d.**

Recurrent herpes simplex virus (HSV) encephalitis is exceedingly rare. Postinfectious encephalitis has been reported in patients recovering from HSV encephalitis, as well as a few other herpesvirus central nervous system infections. Although antibodies to N-methyl-D-aspartate receptor are the most common, other antibodies, including unclassified neural antibodies, have been described. Symptoms can respond to immunotherapy (but not surgery), so a high index of suspicion is necessary.

II.20. **Answer c.**

The clinical scenario, exposure history, imaging studies, and normal cerebrospinal fluid (CSF) parameters could be consistent with influenza-associated encephalopathy but not classic multiple sclerosis. Polymerase chain reaction (PCR) testing for influenza is most sensitive. However, there is little role for CSF testing in this setting because direct infection of the central nervous system is not thought to be the main pathophysiologic mechanism and it rarely gives positive results. A positive nasopharyngeal PCR result in the right clinical scenario confirms the diagnosis.

II.21. **Answer b.**
Gait instability and diplopia are the most common symptoms associated with KLHL11 (kelch like family member 11) autoimmunity. Vertigo, tinnitus, and hearing loss can occur; in some cases these can precede incoordination or oculomotor manifestations by weeks to months. Seizures and encephalopathy can also occur but are less common. Faciobrachial dystonic spells are specific for anti–leucine-rich, glioma-inactivated protein 1 encephalitis. Neuropsychiatric dysfunction is a general feature of many brain diseases. Meningoencephalomyelitis is the phenotype most associated with autoimmune glial fibrillary acidic protein astrocytopathy.

II.22. **Answer d.**
Testicular germ cell tumors are found on cancer screening in the majority of patients with KLHL11 (kelch like family member 11) autoimmunity; in some cases, these were extratesticular. This supports the need for full-body positron emission tomography if testicular ultrasonography is normal. Small cell lung cancer, adenocarcinoma of the breast, and thymoma can be seen with various other autoantibodies, but none have been described to be associated with KLHL11. Prostate adenocarcinoma is not typically associated with paraneoplastic neurologic syndromes.

II.23. **Answer c.**
In the original and subsequent reports of IgLON family member 5 (IgLON5) autoimmunity syndrome, rapid eye movement (REM) sleep behavior disorder, typified by dream enactment behaviors, and polysomnographic REM sleep without atonia are the most frequent parasomnias described. Although the other disorders listed could possibly occur in IgLON5 autoimmunity as in any patient, they are not typical of the disorder, nor have these yet been reported to occur.

II.24. **Answer e.**
IgLON proteins comprise a family of 5 cell-adhesion proteins that are thought to be involved in growth of neurons and their connectivity and may have roles in maturation and maintenance of the blood-brain barrier. Antibodies against IgLON family member 5 have been found to be associated with autoimmunity and possible neurodegeneration.

II.25. **Answer b.**
Ataxia may be the presenting neurologic phenotype for autoimmunity to any of the neural antibody choices listed. However, Purkinje cell cytoplasmic antibody type 1 is the only one with a strong association with cancers of the breast and gynecologic tract.

II.26. **Answer d.**
Ataxia may be the presenting neurologic phenotype for autoimmunity to any of the neural antibody choices listed. Glutamic acid decarboxylase 65-kDa isoform–immunoglobulin G antibody is the only one also associated with stiff-person syndrome, including patients with an ataxia–stiff-person syndrome overlap syndrome.

II.27. **Answer d.**
Unlike patients with paraneoplastic disorders, patients with chorea in the setting of systemic lupus erythematosus typically have remission with corticosteroid therapy. These patients do not have neuronal antibodies detected, and the context is nonparaneoplastic.

II.28. **Answer a.**
Patients with collapsin-response mediator protein 5–immunoglobulin G antibody are typically smokers with small cell lung carcinoma but are poorly responsive to immunotherapy and have a poor neurologic and cancer prognosis. Purkinje cell cytoplasmic antibody type 1 is a biomarker of breast or gynecologic adenocarcinoma in women with paraneoplastic cerebellar ataxia.

II.29. **Answer c.**
Although glycine receptor α1 subunit–immunoglobulin G may be detected in patients with diverse neurologic problems, its clinical significance is unclear outside the context of the stiff-person syndrome spectrum (including classic forms, progressive encephalomyelitis with rigidity and myoclonus, and stiff-limb syndrome).

II.30. **Answer a.**
Recognized clinical autoimmune associations of glutamic acid decarboxylase 65-kDa isoform–immunoglobulin G antibody include central nervous system disorders (encephalitis, epilepsy, ataxia, stiff-person syndrome, chorea, and myelopathy) and certain nonneurologic autoimmune diseases (type 1 diabetes, autoimmune thyroid disease, and pernicious anemia).

II.31. **Answer d.**
Faciobrachial dystonic spells are most commonly a manifestation of leucine-rich, glioma-inactivated protein 1 autoimmunity. Progressive encephalomyelitis with rigidity and myoclonus (PERM) is considered a variant of stiff-person syndrome, characterized by central nervous system hyperexcitability with exaggerated startle, muscle rigidity, and painful spasms. Patients with PERM may also have ophthalmalgia, ptosis, dysphagia, dysarthria, autonomic dysfunction, seizures, and respiratory events.

II.32. **Answer c.**
Although glutamic acid decarboxylase 65-kDa isoform (GAD65) and dipeptidyl-peptidase-like protein-6 antibodies are associated with central nervous system hyperexcitability syndromes, the presence of glycine receptor α1 subunit–immunoglobulin G (IgG) is associated with a higher rate of response to immunosuppression compared with stiff-person syndrome spectrum disorders associated with GAD65-IgG alone. Antibodies targeting the N-methyl-D-aspartate receptor or leucine-rich, glioma-inactivated

protein 1 are not associated with progressive encephalomyelitis with rigidity and myoclonus.

II.33. Answer b.

The sensory abnormalities starting at a spinal cord level and extending into the saddle area are suggestive of transverse myelitis. Her examination is notable for symmetric weakness and upper motor neuron signs of hyperreflexia and positive Babinski sign. Areflexia is usual in neuropathies. Mononeuritis multiplex has an asymmetric distribution of symptoms and signs. Aseptic meningitis is predominated by pain and meningeal signs alone.

II.34. Answer c.

Antiphospholipid antibody is associated with chorea and venous thromboses, as well as recurrent spontaneous abortions. Aquaporin-4 antibody is associated with relapsing transverse myelitis and optic neuritis. Antiribosomal P antibody is associated with neuropsychiatric symptoms. Antinuclear antibody is a nonspecific autoimmune marker. N-methyl-D-aspartate receptor antibody is associated with autoimmune encephalitis.

II.35. Answer d.

Although spinal cord magnetic resonance imaging findings may be normal in approximately one-third of cases, the presence of a longitudinally extensive (3 or more contiguous vertebral segments), tract-specific, T2-hyperintense signal along the dorsal or lateral columns that enhances in a similar tract-specific pattern after gadolinium is suggestive of a paraneoplastic myelopathy. The absence of gadolinium enhancement is more consistent with vitamin B_{12} deficiency. Multiple, short, and peripherally located T2-hyperintense lesions are typically observed in multiple sclerosis.

II.36. Answer c.

Small cell lung carcinoma and breast adenocarcinoma are the most common oncologic accompaniments of paraneoplastic myelopathies. Collapsin-response mediator protein 5–immunoglobulin G (IgG) and amphiphysin-IgG are the most commonly detected neural autoantibodies. Teratoma is less frequently encountered with glial fibrillary acidic protein-IgG–associated myelopathy. Astrocytoma and ependymoma are causes of neoplastic (rather than paraneoplastic) myelopathies. Melanoma and prostate cancer can metastasize to spine but are seldom reported with paraneoplastic myelopathies.

II.37. Answer d.

Asymmetrical sensory loss and sensory ataxia are clinical features suggestive of dorsal root ganglion involvement. Distal paresthesia and numbness associated with sicca symptoms can also be neurologic complications of Sjögren syndrome. However, the neuropathy phenotype is more suggestive of symmetric sensory polyneuropathy.

II.38. Answer d.

In a study of 92 patients with Sjögren syndrome–associated neuropathy, patients with multiple mononeuropathy and cranial neuropathy showed the most favorable response to corticosteroid therapy. Only 18% of patients with sensory ataxic neuropathy or sensory ganglionopathy responded to corticosteroid treatment. The rates of favorable response to intravenous immunoglobulin therapy among patients with polyradiculoneuropathy, painful sensory neuropathy without sensory ataxia, and sensory ataxic neuropathy were 100%, 67%, and 23%, respectively.

II.39. Answer c.

Collapsin-response mediator protein 5 (CRMP5) antibodies have been associated with paraneoplastic myeloneuropathy. Patients with CRMP5–immunoglobulin G–associated myeloneuropathy syndromes typically have progressive, asymmetric, sensorimotor deficits in all limbs, often with severe neuropathic pain and myelopathic features (extensor plantar reflex, marked sensory ataxia secondary to dorsal column involvement, and bowel or bladder incontinence). Unexplained weight loss is another clue to a paraneoplastic cause.

II.40. Answer a.

Collapsin-response mediator protein 5 (CRMP5) antibodies are strongly associated with cancer. Small cell lung cancer and thymomas are the most common cancer associations. Ongoing surveillance is mandatory if cancer is not found during initial evaluation. Immunotherapies are usually given in combination with oncologic treatments, and some patients have clinical improvement and stabilization, but response is often partial. CRMP5–immunoglobulin G–associated polyradiculoneuropathies typically show axonal features on electrodiagnostic testing.

II.41. Answer b.

In the largest series of patients to date, if cognitive examination findings are available, abnormalities are detected, even in patients with primarily neuropathy. Small cell lung carcinoma is seen in the majority of affected patients. Most patients are without pain.

II.42. Answer a.

Paraneoplastic neuropathies have diverse presentations including classical sensory neuronopathy and other neuropathy forms. The key clinical clue is the subacute evolution of symptoms over days to weeks. Insidiously progressive neuropathies usually have a hereditary cause. Carpal tunnel syndrome and tarsal tunnel syndrome are focal disorders caused by nerve entrapment. Spinal stenosis is a nonparaneoplastic cause of radiculopathies.

II.43. Answer e.

Chronic inflammatory demyelinating polyradiculoneuropathy is one of the most common inflammatory neuropathies that usually causes distal and proximal weakness (polyradiculoneuropathy), imbalance, large fiber–predominant sensation loss on examination, and demyelinating features on nerve conduction studies. It is very rarely associated with malignancy and is a treatable neuropathy.

II.44. Answer d.

Severe autonomic dysfunction and dyspnea are very rarely encountered in chronic inflammatory demyelinating polyradiculoneuropathy. Severe dysautonomia suggests amyloidosis, Sjögren syndrome, sarcoidosis, or a paraneoplastic syndrome. In neuropathies, dyspnea can occur owing to neuromuscular respiratory weakness or concomitant cardiac and/or pulmonary involvement. When dyspnea occurs, it should raise the possibility of POEMS syndrome (*p*olyneuropathy, *o*rganomegaly, *e*ndocrinopathy, *M* component, *s*kin changes), sarcoidosis, amyloidosis, or a connective tissue disease.

II.45. Answer a.

Patients with contactin-associated protein 2–immunoglobulin G autoimmunity have an immunotherapy-responsive disorder that is frequently but not always associated with seizures, encephalopathy, and cognitive involvement. These are more common in persons with older age of onset. Both immunotherapy and membrane-stabilizing drugs can assist in control of pain.

II.46. Answer b.

The strongest cancer association with contactin-associated protein 2–immunoglobulin G (IgG) is thymoma, and that association has been highest in persons with both that autoantibody and coexisting leucine-rich, glioma-inactivated protein 1-IgG autoimmunity. There are no data indicating that it is more common in persons with pain, more aggressive cancer, or common hematologic cancers.

II.47. Answer b.

The findings are those of autoimmune autonomic ganglionopathy due to antibodies against the ganglionic-type nicotinic acetylcholine receptors containing the α3 subunit. The α1 subunits are present at the neuromuscular junction and are the target in myasthenia gravis. Muscarinic M3 receptor antibodies have been described in Sjögren syndrome but are unlikely to result in orthostatic hypotension. Antibodies against the auxiliary dipeptidyl-peptidase-like protein-6 subunit of the Kv4.2 channel have been associated with autonomic hyperactivity and diarrhea. There is no known L-type channel–associated autoimmunity affecting autonomic function.

II.48. Answer a.

Intestinal pseudo-obstruction may be the sole autonomic manifestation of a paraneoplastic disorder, typically in the setting of small cell lung carcinoma. The most commonly associated antibody is antineuronal nuclear antibody type 1 (anti-Hu). Classic neurologic accompaniments of the other antibodies include brainstem or limbic encephalitis (anti-Ma2), diverse central nervous system and peripheral nervous system manifestations (antiamphiphysin), cerebellar ataxia (anti-Yo), and brainstem encephalitis and opsoclonus-myoclonus syndrome (anti-Ri).

II.49. Answer e.

After exclusion of alternative diagnoses, patients with severe, refractory symptoms of autoimmune gastrointestinal dysmotility can be considered for a trial of immunosuppressive therapy, even if they are seronegative for related neural-specific antibodies. A favorable response to a 6- to 12-week trial, defined by marked improvement on objective testing, can support the diagnosis of an autoimmune process. Gastrointestinal dysmotility can be encountered in patients with Ehlers-Danlos syndrome (who also have hypermobile joints). Because Ehlers-Danlos syndrome is a hereditary, rather than autoimmune, disorder, an immunotherapy trial is not warranted.

II.50. Answer a.

Antineuronal nuclear antibody type 1 (anti-Hu) is associated with small cell carcinomas, pediatric neuroblastoma, or thymoma. Symptom onset is often acute or subacute. This typically responds poorly to immunotherapy. Dipeptidyl-peptidase-like protein-6 (DPPX)–immunoglobulin G (IgG) is frequently associated with autoimmune gastrointestinal dysmotility (AGID) and gastrointestinal tract symptoms. DPPX-IgG is not typically associated with small cell carcinoma but can be associated with hematologic cancers such as B-cell lymphomas. *N*-methyl-D-aspartate receptor (NMDAR)-IgG, leucine-rich, glioma-inactivated protein 1 (LGI1)-IgG, and contactin-associated protein 2 (CASPR2)-IgG autoantibodies can be associated with autoimmune dysautonomia but less frequently manifest with AGID. These are also not typically paraneoplastic or associated with small cell carcinoma. When associated with neoplasm, NMDAR-IgG is more commonly associated with an ovarian teratoma; LGI1-IgG and CASPR2-IgG are associated with thymoma.

II.51. Answer b.

Patients with thymoma are acetylcholine receptor (AChR) binding antibody positive but are usually also positive for a profile of other thymoma antigen–directed immunoglobulin Gs, such as modulating AChR and striational antibodies. Muscle-specific tyrosine kinase and low-density lipoprotein receptor-related protein 4 antibodies are not known to have neoplastic accompaniments.

II.52. Answer c.

Rituximab is favored by many clinicians, but this preference is based on class IV evidence. In the absence of randomized clinical trial evidence, mycophenolate mofetil, azathioprine, and cyclosporine are reasonable considerations for long-term immunotherapy in muscle-specific tyrosine kinase–immunoglobulin G myasthenia gravis.

II.53. Answer d.

The most common cancer found in patients with Lambert-Eaton myasthenic syndrome is small cell lung carcinoma. Patients with negative findings on conventional computed tomography (CT) should undergo positron emission tomography/CT, especially if they have known risk factors for cancer.

II.54. Answer a.

Antibodies to the voltage-gated calcium channel, particularly of P/Q type, are commonly detected in the serum of patients with Lambert-Eaton myasthenic syndrome. Coexistence of SOX1 (sex-determining region Y-box 1)–immunoglobulin G in paraneoplastic cases increases the likelihood of small cell carcinoma.

II.55. Answer a.

Anti–signal recognition particle and anti–3-hydroxy-3-methylglutaryl–coenzyme A reductase (HMGCR) antibodies are identified in 60% of patients with necrotizing autoimmune myopathy (NAM). Anti-HMGCR antibody–associated NAM can occur with or without prior statin exposure. Anti–transcription intermediary factor 1-γ antibodies are highly specific to dermatomyositis, not NAM. In NAM, muscle biopsy shows various stages of necrotic fibers with no or minimal inflammatory exudate. Perifascicular atrophy is the canonical finding of dermatomyositis, not NAM. Rimmed vacuoles and congophilic deposits are not pathologic hallmarks of NAM but can be observed in inclusion body myositis and certain hereditary myopathies. For patients with NAM taking statins, discontinuation of the statin alone does not halt the progression of weakness, and aggressive immunomodulatory therapy is necessary.

II.56. Answer c.

Although signal recognition particle antibody–mediated necrotizing autoimmune myopathy (NAM) has reportedly occurred as a paraneoplastic disorder, the incidence of cancer in this subset of NAM is not different than that observed in the general population. In contrast, patients with seronegative and 3-hydroxy-3-methylglutaryl–coenzyme A reductase antibody–mediated NAM have a higher incidence of cancer than in the general population.

II.57. Answer b.

Dermatomyositis is an idiopathic inflammatory myopathy characterized by perifascicular pathologic findings, including perifascicular muscle atrophy, necrosis, and regeneration and sarcolemmal overexpression of myxovirus resistance protein A. The inflammatory reaction is perivascular.

II.58. Answer a.

Nuclear matrix protein 2 (NXP-2) autoantibodies are considered specific to dermatomyositis. Compared with other dermatomyositis-specific antibodies, anti-NXP-2 and anti–transcriptional intermediary factor-1γ antibodies are associated with a higher risk of cancer.

II.59. Answer d.

Neurologic complications have been described with all immune checkpoint inhibitors (ICIs). In any cancer patient with a neurologic complication, the medication list should be checked for an ICI.

II.60. Answer b.

This presentation is compatible with immune checkpoint inhibitor (ICI)-related myopathy that can be associated with cardiomyopathy. The ICI treatment should be discontinued because the patient has generalized weakness and should be withheld at least until potential cardiac involvement is excluded. First-line treatment would be corticosteroids; in cases of lack of response or aggravation, plasma exchange or intravenous immunoglobulin could be considered.

II.61. Answer e.

The occurrence of striational antibodies is highest in patients with thymoma with a diagnosis of myasthenia gravis. This occurs in ≈75% of such cases. In contrast, less than 30% of those with thymoma without myasthenia gravis have striational antibodies at any titer. Striational antibodies are not known to have an association with congenital myasthenic syndrome or necrotizing autoimmune myopathy. Lambert-Eaton myasthenic syndrome has only a weak association with striational antibodies (≈5% of cases are positive).

II.62. Answer c.

Testing for an antibody with low clinical specificity outside of the correct clinical context will result in low positive predictive value. Clinical sensitivity and specificity are not affected by the testing population. Clinical specificity has minimal effect on the negative predictive value.

SECTION II (CASES 22-52) SUGGESTED READING

Adamus G, Chew EY, Ferris FL, Klein ML. Prevalence of anti-retinal autoantibodies in different stages of age-related macular degeneration. BMC Ophthalmol. 2014 Dec 8;14:154.

The American College of Rheumatology nomenclature and case definitions for neuropsychiatric lupus syndromes. Arthritis Rheum. 1999 Apr;42(4):599–608.

Armangue T, Spatola M, Vlagea A, Mattozzi S, Carceles-Cordon M, Martinez-Heras E, et al; Spanish Herpes Simplex Encephalitis Study Group. Frequency, symptoms, risk factors, and outcomes of autoimmune encephalitis after herpes simplex encephalitis: a prospective observational study and retrospective analysis. Lancet Neurol. 2018 Sep;17(9):760-72. Epub 2018 Jul 23.

Aurangzeb S, Symmonds M, Knight RK, Kennett R, Wehner T, Irani SR. LGI1-antibody encephalitis is characterised by frequent, multifocal clinical and subclinical seizures. Seizure. 2017 Aug;50:14-7. Epub 2017 May 30.

Bhat A, Naguwa S, Cheema G, Gershwin ME. The epidemiology of transverse myelitis. Autoimmun Rev. 2010 Mar;9(5):A395-9. Epub 2009 Dec 24.

Bortoluzzi A, Scire CA, Bombardieri S, Caniatti L, Conti F, De Vita S, et al; Study Group on Neuropsychiatric Systemic Lupus Erythematosus of the Italian Society of Rheumatology. Development and validation of a new algorithm for attribution of neuropsychiatric events in systemic lupus erythematosus. Rheumatology (Oxford). 2015 May;54(5):891-8. Epub 2014 Oct 21.

Brune AJ, Gold DR. Acute visual disorders: what should the neurologist know? Semin Neurol. 2019 Feb;39(1):53-60. Epub 2019 Feb 11.

Camdessanche JP, Jousserand G, Ferraud K, Vial C, Petiot P, Honnorat J, et al. The pattern and diagnostic criteria of sensory neuronopathy: a case-control study. Brain. 2009 Jul;132(Pt 7):1723-33. Epub 2009 Jun 8.

Castillo P, Woodruff B, Caselli R, Vernino S, Lucchinetti C, Swanson J, et al. Steroid-responsive encephalopathy associated with autoimmune thyroiditis. Arch Neurol. 2006 Feb;63(2):197–202.

Chan KH, Lachance DH, Harper CM, Lennon VA. Frequency of seronegativity in adult-acquired generalized myasthenia gravis. Muscle Nerve. 2007 Nov;36(5):651–8.

Choi Decroos E, Hobson-Webb LD, Juel VC, Massey JM, Sanders DB. Do acetylcholine receptor and striated muscle antibodies predict the presence of thymoma in patients with myasthenia gravis? Muscle Nerve. 2014 Jan;49(1):30-4. Epub 2013 Jul 17.

Clardy SL, Lennon VA, Dalmau J, Pittock SJ, Jones HR Jr, Renaud DL, et al. Childhood onset of stiff-man syndrome. JAMA Neurol. 2013 Dec;70(12):1531–6.

Cohen DA, Bhatti MT, Pulido JS, Lennon VA, Dubey D, Flanagan EP, et al. Collapsin response-mediator protein 5-associated retinitis, vitritis, and optic disc edema. Ophthalmology. 2020 Feb;127(2):221-9. Epub 2019 Sep 20.

Crisp SJ, Balint B, Vincent A. Redefining progressive encephalomyelitis with rigidity and myoclonus after the discovery of antibodies to glycine receptors. Curr Opin Neurol. 2017 Jun;30(3):310–6.

Cross SA, Salomao DR, Parisi JE, Kryzer TJ, Bradley EA, Mines JA, et al. Paraneoplastic autoimmune optic neuritis with retinitis defined by CRMP-5-IgG. Ann Neurol. 2003 Jul;54(1):38–50.

Cutsforth-Gregory JK, McKeon A, Coon EA, Sletten DM, Suarez M, Sandroni P, et al. Ganglionic antibody level as a predictor of severity of autonomic failure. Mayo Clin Proc. 2018 Oct;93(10):1440-7. Epub 2018 Aug 28.

Dalmau J, Armangue T, Planaguma J, Radosevic M, Mannara F, Leypoldt F, et al. An update on anti-NMDA receptor encephalitis for neurologists and psychiatrists: mechanisms and models. Lancet Neurol. 2019 Nov;18(11):1045-57. Epub 2019 Jul 17.

Dalmau J, Graus F. Antibody-mediated encephalitis. N Engl J Med. 2018 Mar 1;378(9):840–51.

Dubey D, Britton J, McKeon A, Gadoth A, Zekeridou A, Lopez Chiriboga SA, et al. Randomized placebo-controlled trial of intravenous immunoglobulin in autoimmune LGI1/CASPR2 epilepsy. Ann Neurol. 2020 Feb;87(2):313-23. Epub 2019 Dec 14.

Dubey D, Hinson SR, Jolliffe EA, Zekeridou A, Flanagan EP, Pittock SJ, et al. Autoimmune GFAP astrocytopathy: prospective evaluation of 90 patients in 1 year. J Neuroimmunol. 2018 Aug 15;321:157-63. Epub 2018 Apr 27.

Dubey D, Lennon VA, Gadoth A, Pittock SJ, Flanagan EP, Schmeling JE, et al. Autoimmune CRMP5 neuropathy phenotype and outcome defined from 105 cases. Neurology. 2018 Jan 9;90(2):e103-10. Epub 2017 Dec 8.

Dubey D, Wilson MR, Clarkson B, Giannini C, Gandhi M, Cheville J, et al. Expanded clinical phenotype, oncological associations, and immunopathologic insights of paraneoplastic kelch-like protein-11 encephalitis. JAMA Neurol. 2020 Aug 3;77(11):1-10. Epub ahead of print.

Dyck PJB, Tracy JA. History, diagnosis, and management of chronic inflammatory demyelinating polyradiculoneuropathy. Mayo Clin Proc. 2018 Jun;93(6):777–93.

Escudero D, Guasp M, Arino H, Gaig C, Martinez-Hernandez E, Dalmau J, et al. Antibody-associated CNS syndromes without signs of inflammation in the elderly. Neurology. 2017 Oct 3;89(14):1471-5. Epub 2017 Sep 6.

Fang B, McKeon A, Hinson SR, Kryzer TJ, Pittock SJ, Aksamit AJ, et al. Autoimmune glial fibrillary acidic protein astrocytopathy: a novel meningoencephalomyelitis. JAMA Neurol. 2016 Nov 1;73(11):1297–1307.

Flanagan EP, Drubach DA, Boeve BF. Autoimmune dementia and encephalopathy. Handb Clin Neurol. 2016;133:247–67.

Flanagan EP, Hinson SR, Lennon VA, Fang B, Aksamit AJ, Morris PP, et al. Glial fibrillary acidic protein immunoglobulin G as biomarker of autoimmune astrocytopathy: analysis of 102 patients. Ann Neurol. 2017 Feb;81(2):298–309.

Flanagan EP, McKeon A, Lennon VA, Boeve BF, Trenerry MR, Tan KM, et al. Autoimmune dementia: clinical course and predictors of immunotherapy response. Mayo Clin Proc. 2010 Oct;85(10):881–97.

Flanagan EP, McKeon A, Lennon VA, Kearns J, Weinshenker BG, Krecke KN, et al. Paraneoplastic isolated myelopathy: clinical course and neuroimaging clues. Neurology 2011 Jun 14;76:2089–95.

Flanagan EP, Saito YA, Lennon VA, McKeon A, Fealey RD, Szarka LA, et al. Immunotherapy trial as diagnostic test in evaluating patients with presumed autoimmune gastrointestinal dysmotility. Neurogastroenterol Motil. 2014 Sep;26(9):1285-97. Epub 2014 Jul 20.

Fox AR, Gordon LK, Heckenlively JR, Davis JL, Goldstein DA, Lowder CY, et al. Consensus on the diagnosis and management of nonparaneoplastic autoimmune retinopathy using a modified delphi approach. Am J Ophthalmol. 2016 Aug;168:183-90. Epub 2016 May 20.

Gadoth A, Pittock SJ, Dubey D, McKeon A, Britton JW, Schmeling JE, et al. Expanded phenotypes and outcomes among 256 LGI1/CASPR2-IgG-positive patients. Ann Neurol. 2017 Jul;82(1):79–92.

Gaig C, Graus F, Compta Y, Hogl B, Bataller L, Bruggemann N, et al. Clinical manifestations of the anti-IgLON5 disease. Neurology. 2017 May 2;88(18):1736-43. Epub 2017 Apr 5.

Gelpi E, Hoftberger R, Graus F, Ling H, Holton JL, Dawson T, et al. Neuropathological criteria of anti-IgLON5-related tauopathy. Acta Neuropathol. 2016 Oct;132(4):531-43. Epub 2016 Jun 29.

Gibbons CH, Freeman R. Antibody titers predict clinical features of autoimmune autonomic ganglionopathy. Auton Neurosci. 2009 Mar 12;146(1-2):8-12. Epub 2009 Jan 13.

Gilhus NE, Skeie GO, Romi F, Lazaridis K, Zisimopoulou P, Tzartos S. Myasthenia gravis: autoantibody characteristics and their implications for therapy. Nat Rev Neurol. 2016 May;12(5):259-68. Epub 2016 Apr 22.

Goodman BP. Diagnostic approach to myeloneuropathy. Continuum (Minneap Minn). 2011 Aug;17(4):744–60.

Grange L, Dalal M, Nussenblatt RB, Sen HN. Autoimmune retinopathy. Am J Ophthalmol. 2014 Feb;157(2):266-72.e1. Epub 2013 Sep 29.

Griffin JW, Cornblath DR, Alexander E, Campbell J, Low PA, Bird S, et al. Ataxic sensory neuropathy and dorsal root ganglionitis associated with Sjögren's syndrome. Ann Neurol. 1990 Mar;27(3):304–15.

Harper CM, Lennon VA. Lambert-Eaton syndrome. In: Kaminshi H, Kusner L, editors. Myasthenia gravis and related disorders, 3rd ed. New York (NY): Humana Press, Cham/Springer; c2018. p. 221-37. (Current Clinical Neurology book series).

Hinson SR, Lopez-Chiriboga AS, Bower JH, Matsumoto JY, Hassan A, Basal E, et al. Glycine receptor modulating antibody predicting treatable stiff-person spectrum disorders. Neurol Neuroimmunol Neuroinflamm. 2018 Jan 23;5(2):e438.

Hoftberger R, van Sonderen A, Leypoldt F, Houghton D, Geschwind M, Gelfand J, et al. Encephalitis and AMPA receptor antibodies: novel findings in a case series of 22 patients. Neurology. 2015 Jun 16;84(24):2403-12. Epub 2015 May 15.

Honorat JA, Komorowski L, Josephs KA, Fechner K, St Louis EK, Hinson SR, et al. IgLON5 antibody: neurological accompaniments and outcomes in 20 patients. Neurol Neuroimmunol Neuroinflamm. 2017 Jul 18;4(5):e385.

Honorat JA, McKeon A. Autoimmune movement disorders: a clinical and laboratory approach. Curr Neurol Neurosci Rep. 2017 Jan;17(1):4.

Irani SR, Gelfand JM, Bettcher BM, Singhal NS, Geschwind MD. Effect of rituximab in patients with leucine-rich, glioma-inactivated 1 antibody-associated encephalopathy. JAMA Neurol. 2014 Jul 1;71(7):896–900.

Jones AL, Flanagan EP, Pittock SJ, Mandrekar JN, Eggers SD, Ahlskog JE, et al. Responses to and outcomes of treatment of autoimmune cerebellar ataxia in adults. JAMA Neurol. 2015 Nov;72(11):1304–12.

Kassardjian CD, Lennon VA, Alfugham NB, Mahler M, Milone M. Clinical features and treatment outcomes of necrotizing autoimmune myopathy. JAMA Neurol. 2015 Sep;72(9):996–1003.

Klein CJ. Autoimmune-mediated peripheral neuropathies and autoimmune pain. Handb Clin Neurol. 2016;133:417–46.

Klein CJ, Lennon VA, Aston PA, McKeon A, Pittock SJ. Chronic pain as a manifestation of potassium channel-complex autoimmunity. Neurology. 2012 Sep 11;79(11):1136-44. Epub 2012 Aug 15.

Kunchok A, Zekeridou A, McKeon A. Autoimmune glial fibrillary acidic protein astrocytopathy. Curr Opin Neurol. 2019 Jun;32(3):452-8

Lopez-Chiriboga AS, Komorowski L, Kumpfel T, Probst C, Hinson SR, Pittock SJ, et al. Metabotropic glutamate receptor type 1 autoimmunity: clinical features and treatment outcomes. Neurology. 2016 Mar 15;86(11):1009-13. Epub 2016 Feb 17.

Lucchinetti CF, Kimmel DW, Lennon VA. Paraneoplastic and oncologic profiles of patients seropositive for type 1 antineuronal nuclear autoantibodies. Neurology. 1998 Mar;50(3):652–7.

Makarious D, Horwood K, Coward JIG. Myasthenia gravis: an emerging toxicity of immune checkpoint inhibitors. Eur J Cancer. 2017 Sep;82:128-36. Epub 2017 Jun 27.

Mammen AL, Allenbach Y, Stenzel W, Benveniste O; ENMC 239th Workshop Study Group. 239th ENMC International Workshop: Classification of Dermatomyositis, Amsterdam, the Netherlands, 14-16 December 2018. Neuromuscul Disord. 2020 Jan;30(1):70-92. Epub 2019 Oct 25.

Mammen AL. Statin-associated autoimmune myopathy. N Engl J Med. 2016 Feb 18;374(7):664–9.

Mandel-Brehm C, Dubey D, Kryzer TJ, O'Donovan BD, Tran B, Vazquez SE, et al. Kelch-like protein 11 antibodies in seminoma-associated paraneoplastic encephalitis. N Engl J Med. 2019 Jul 4;381(1):47–54.

Mariampillai K, Granger B, Amelin D, Guiguet M, Hachulla E, Maurier F, et al. Development of a new classification system for idiopathic inflammatory myopathies based on clinical manifestations and myositis-specific autoantibodies. JAMA Neurol. 2018 Dec 1;75(12):1528–37.

Mathey EK, Park SB, Hughes RA, Pollard JD, Armati PJ, Barnett MH, et al. Chronic inflammatory demyelinating polyradiculoneuropathy: from pathology to phenotype. J Neurol Neurosurg Psychiatry. 2015 Sep;86(9):973-85. Epub 2015 Feb 12.

McKeon A. Autoimmune encephalopathies and dementias. Continuum (Minneap Minn). 2016 Apr;22(2, Dementia):538–58.

McKeon A. Immunotherapeutics for autoimmune encephalopathies and dementias. Curr Treat Options Neurol. 2013 Dec;15(6):723–37.

McKeon A, Benarroch EE. Autoimmune autonomic disorders. Handb Clin Neurol. 2016;133:405–16.

McKeon A, Lennon VA, LaChance DH, Klein CJ, Pittock SJ. Striational antibodies in a paraneoplastic context. Muscle Nerve. 2013 Apr;47(4):585-7. Epub 2013 Mar 5.

McKeon A, Lennon VA, Pittock SJ, Kryzer TJ, Murray J. The neurologic significance of celiac disease biomarkers. Neurology. 2014 Nov 11;83(20):1789-96. Epub 2014 Sep 26.

McKeon A, Robinson MT, McEvoy KM, Matsumoto JY, Lennon VA, Ahlskog JE, et al. Stiff-man syndrome and variants: clinical course, treatments, and outcomes. Arch Neurol. 2012 Feb;69(2):230–8.

Milone M. Diagnosis and management of immune-mediated myopathies. Mayo Clin Proc. 2017 May;92(5):826–37.

Mittal MK, Rabinstein AA, Hocker SE, Pittock SJ, Wijdicks EF, McKeon A. Autoimmune encephalitis in the ICU: analysis of phenotypes, serologic findings, and outcomes. Neurocrit Care. 2016 Apr;24(2):240–50.

Mori K, Iijima M, Koike H, Hattori N, Tanaka F, Watanabe H, et al. The wide spectrum of clinical manifestations in Sjögren's syndrome-associated neuropathy. Brain. 2005 Nov;128(Pt 11):2518-34. Epub 2005 Jul 27.

Moss HE, Liu GT, Dalmau J. Glazed (vision) and confused. Surv Ophthalmol. 2010 Mar-Apr;55(2):169-73. Epub 2009 Oct 4.

Okuno H, Yahata Y, Tanaka-Taya K, Arai S, Satoh H, Morino S, et al. Characteristics and outcomes of influenza-associated encephalopathy cases among children and adults in Japan, 2010-2015. Clin Infect Dis. 2018 Jun 1;66(12):1831–7.

O'Toole O, Lennon VA, Ahlskog JE, Matsumoto JY, Pittock SJ, Bower J, et al. Autoimmune chorea in adults. Neurology. 2013 Mar 19;80(12):1133-44. Epub 2013 Feb 20.

Pittock SJ, Lennon VA, de Seze J, Vermersch P, Homburger HA, Wingerchuk DM, et al. Neuromyelitis optica and non organ-specific autoimmunity. Arch Neurol. 2008 Jan;65(1):78–83.

Postuma RB, Iranzo A, Hu M, Hogl B, Boeve BF, Manni R, et al. Risk and predictors of dementia and parkinsonism in idiopathic REM sleep behaviour disorder: a multicentre study. Brain. 2019 Mar 1;142(3):744–59.

Rahimy E, Sarraf D. Paraneoplastic and non-paraneoplastic retinopathy and optic neuropathy: evaluation and management. Surv Ophthalmol. 2013 Sep-Oct;58(5):430–58.

Sabater L, Gaig C, Gelpi E, Bataller L, Lewerenz J, Torres-Vega E, et al. A novel non-rapid-eye movement and rapid-eye-movement parasomnia with sleep breathing disorder associated with antibodies to IgLON5: a case series, characterisation of the antigen, and postmortem study. Lancet Neurol. 2014 Jun;13(6):575-86. Epub 2014 Apr 3. Erratum in: Lancet Neurol. 2015 Jan;14(1):28.

Sanders DB, Wolfe GI, Benatar M, Evoli A, Gilhus NE, Illa I, et al. International consensus guidance for management of myasthenia gravis: executive summary. Neurology. 2016 Jul 26;87(4):419-25. Epub 2016 Jun 29.

Sechi E, Markovic SN, McKeon A, Dubey D, Liewluck T, Lennon VA, et al. Neurologic autoimmunity and immune checkpoint inhibitors: autoantibody profiles and outcomes. Neurology. 2020 Oct 27;95(17):e2442-52. Epub 2020 Aug 13.

Sheikh SI, Amato AA. The dorsal root ganglion under attack: the acquired sensory ganglionopathies. Pract Neurol. 2010 Dec;10(6):326–34.

Skjei KL, Lennon VA, Kuntz NL. Muscle specific kinase autoimmune myasthenia gravis in children: a case series. Neuromuscul Disord. 2013 Nov;23(11):874-82. Epub 2013 Aug 7.

St Louis EK, Boeve BF. REM sleep behavior disorder: diagnosis, clinical implications, and future directions. Mayo Clin Proc. 2017 Nov;92(11):1723-36. Epub 2017 Nov 1.

Thompson J, Bi M, Murchison AG, Makuch M, Bien CG, Chu K, et al; Faciobrachial Dystonic Seizures Study Group. The importance of early immunotherapy in patients with faciobrachial dystonic seizures. Brain. 2018 Feb 1;141(2):348–56.

Titulaer MJ, Lang B, Verschuuren JJ. Lambert-Eaton myasthenic syndrome: from clinical characteristics to therapeutic strategies. Lancet Neurol. 2011 Dec;10(12):1098–107.

Titulaer MJ, McCracken L, Gabilondo I, Armangue T, Glaser C, Iizuka T, et al. Treatment and prognostic factors for long-term outcome in patients with anti-NMDA receptor encephalitis: an observational cohort study. Lancet Neurol. 2013 Feb;12(2):157-65. Epub 2013 Jan 3.

Tobin WO, Lennon VA, Komorowski L, Probst C, Clardy SL, Aksamit AJ, et al. DPPX potassium channel antibody: frequency, clinical accompaniments, and outcomes in 20 patients. Neurology. 2014 Nov 11;83(20):1797-803. Epub 2014 Oct 15.

Vernino S, Low PA, Fealey RD, Stewart JD, Farrugia G, Lennon VA. Autoantibodies to ganglionic acetylcholine receptors in autoimmune autonomic neuropathies. N Engl J Med. 2000 Sep 21;343(12):847–55.

Winston N, Vernino S. Autoimmune autonomic ganglionopathy. Front Neurol Neurosci. 2009;26:85-93. Epub 2009 Apr 6.

Wolfe GI, Kaminski HJ, Aban IB, Minisman G, Kuo HC, Marx A, et al; MGTX Study Group. Randomized trial of thymectomy in myasthenia gravis. N Engl J Med. 2016 Aug 11;375(6):511-22. Erratum in: N Engl J Med. 2017 May 25;376(21):2097. [Dosage error in article text].

Xu M, Bennett DLH, Querol LA, Wu LJ, Irani SR, Watson JC, et al. Pain and the immune system: emerging concepts of IgG-mediated autoimmune pain and immunotherapies. J Neurol Neurosurg Psychiatry. 2020 Feb;91(2):177-88. Epub 2018 Sep 17.

Zalewski NL, Flanagan EP. Autoimmune and paraneoplastic myelopathies. Semin Neurol. 2018 Jun;38(3):278-89. Epub 2018 Jul 16.

Zekeridou A, Lennon VA. Neurologic autoimmunity in the era of checkpoint inhibitor cancer immunotherapy. Mayo Clin Proc. 2019 Sep;94(9):1865-78. Epub 2019 Jul 26.

Section III

OTHER INFLAMMATORY CNS DISORDERS AND NEUROIMMUNOLOGIC MIMICS QUESTIONS AND ANSWERS

SECTION III (CASES 53-83) QUESTIONS

MULTIPLE CHOICE (CHOOSE THE BEST ANSWER)

III.1. Neurosarcoidosis most commonly causes clinical symptoms by involving which cranial nerve?
   a. Optic (CNII)
   b. Oculomotor (CNIII)
   c. Trochlear (CNIV)
   d. Abducens (CNVI)
   e. Facial (CNVII)

III.2. What is the best treatment for newly diagnosed sarcoid optic neuropathy?
   a. High-dose oral corticosteroids for 5 days
   b. High-dose intravenous corticosteroids for 5 days
   c. Intermittent intravenous corticosteroids
   d. High-dose intravenous corticosteroids for 5 days, followed by high-dose oral corticosteroids for 3 months, followed by a slow taper
   e. Plasma exchange

III.3. Which of the following is *not* a typical sign/symptom of sarcoid optic neuropathy?
   a. Decreased color vision over months
   b. Sudden total loss of vision in 1 eye
   c. Decreased visual acuity over weeks
   d. Optic disc edema on examination
   e. Afferent pupillary defect on examination

III.4. In which of the following anatomical sites are lesions commonly seen in patients with Susac syndrome?
   a. Periaqueductal gray
   b. Septum pellucidum
   c. Corpus callosum
   d. Thalamus
   e. Visual cortex

III.5. What is the proposed pathomechanism of Susac syndrome?
   a. Inflammatory demyelination
   b. Autoimmune endotheliopathy
   c. Thromboembolism
   d. Infectious vasculitis
   e. Mitochondrial dysfunction

III.6. Which of the following is *least* helpful in distinguishing a leukodystrophy from multiple sclerosis?
   a. Subcortical U-fiber sparing
   b. Tract-specific signal abnormality in the spinal cord
   c. Highly symmetric cerebral white matter abnormalities
   d. White matter lesions involving the corpus callosum
   e. Presence of demyelinating peripheral neuropathy

III.7. Which of the following is *not* a major magnetic resonance imaging diagnostic criterion for LBSL (leukoencephalopathy with brainstem and spinal cord involvement and lactate elevation)?
   a. Signal abnormalities in the cerebral white matter that relatively spare the U fibers
   b. Signal abnormalities in the dorsal columns and lateral corticospinal tracts of the spinal cord
   c. Signal abnormalities in the pyramids of the medulla oblongata
   d. Increased lactate levels of abnormal cerebral white matter on magnetic resonance spectroscopy

III.8. Which genetic abnormality is found in hereditary forms of diffuse leukoencephalopathy with axonal spheroids?
   a. *NOTCH3* sequence variation
   b. Lamin B1 gene duplication
   c. *C9ORF72* repeat expansion
   d. Colony-stimulating factor 1 receptor sequence variation
   e. CAG trinucleotide expansion

III.9. When magnetic resonance imaging diffusion restriction is identified in diffuse leukoencephalopathy with axonal spheroids, where is it found?
   a. Subcortical white matter
   b. Cortical ribbon
   c. Cervical spinal cord
   d. Thoracic spinal cord
   e. Basal ganglia

III.10. A patient receiving rituximab for diffuse large B-cell lymphoma seeks care for 3 days of headache, malaise, and fever. She has seizures while in the emergency department. Cerebrospinal fluid (CSF) analysis shows a mildly increased protein concentration and 126 total nucleated cells/μL with 42% polymorphonuclear cells. Magnetic resonance imaging shows asymmetric T2 hyperintensities in the thalamus and basal ganglia. West Nile virus (WNV) is strongly suspected as the cause. Which statement is most accurate regarding WNV testing?

a. CSF polymerase chain reaction (PCR) is the most sensitive test for WNV

b. Serum and CSF serologic studies are sufficient in this setting

c. CSF viral culture is most useful in this setting

d. WNV serologic and PCR studies should be obtained together because serology may be falsely negative in the setting of rituximab therapy

e. CSF WNV immunoglobulin G positivity is diagnostic

III.11. A 72-year-old man is brought to the emergency department for confusion. He is noted to be febrile, encephalopathic, and aphasic. While undergoing computed tomography, he has a witnessed focal seizure with right arm tonic-clonic jerking followed by secondary generalization. Cerebrospinal fluid analysis shows a protein concentration of 123 mg/dL, 120 total nucleated cells/μL (mostly lymphocytes), and normal glucose value. He is started on broad-spectrum antibiotics and acyclovir. The next morning he continues to spike fevers and remains somnolent and poorly communicative. Magnetic resonance imaging (MRI) of the head shows fluid-attenuated inversion recovery signal change and swelling in his left greater than right mesiotemporal and orbitofrontal regions. Polymerase chain reaction (PCR) testing for herpes simplex virus (HSV) is negative. What is the best next step?

a. Discontinue acyclovir because the patient does not have HSV encephalitis

b. Continue acyclovir and repeat cerebrospinal fluid (CSF) PCR for HSV

c. Initiate ganciclovir for suspected human herpesvirus-6 encephalitis

d. Initiate intravenous immunoglobulin for suspected autoimmune encephalitis

e. Obtain continued electroencephalography because the changes on MRI likely reflect ongoing nonconvulsive seizure activity

III.12. Typical clinical features of MELAS syndrome include:

a. Mitochondrial inheritance, encephalopathy, lactic acidosis, and tension headaches

b. Mitochondrial inheritance, encephalopathy, lactic acidosis, and stroke-like episodes

c. Paternal inheritance, encephalopathy, lactic acidosis, and stroke-like episodes

d. X-linked inheritance, encephalopathy, lactic acidosis, and stroke-like episodes

e. X-linked inheritance, lactic acidosis, and migraine headaches

III.13. Typical central nervous system magnetic resonance imaging findings in mitochondrial disorders include:

a. Mesial temporal abnormalities

b. Corpus callosal lesions

c. Spinal cord lesions

d. Large cortical and juxtacortical neocortical findings that may come and go

e. Small cortical and juxtacortical neocortical findings, with subsequent atrophy

III.14. Which of the following tests has the highest sensitivity and specificity for sporadic Creutzfeldt-Jakob disease?

a. Periodic sharp wave complexes on electroencephalography

b. Positive real-time quaking-induced conversion findings in cerebrospinal fluid (CSF)

c. Increased 14-3-3 protein level in CSF

d. Cortical ribbon sign on magnetic resonance imaging

e. Increased neuron-specific enolase level in CSF

III.15. Which of the following magnetic resonance imaging findings has the highest sensitivity and specificity for sporadic Creutzfeldt-Jakob disease?

a. Increased cortical ribbon and deep nuclear signal on diffusion-weighted imaging

b. Cortical ribbon sign

c. Increased cortical ribbon and deep nuclear signal on T2/fluid-attenuated inversion recovery imaging

d. Caudate head enhancement, T1, post gadolinium

e. Hockey stick sign

III.16. Autoimmune central nervous system disorders usually present with onset that is:

a. Hyperacute (over seconds to minutes)

b. Acute (over hours to days)

c. Subacute (over days to weeks)

d. Chronic (over months)

e. Insidiously progressive (over years)

III.17. Which of the following findings on head magnetic resonance imaging may help identify ischemic stroke?

a. Bright on diffusion-weighted imaging (DWI) only

b. Bright on DWI, bright on apparent diffusion coefficient (ADC)

c. Dark on DWI, dark on ADC

d. Bright on DWI, dark on ADC

e. Dark on DWI, bright on ADC

III.18. Which of the following cerebrospinal fluid (CSF) findings may be suggestive of primary angiitis of the central nervous system?

a. Low glucose value

b. Neutrophilic pleocytosis

c. Oligoclonal bands

d. Lymphocytic pleocytosis

e. Increased CSF pressure

III.19. Which is the standard induction treatment for primary angiitis of the central nervous system?

a. Thrombolysis and blood pressure control

b. Intravenous immunoglobulin

c. Glucocorticoids and cyclophosphamide

d. Azathioprine

e. Methotrexate

III.20. An older woman with cognitive dysfunction and lobar intracerebral hemorrhage underwent a brain biopsy that showed a vasculitic, transmural, granulomatous infiltrate of blood vessels containing extensive

amyloid-β peptide deposition. Which of the following is consistent with these findings?
   a. Cerebral amyloid angiopathy (CAA)
   b. CAA-related inflammation
   c. Amyloid-β-related angiitis
   d. Central nervous system vasculitis
   e. Susac syndrome

III.21. Which of the following can be an initial manifestation of amyloid-β-related angiitis?
   a. Seizures
   b. Optic neuritis
   c. Neuropathy
   d. Parkinsonism
   e. Depression

III.22. Which of the following extra-axial sites is most likely to be involved by lymphoma in a patient with primary central nervous system lymphoma?
   a. Vitreous
   b. Cerebrospinal fluid
   c. Bone marrow
   d. Mediastinal lymph nodes
   e. Liver

III.23. In an otherwise healthy patient with pathologically confirmed primary central nervous system lymphoma, which of the following is most appropriate as first-line therapy?
   a. Methotrexate
   b. Whole-brain radiotherapy
   c. Intrathecal rituximab
   d. Hematopoietic stem cell transplant
   e. Chimeric antigen receptor T-cell therapy

III.24. A 66-year-old man has encephalopathy, seizures, and weight loss. Careful evaluations show no lymphadenopathy or skin lesions but increased lactate dehydrogenase level and pancytopenia. Magnetic resonance imaging shows patchy T2 hyperintensities throughout the brain and spinal cord. Computed tomography of the chest, abdomen, and pelvis is normal. Bone marrow biopsy shows decreased cellularity but no malignant cells. Intravascular lymphoma is suspected. Which of the following studies is most likely to confirm this diagnosis?
   a. Cerebrospinal fluid analysis
   b. Electroencephalography
   c. Random skin biopsy
   d. Electromyography
   e. Peripheral blood smear

III.25. When treating intravascular lymphoma, which of the following chemotherapeutic agents would be expected to have the greatest effect on central nervous system lesion burden?
   a. Rituximab
   b. Methotrexate
   c. Doxorubicin
   d. Cyclophosphamide
   e. Vincristine

III.26. The differential diagnosis for a mass emanating from the corpus callosum includes:
   a. Lymphoma, glioma, brain abscess, and chloroma (myeloid neoplastic infiltration)
   b. Glioma, demyelination, brain abscess, and lymphoma
   c. Demyelination, glioma, brain abscess, and chloroma
   d. Chloroma, lymphoma, demyelination, and glioma
   e. Chloroma, demyelination, glioma, and immunoglobulin G4 disease

III.27. Which of the following clinical features argues against a diagnosis of limbic encephalitis?
   a. Absence of delirium
   b. Seizures
   c. Movement disorders
   d. Psychosis
   e. Fever

III.28. Which radiographic feature is most consistent with a diagnosis of limbic encephalitis?
   a. Intense T1-weighted, postcontrast-enhancing lesions
   b. Bilateral, mesial temporal lobe, T2/fluid-attenuated inversion recovery–hyperintense lesions
   c. Presence of restricted diffusion
   d. Areas of microhemorrhage
   e. Temporal lobe neocortex involvement

III.29. Characteristic clinical and testing features of Behçet syndrome include which of the following?
   a. Ulcers restricted to the mouth, meningitis, *HLA-B51* positivity, and Middle Eastern, Eastern Mediterranean, or Asian ancestry
   b. Oral and genital ulcers, myelitis, *HLA-B51* positivity, and Middle Eastern, Eastern Mediterranean, or Asian ancestry
   c. Oral and genital ulcers, meningitis, *HLA-B51* positivity, and Middle Eastern, Eastern Mediterranean, or Asian ancestry
   d. Oral and genital ulcers, myelitis, *HLA-B27* positivity, and Middle Eastern, Eastern Mediterranean, or Asian ancestry
   e. Oral and genital ulcers, meningitis, *HLA-B51* positivity, and Irish ancestry

III.30. A 35-year-old man with Behçet syndrome has a history of oral ulcers and inflammatory mucositis of the bowel, currently well controlled on azathioprine. He then has acute-onset bidirectional diplopia associated with enhancing lesions in the pontomesencephalic junction. Which of the following is the most appropriate course of treatment for this patient?
   a. Acute intravenous methylprednisolone (IVMP) 1 g/d (3-5 days) followed by oral prednisone and continued azathioprine
   b. Acute IVMP 1 g/d (3-5 days) and continued azathioprine
   c. Oral prednisone and continued azathioprine
   d. Acute IVMP 1 g/d (3-5 days) followed by oral prednisone, then switching to a tumor necrosis factor (TNF)-α inhibitor

e. Acute IVMP 1 g/d (3-5 days), then switching to a TNF-α inhibitor

III.31. Characteristic clinical features of Vogt-Koyanagi-Harada syndrome include which of the following?
a. Anterior uveitis, hearing loss, aseptic meningitis, skin changes
b. Panuveitis, oral and genital ulceration, aseptic meningitis, skin changes
c. Panuveitis, hearing loss, peripheral neuropathy, skin changes
d. Panuveitis, hearing loss, aseptic meningitis, skin changes
e. Panuveitis, oral and genital ulcers, hearing loss, aseptic meningitis

III.32. Which medications are commonly used in chronic immunotherapy for noninfectious uveomeningeal syndromes?
a. Corticosteroids
b. Rituximab
c. Tumor necrosis factor-α inhibitors
d. Corticosteroids and rituximab
e. Corticosteroids and tumor necrosis factor-α inhibitors

III.33. Which of the following magnetic resonance imaging findings is most suggestive of CLIPPERS (chronic lymphocytic inflammation with pontine perivascular enhancement responsive to steroids)?
a. Clinical improvement with corticosteroids
b. Minimal T2/fluid-attenuated inversion recovery abnormality
c. Pial enhancement
d. Asymmetric enhancement
e. Increased cerebrospinal fluid pressure

III.34. Which of the following clinical features is *not* typical of CLIPPERS (chronic lymphocytic inflammation with pontine perivascular enhancement responsive to steroids)?
a. Seizures
b. Pseudobulbar affect
c. Spasticity
d. Ataxia
e. Cognitive impairment

III.35. Which of the following drugs or class of drugs used to treat connective tissue disease and inflammatory bowel disease have been implicated in central nervous system inflammation?
a. Sulfasalazine
b. Anti-CD20
c. Tumor necrosis factor-α inhibitors
d. Azathioprine
e. Mycophenolate mofetil

III.36. A 32-year-old woman with a history of rheumatoid arthritis had a 4-day history of bilateral lower limb numbness and unsteady gait. There was asymmetric pyramidal weakness affecting the right leg flexors, with bilateral brisk reflexes and right extensor plantar response. Sensory examination showed reduced vibration sense at the right toe and reduced pinprick on the left leg to the mid abdomen. Magnetic resonance imaging of the spine showed multiple, short-segment, T2-hyperintense lesions at T4, T6, and T7, with contrast enhancement of the T6 lesion. Which of her medications should be reviewed?
a. Hydroxychloroquine
b. Ibuprofen
c. Pantoprazole
d. Vitamin D
e. Etanercept

III.37. A 50-year-old man sought care for new-onset tonic-clonic seizures. He had no history of head trauma, epilepsy, or recent infections and no family history of epilepsy. At his first visit, the neurologic examination was unremarkable. Electroencephalography findings were normal. Brain magnetic resonance imaging (MRI) showed patchy, gadolinium-enhancing, T2 hyperintensity in the left temporo-occipital lobes. Cerebrospinal fluid (CSF) examination was unremarkable; no neuronal autoantibody was detected in the CSF or serum. Chest radiography and spine MRI were normal. What is the best next step in diagnosis for this patient?
a. Start immunotherapy
b. Perform brain biopsy
c. Repeat CSF testing
d. Begin antiseizure therapy
e. Use an expectative approach

III.38. A brain biopsy for the above patient showed parenchymal and perivascular CD3 T-lymphocytic infiltration, no granulomas, and no evidence of infections or neoplasm. Corticosteroids with taper are started, with mycophenolate mofetil as a steroid-sparing agent. How long should the patient continue on immunosuppression?
a. One month
b. Indefinitely
c. Until the patient becomes asymptomatic
d. Per physician judgment, with typical 3 to 5 years' duration after the last clinical relapse
e. Until adverse effects develop

III.39. What is the most common neurologic manifestation of HaNDL syndrome (transient headache and neurologic deficits with cerebrospinal fluid lymphocytosis)?
a. Acute confusional state
b. Aphasia
c. Motor deficits
d. Sensory symptoms
e. Visual symptoms

III.40. Which of the following diagnostic studies may be abnormal (in addition to cerebrospinal fluid lymphocytic pleocytosis) in a patient with HaNDL syndrome (transient headache and neurologic deficits with cerebrospinal fluid lymphocytosis)?
a. Magnetic resonance imaging of the brain with and without contrast

b. Electroencephalography

c. Cerebral angiography

d. Erythrocyte sedimentation rate

e. Computed tomography of the head without contrast

III.41. Which of the following imaging modalities is preferred for evaluation of possible histiocytosis?

a. Brain magnetic resonance imaging

b. Bone scan

c. Long-bone radiography

d. Positron emission tomography/computed tomography (PET/CT) from orbits to thighs

e. PET/CT from vertex to toes

III.42. Which of the following features is not typical of central nervous system histiocytosis?

a. Diabetes insipidus

b. Optic neuritis

c. Persistent gadolinium enhancement on magnetic resonance imaging

d. Ataxia

e. Myelopathy

III.43. Seizures occurring after stroke and internal carotid artery stenting could be caused by which of the following?

a. Reperfusion injury, stroke-related injury, intracerebral hemorrhage, or demyelinating disease

b. Demyelinating disease, stroke-related injury, intracerebral hemorrhage, or retained foreign-body material

c. Reperfusion injury, stroke-related injury, intracerebral hemorrhage, or retained foreign-body material

d. Reperfusion injury, stroke-related injury, demyelinating disease, or retained foreign-body material

e. Reperfusion injury, demyelinating disease, intracerebral hemorrhage, or retained foreign-body material

III.44. A 35-year-old woman has a 6-month history of pain and clumsiness in the right upper extremity. Gait demonstrates circumduction of the right leg. She has a change in sensation with pinprick near the base of her neck. Imaging shows an expansile lesion restricted to the lower cervical cord with gadolinium enhancement and a syrinx. Which of the following is the most likely diagnosis?

a. Diffuse astrocytoma

b. Glioma with histone H3 K27M sequence variation

c. Ependymoma

d. Glioblastoma

e. Spinal cord metastases

III.45. A 61-year-old man had a 2-year history of brief episodes of imbalance that would come and go, each lasting about 1 second. He then noted "dryness" and an inability to close his right eye. His wife noted that the right side of his face was weak. He was initially diagnosed with Bell palsy pain, but because of his imbalance he underwent brain magnetic resonance imaging, which showed abnormal hyperintensity within the brainstem and upper cervical spine, without abnormal contrast enhancement. He was treated with 5 days of high-dose intravenous corticosteroids, with improvement of his right facial weakness. Follow-up imaging showed persistence of the expansile T2-hyperintense lesion within the dorsal pons, medulla, and cervical spinal cord. On evaluation, he reported parageusia on the right side of his tongue. What is the most likely diagnosis?

a. Diffuse astrocytoma

b. Pilocytic astrocytoma

c. Ependymoma

d. Glioblastoma

e. Metastasis

III.46. Which of the following gadolinium enhancement patterns on spine magnetic resonance imaging accompanying a myelopathy is most suggestive of spinal cord neurosarcoidosis?

a. Dorsal subpial enhancement with or without accompanying trident sign

b. The rim and flame sign

c. A transverse band/pancake enhancement pattern

d. A missing piece of enhancement

e. A ring of enhancement

III.47. Which of the following is the mainstay of treatment of spinal cord neurosarcoidosis?

a. A single short course of intravenous (IV) corticosteroids

b. Plasma exchange

c. Prolonged high-dose oral corticosteroids with or without preceding high-dose IV corticosteroids

d. Fingolimod

e. Natalizumab

III.48. At which level is spinal cord T2-hyperintense signal most often seen in patients with spinal dural arteriovenous fistula?

a. Cervical

b. Low thoracic

c. Mid thoracic

d. Conus

e. Cervicomedullary junction

III.49. Which treatment may contribute to substantial worsening of deficits in patients with a spinal dural arteriovenous fistula?

a. Plasma exchange

b. Corticosteroids

c. Intravenous immunoglobulin

d. Angiotensin-converting enzyme inhibitor

e. Surgery

III.50. In spontaneous spinal cord infarction, how quickly should severe acute myelopathy deficits accrue?

a. Within 10 minutes

b. Within 4 hours

c. Within 8 hours

d. Within 12 hours

e. Within 24 hours

III.51. A 65-year-old woman seeks care for acute chest pain radiating to the back, followed by rapid lower extremity weakness and numbness, reaching nadir within 12 hours. Which of the following should be done first?
a. Magnetic resonance imaging of the spine
b. Computed tomography (CT) angiography of the chest
c. Cerebrospinal fluid examination
d. Serum antibody testing
e. CT of the spine

III.52. Which specific magnetic resonance imaging characteristics suggest recent hematomyelia, as opposed to an alternative cause of myelopathy?
a. Longitudinally extensive T2-hyperintense signal
b. Gadolinium enhancement
c. T2 hypointensity and T1 hyperintensity before gadolinium administration
d. T1 hypointensity
e. Flow voids

III.53. What is the most common cause of hematomyelia?
a. Trauma
b. Coagulopathy
c. Cavernous malformation
d. Arteriovenous malformation
e. Dural arteriovenous fistula

III.54. Which of the following gadolinium enhancement patterns on spine magnetic resonance imaging is most suggestive of cervical spondylotic myelopathy?
a. Dorsal subpial enhancement with or without an accompanying trident sign
b. The rim and flame sign
c. A transverse band/pancakelike enhancement pattern
d. A missing piece of enhancement
e. A ring of enhancement

III.55. After successful cervical decompression surgery, how long does it typically take the enhancement associated with cervical spondylotic myelopathy to resolve completely?
a. Immediately
b. Less than 1 week
c. Less than 1 month
d. 1 to 2 years
e. More than 2 years

III.56. Which of the following is not a possible cause of a myeloneuropathy?
a. Vitamin B$_{12}$ deficiency
b. HIV

c. Copper deficiency
d. Nitrous oxide toxicity
e. Pyridoxine deficiency

III.57. Which of the following measures is most specific for pernicious anemia?
a. Intrinsic factor antibodies
b. Parietal cell antibodies
c. Increased gastrin levels
d. Increased methylmalonic acid levels
e. Increased homocysteine levels

III.58. Which of the following features is most suggestive of a noninflammatory myelopathy in a patient with a longitudinally extensive T2 lesion on spinal cord magnetic resonance imaging (MRI)?
a. Myelin oligodendrocyte glycoprotein–immunoglobulin G (IgG) positivity
b. Aquaporin-4-IgG positivity
c. Insidious progression after spine surgery
d. Paraplegia
e. Absence of flow voids on sagittal MRI

III.59. Which of the following accompanying disorders is *not* a cause of chronic adhesive arachnoiditis?
a. Trauma
b. Prior spine surgery
c. Nontraumatic subarachnoid hemorrhage
d. Neuromyelitis optica spectrum disorders
e. Iophendylate contrast administration

III.60. A 70-year-old man has subacute onset of headache, altered mental status, short-term memory loss, fever, and pneumonia. Cerebrospinal fluid analysis shows slight pleocytosis (10 white blood cells/µL) and increased protein levels. Which of the following are the most probable involved pathogens?
a. Influenza virus A or B
b. *Legionella pneumophila* or severe acute respiratory syndrome coronavirus 2
c. *Streptococcus pneumoniae* or *Streptococcus agalactiae*
d. *Listeria monocytogenes* or *Neisseria meningitidis*
e. *Escherichia coli* or *Haemophilus influenzae*

III.61. Which of the following criteria characterize possible autoimmune encephalitis?
a. Subacute onset of working memory deficit and altered mental status
b. Acute vision loss
c. Lower limb weakness and sensory loss
d. Extrapyramidal signs
e. Peripheral neuropathy

III.1.   Answer e.

The cranial nerve most frequently affected by neurosarcoidosis is the facial nerve; this presents with facial palsy in up to 50% of patients with neurosarcoidosis. However, most patients with facial nerve palsy due to neurosarcoidosis have other neurologic manifestations of the disease. The optic nerve is the second most common cranial nerve to be involved by neurosarcoidosis.

III.2.   Answer d.

Currently, the optimal treatment for sarcoid optic neuropathy is high-dose intravenous (IV) corticosteroids, followed by a prolonged course of high-dose oral corticosteroids with a slow taper. Intermittent IV corticosteroids or short courses of IV or oral corticosteroids are not sufficient. Plasma exchange is not a recommended treatment for sarcoid optic neuropathy. Steroid-sparing immunotherapies such as methotrexate may be used in conjunction with corticosteroids in those intolerant of corticosteroids or in those who have relapses off of corticosteroids. Infliximab is emerging as a potential alternative to corticosteroids in patients with neurosarcoidosis.

III.3.   Answer b.

Sudden loss of vision is atypical for sarcoid optic neuropathy, which is usually insidious in onset and causes progressive decrease in visual acuity and color vision over weeks to months. Sarcoid optic neuropathy may present with optic disc swelling and relative afferent pupillary defect. Causes of sudden unilateral vision loss may include optic nerve ischemia or trauma.

III.4.   Answer c.

Central corpus callosum lesions, which have been described as snowballs or spokes, are common in Susac syndrome and are considered pathognomonic for the disease. Lesions of the periaqueductal gray are commonly present in patients with Wernicke encephalopathy. Thalamic lesions can be seen in patients with prion disease. The septum pellucidum separates the 2 lateral ventricles.

III.5.   Answer b.

Susac syndrome is believed to be an autoimmune disease targeting vascular endothelial cells, although this remains unproved. There is no current evidence to support an infectious vasculitis pathogenesis. Multiple sclerosis and neuromyelitis optica spectrum disorder are examples of inflammatory demyelinating diseases. Thromboembolic disease is the underlying cause of a cerebrovascular accident.

III.6.   Answer d.

White matter lesions involving the corpus callosum can be seen in leukodystrophies and in multiple sclerosis (MS). The other choices may be a diagnostic clue to a leukodystrophy rather than MS.

III.7.   Answer d.

Increased lactate levels of abnormal cerebral white matter on magnetic resonance spectroscopy is a supportive magnetic resonance imaging (MRI) criterion for LBSL (leukoencephalopathy with brainstem and spinal cord involvement and lactate elevation) but is not required for MRI-based diagnosis. The other choices are all major MRI criteria and should all be present to make an MRI-based diagnosis of LBSL.

III.8.   Answer d.

Sequence variations in the colony-stimulating factor 1 receptor gene are found in hereditary forms of diffuse leukoencephalopathy with axonal spheroids. *NOTCH3* sequence variations are found in patients with CADASIL syndrome (cerebral autosomal dominant arteriopathy with subcortical infarcts and leukoencephalopathy). Lamin B1 gene duplication is seen in adult-onset autosomal dominant leukodystrophy. *C9ORF72* repeat expansion occurs in frontotemporal dementia and amyotrophic lateral sclerosis syndromes. CAG trinucleotide expansion is found in neurologic disorders including Huntington disease.

III.9.   Answer a.

Patients with more acute deterioration and diffuse leukoencephalopathy with axonal spheroids may have subcortical diffusion restriction. Cortical diffusion restriction is seen in neuronal intranuclear inclusion disease. Spinal cord abnormalities, including any diffusion restriction, is not seen in sporadic, adult-onset, diffuse leukoencephalopathy with axonal spheroids. Basal ganglia diffusion abnormalities may be seen in prion disorders such as Creutzfeldt-Jakob disease.

III.10.   Answer d.

In the vast majority of patients, the detection of immunoglobulin M antibodies to West Nile virus (WNV) in the cerebrospinal fluid establishes the diagnosis. Immunoglobulin G positivity, however, cannot be used to establish the diagnosis of acute meningoencephalitis. Although highly specific, polymerase chain reaction (PCR) for WNV is insensitive because active viral replication occurs early in the course of disease. Serologic assays, however, may be falsely negative in immunocompromised patients. Viremia also tends to be more prolonged in these patients, so obtaining both serologic and PCR testing is recommended.

III.11.   Answer b.

Radiographically, herpes simplex virus (HSV) encephalitis shows markedly asymmetric, but usually bilateral, T2-weighted fluid-attenuated inversion recovery hyperintensity and swelling in the medial temporal lobes, insular cortices, and orbitofrontal lobes. Although cerebrospinal fluid (CSF) polymerase chain reaction (PCR) for HSV is highly sensitive and specific, it can be negative if obtained acutely. Repeated CSF examination 24 to 72 hours after the first test is usually diagnostic. Acyclovir should be continued until this diagnosis has been ruled out with a second CSF PCR test for HSV.

III.12. Answer b.

MELAS syndrome (mitochondrial encephalopathy, lactic acidosis, and stroke-like episodes) is a maternally inherited mitochondrial disorder (not somatically X-linked). Migraine history (not tension headaches) is common in MELAS syndrome.

III.13. Answer d.

Patients with mitochondrial cytopathic processes such as mitochondrial encephalopathy, lactic acidosis, and stroke-like episodes may have normal imaging findings at times, or they may have large neocortical abnormalities that are nonenhancing. They also sometimes have abnormalities on diffusion-weighted imaging, although without true diffusion restriction (normal or hyperintense lesions on apparent diffusion coefficient imaging). These lesions may fluctuate in size and even migrate from one hemisphere to the next. Mesial temporal abnormalities are typical of limbic encephalitis. Corpus callosal lesions, spinal cord lesions, and small cortical and juxtacortical neocortical findings, with subsequent atrophy, are encountered in multiple sclerosis.

III.14. Answer b.

Real-time quaking-induced conversion is a highly sensitive and specific assay for sporadic Creutzfeldt-Jakob disease (CJD), as well as other forms of prion disease. The other answer choices are commonly encountered in patients with CJD but are not as specific. In addition, electroencephalographic abnormalities vary throughout the disease course, and periodic sharp wave complexes may not arise until late in the illness.

III.15. Answer a.

The combination of cortical ribbon sign and basal ganglial/thalamic nuclear hyperintensity on diffusion-weighted imaging has approximately 90% sensitivity and specificity for sporadic Creutzfeldt-Jakob disease (sCJD). These findings on fluid-attenuated inversion recovery imaging are also highly specific, but they lack sensitivity. Cortical ribbon sign occurring in isolation may also occur in some autoimmune and mitochondrial encephalopathies. Postgadolinium enhancement is not a feature of sCJD. Hyperintensity of the pulvinar and dorsolateral thalamic nuclei (hockey stick sign) may occur in sCJD but is more characteristic of variant CJD.

III.16. Answer c.

Autoimmune central nervous system (CNS) disorders usually have subacute onset, although there are some exceptions, such as IgLON family member 5–antibody related CNS disorders, which may have a more chronic, progressive course. Brain infections and demyelinating disease episodes may present subacutely. Stroke is the classic cause of a hyperacute neurologic presentation, although occasionally the history given will suggest a subacute clinical course. Neurodegenerative diseases such as Alzheimer disease have an insidious progressive course.

III.17. Answer d.

Evaluating diffusion-weighted imaging (DWI) (hyperintense or bright) and apparent diffusion coefficient (ADC) (hypointense or dark) sequences, in addition to T2 and T1 postgadolinium images can assist in evaluating for the possibility of subacute infarction. Ischemic strokes tend to be bright on DWI and dark on ADC (diffusion restriction). Brain abscesses may have a similar appearance on DWI and ADC but also demonstrate diffuse T2 hyperintensity and ring enhancement. Brain tumors tend to be bright on both DWI and ADC.

III.18. Answer d.

Cerebrospinal fluid findings are abnormal in 80% to 90% of patients with primary angiitis of the central nervous system, showing an aseptic meningitis pattern with lymphocytic pleocytosis, increased protein concentration, and normal glucose value. Oligoclonal bands are frequently detected in patients with multiple sclerosis. Neutrophilic pleocytosis would be suggestive of a suppurative meningitis, whereas low glucose value may be seen with suppurative, tuberculous, and fungal infections, sarcoidosis, and meningeal dissemination of tumors.

III.19. Answer c.

The standard induction treatment of primary angiitis of the central nervous system is corticosteroids and cyclophosphamide. After induction, other agents such as azathioprine and mycophenolate mofetil are frequently used. Rituximab has been used in small cohorts of patients, with apparent benefit.

III.20. Answer c.

Patients with amyloid-β-related angiitis have distinct pathologic findings, with both vasculitic (angiopathic) changes and amyloid-β peptide deposition. None of the other choices have all of these features.

III.21. Answer a.

Common initial manifestations of amyloid-β-related angiitis (ABRA) include cerebral hemorrhage, ischemic stroke, headache, and encephalopathy, along with seizures. Optic neuritis, parkinsonism, and neuropathy are not clinical features associated with ABRA. Depression can occur as a long-term consequence of any brain illness.

III.22. Answer b.

Cerebrospinal fluid involvement is more common than vitreous involvement by primary central nervous system lymphoma. Visceral, lymph node, and bone marrow involvement is rare at the time of diagnosis.

III.23. Answer a.

Methotrexate-based chemotherapy is the most appropriate initial therapy for primary central nervous system lymphoma (PCNSL). Chimeric antigen receptor T-cell therapy is considered investigational for PCNSL. Whole-brain irradiation is associated with substantial toxicity and is usually avoided unless the PCNSL is refractory to chemotherapy. There is no role for intrathecal rituximab.

III.24. **Answer c.**

An accurate diagnosis of intravascular lymphoma requires pathologic confirmation. Random skin biopsy, even in the absence of cutaneous abnormalities, has been shown to confirm the diagnosis of intravascular lymphoma in a large percentage of patients and can be especially useful if investigations do not identify a specific biopsy target. Cerebrospinal fluid and peripheral blood smear abnormalities are typically nonspecific and rarely demonstrate malignant cells. Electroencephalography and electromyography may demonstrate electrophysiologic sequelae of intravascular lymphoma involvement, but these findings would be nonspecific.

III.25. **Answer b.**

In cases of intravascular lymphoma with central nervous system (CNS) involvement, a chemotherapy regimen with adequate CNS penetration is necessary. High-dose methotrexate administered systemically can achieve adequate CNS concentrations. The other answer choices are medications from the R-CHOP regimen, which is frequently used in the treatment of intravascular lymphoma but does not alone adequately address CNS involvement.

III.26. **Answer b.**

Lymphoma, glioma, demyelinating disease, and brain abscesses can all have corpus callosal origin. In contrast, chloromas (myeloid neoplastic infiltration) and immunoglobulin G4 disease usually have an intradural extraparenchymal origin.

III.27. **Answer a.**

Focal neurologic deficits without delirium argue against a diagnosis of limbic encephalitis. Mesial temporal lobe involvement frequently leads to seizures, regardless of cause. Movement disorders such as chorea, dystonia, and stereotypies are common in limbic encephalitis, particularly anti-N-methyl-D-aspartate receptor encephalitis. Psychosis is frequent in limbic encephalitis, and fever occurs frequently in infectious and, occasionally, in autoimmune causes of limbic encephalitis.

III.28. **Answer b.**

Bilateral mesial temporal lobe involvement is common in limbic encephalitis, occurring in up to 60% of cases. Although patchy gadolinium enhancement can occur in limbic encephalitis, intensely enhancing lesions would be more suggestive of a high-grade neoplasm. Restricted diffusion, microhemorrhages, and neocortex involvement are rare in limbic encephalitis and suggest other diagnoses.

III.29. **Answer c.**

HLA-B27 positivity is associated with reactive arthritis and ankylosing spondylitis, whereas *HLA-B51* positivity can be associated with Behçet syndrome. Meningitis, rather than myelitis, is typical of Behçet syndrome. Classic Behçet syndrome ancestry in the Western World is Turkish, although this disease occurs among patients of descent from other Middle Eastern and Asian countries.

III.30. **Answer d.**

This patient has not responded to azathioprine and has 3 factors for poor prognosis: being male, having gastrointestinal tract involvement, and having neurologic involvement. Therefore, a switch to tumor necrosis factor (TNF)-α inhibitor therapy is indicated on the basis of open-label studies. Acute corticosteroid treatment as a bridge until TNF-α inhibitor therapy becomes effective is also recommended. The duration of continued treatment with oral prednisone is unclear and should be individualized to the patient and physician preference.

III.31. **Answer d.**

Oral and genital ulceration is classically associated with Behçet syndrome, not Vogt-Koyanagi-Harada syndrome (VKH). Aseptic meningitis, panuveitis, hearing loss, and skin changes (and not neuropathy or anterior uveitis) are characteristic of VKH.

III.32. **Answer e.**

A common mechanism seemingly shared by some of the uveomeningeal syndromes such as Behçet syndrome, Vogt-Koyanagi-Harada syndrome, and inflammatory bowel disease involves the tumor necrosis factor (TNF)-α pathway. Ultimately, all of these disorders benefit from corticosteroids and TNF-α inhibitor use. B-cell depletion therapies (ie, rituximab) have not been shown to benefit uveomeningeal syndromes and therefore are not as commonly used for these syndromes.

III.33. **Answer b.**

Although clinical improvement with corticosteroids is typical of chronic lymphocytic inflammation with pontine perivascular enhancement responsive to steroids (CLIPPERS), it is a nonspecific finding common to many other enhancing brainstem disorders. The presence of pial enhancement, asymmetric enhancement, or increased cerebrospinal fluid pressure is concerning for a neoplastic disorder. Patients with typical CLIPPERS have an area of T2/fluid-attenuated inversion recovery abnormality that is similar in size to the area of postgadolinium enhancement. Because patients with this disorder can sometimes have only small areas of punctate enhancement, magnetic resonance imaging in the absence of gadolinium administration can often be reported as normal.

III.34. **Answer a.**

The presence of seizures is a red flag that should alert the provider to a diagnosis other than chronic lymphocytic inflammation with pontine perivascular enhancement responsive to steroids (CLIPPERS). Other red flags include a lack of substantial clinical or radiologic response to corticosteroids, lack of typical brainstem-predominant findings, progression to severe deficits within days, fever or marked B symptoms, depressed level of consciousness, and any other findings localizing outside the central nervous system.

III.35. Answer c.

Tumor necrosis factor-α inhibitors have been implicated in triggering central nervous system (CNS) demyelinating disease and other inflammatory CNS disorders, although the diseases for which these drugs are US Food and Drug Administration–approved treatments are also risk factors for CNS inflammation. The other drugs are used for treating various inflammatory and autoimmune diseases but are not known to cause inflammation. Azathioprine and mycophenolate mofetil have been linked to lymphoma risk.

III.36. Answer e.

Central nervous system (CNS) demyelination can occur in patients with autoimmune diseases such as rheumatoid arthritis, psoriasis, ankylosing spondylitis, Crohn disease, and ulcerative colitis, and it is possible that both genetics and the underlying autoimmune disease may contribute to this risk. In addition, an association of CNS demyelination with use of etanercept, a tumor necrosis factor-α inhibitor, has been reported in these conditions. Hydroxychloroquine, ibuprofen, and pantoprazole are not known to cause CNS demyelination. Vitamin D deficiency is a population-based risk factor for CNS demyelination.

III.37. Answer b.

Brain biopsy is usually recommended if extensive testing (for autoantibodies, cancer, infectious agents, and other causes) yields no diagnosis and an amenable site (often with gadolinium enhancement) is identified. Starting immunotherapy would make it difficult to rule out some diagnoses such as central nervous system lymphoma. The likelihood that a second cerebrospinal fluid examination would be abnormal is relatively low. Antiseizure therapy is necessary but would not help with the diagnosis.

III.38. Answer d.

There is no consensus for the duration of maintenance immunosuppression. It is recommended to discontinue immunosuppression 3 to 5 years after the last relapse. Patients should be carefully monitored for potential adverse effects.

III.39. Answer d.

The most common neurologic manifestations of HaNDL syndrome (transient headache and neurologic deficits with cerebrospinal fluid lymphocytosis) include sensory symptoms (70%), followed by aphasia (66%), and motor deficits (42%). Visual symptoms are less common, reported in less than 20% of cases, and include decreased vision, homonymous hemianopsia, and photopsias. Rarer presentations include acute confusional state, papilledema, and sixth nerve palsy. Neurologic manifestations often vary from one episode to the next.

III.40. Answer b.

Electroencephalography (EEG) during the symptomatic period in HaNDL syndrome (transient headache and neurologic deficits with cerebrospinal fluid lymphocytosis) is usually abnormal, showing unilateral excessive slowing corresponding to clinical symptoms. In the largest published series, clear EEG abnormalities were found in 30 of 42 patients (71%).

III.41. Answer e.

Positron emission tomography/computed tomography (PET/CT) of the body from vertex to toes is the preferred modality for evaluation of possible histiocytosis. This allows for identification of systemic biopsy targets, including perinephric disease and long-bone disease. Care should be taken not to decalcify tissue before pathologic evaluation because decalcification reduces sensitivity of tissue immunohistochemistry for BRAF staining. Obtaining standard oncologic-protocol PET/CT from orbits to thighs may miss hypermetabolic lesions in the distal femurs, which are typical of Erdheim-Chester disease. Long-bone radiography is not sufficiently sensitive to detect bony lesions in histiocytic disorders. Bone scan is a reasonable imaging modality to detect bone lesions alone, but PET/CT has the added benefit of detecting soft-tissue abnormalities such as perinephric hypermetabolic tissue and lung disease. Brain magnetic resonance imaging is recommended in patients with suspected histiocytic disorders, but only 40% of patients with Erdheim-Chester disease have central nervous system involvement.

III.42. Answer b.

The presence of optic neuritis is a red flag that should alert the provider to a diagnosis other than histiocytosis. Diabetes insipidus is common and can precede diagnosis of central nervous system histiocytosis by up to a decade. Magnetic resonance imaging (MRI) of the brain is normal in half of patients with diabetes insipidus. Persistent gadolinium enhancement on brain and spinal cord MRI is typical of histiocytosis. The cerebellum, brainstem, and spinal cord are commonly involved with Erdheim-Chester disease.

III.43. Answer c.

Reperfusion injury after stenting can lead to focal cerebral disturbance, including seizures. Hemorrhagic conversion of stroke due to natural history, antithrombotic treatment, or both, can result in seizures. Retained embolized polymers into brain parenchyma from a carotid stent can lead to a chronic granulomatous encephalitis, resulting in seizures. This phenomenon is distinct from classical demyelinating diseases, such as multiple sclerosis.

III.44. Answer c.

Ependymoma is the most correct response because it is the most common spinal cord primary neoplasm in adults and typically results in expansile, gadolinium-enhancing lesions on magnetic resonance imaging which can be associated with a syrinx. Surgical resection is the most effective treatment. Gliomas and glioblastomas with the histone H3 K27M sequence variation (H3K27M) are aggressive tumors that can involve the spinal cord. These can also result in expansile, gadolinium-enhancing spinal cord masses, but they are relatively less common than ependymoma. Glioblastomas involving the spinal cord are rare and typically have relatively rapid subacute symptom onset. These tumors frequently exhibit contrast enhancement and carry a poor prognosis. Diffuse astrocytomas are low grade, and, although the time course fits with this clinical scenario, these tumors generally do not have gadolinium enhancement or associated syrinx. H3K27M gliomas are a relatively new entity. This variation is associated with an aggressive refractory course in children, where it is found in most diffuse intrinsic pontine gliomas, but the course in adults may be more indolent. Intramedullary spinal cord metastases without bony disease are very rare.

III.45. Answer a.
Diffuse astrocytomas are of low grade with an indolent course, and symptoms are often present in some manner for years. Diffuse astrocytomas are commonly mistaken for inflammatory, infectious, or cerebrovascular conditions. These tumors generally do not have gadolinium enhancement or an associated syrinx. Symptoms are often less severe than would be predicted by imaging because of their infiltrative nature. Glioma with histone H3 K27M sequence variation would also be possible in this case, because these tumors involve midline structures and are frequently nonenhancing. The radiographic features of this lesion are inconsistent with an ependymoma, which are expansile, gadolinium-enhancing lesions that can be associated with a syrinx. Similarly, glioblastomas involving the spinal cord typically have relatively rapid, subacute symptom onset. These tumors frequently exhibit contrast enhancement, may show central necrosis, and carry a poor prognosis. Pilocytic astrocytomas are typically contrast enhancing and may have a tumor-associated cyst. Intramedullary spinal cord metastases without bony disease are very rare.

III.46. Answer a.
Presence of linear, dorsal, subpial enhancement extending 2 or more vertebral segments on spine magnetic resonance imaging, with or without concurrent central canal enhancement forming a trident appearance on axial postgadolinium spine images, is suggestive of spinal cord neurosarcoidosis. The other gadolinium enhancement patterns are associated with other myelopathies. Rim and flame sign is associated with metastasis, transverse band/pancake enhancement pattern with cervical spondylotic compression, missing piece of enhancement with spinal dural arteriovenous fistula, and a ring of enhancement with neuromyelitis optica spectrum disorders.

III.47. Answer c.
Prolonged high-dose oral prednisone, often with preceding intravenous methylprednisolone, is the mainstay of treatment for spinal cord neurosarcoidosis. Treatment with a short course of intravenous methylprednisolone without prolonged oral prednisone commonly is

associated with early relapse. Plasma exchange, fingolimod, and natalizumab are not recognized treatments of spinal cord neurosarcoidosis.

III.48. Answer d.
About 90% of patients with spinal dural arteriovenous fistula have spinal cord T2-hyperintense signal that extends down into the conus medullaris, due to accumulation of gravity-dependent edema.

III.49. Answer b.
Although immunotherapies (intravenous immunoglobulin, corticosteroids, and plasma exchange) have no role in the treatment of dural arteriovenous fistula, corticosteroids have been documented in multiple case reports and series to be associated with potential severe worsening of deficits, which is most likely secondary to increased venous hypertension. Plasma exchange, by temporarily decreasing systemic blood pressure, may transiently improve symptoms. Surgery is definitive treatment.

III.50. Answer d.
Criteria for spontaneous spinal cord infarction include the rapid onset of severe myelopathic deficits within 12 hours or less.

III.51. Answer b.
Although magnetic resonance imaging of the spine would most likely be ordered early in the evaluation, emergent life-threatening processes must be considered first; thus, computed tomography (CT) angiography of the chest should be performed first because of concern for aortic dissection. Similarly, cerebrospinal fluid examination and antibody testing are not needed acutely before spine imaging. CT of the spine is often obtained first as part of trauma sequences in suspected spinal cord trauma, but the sensitivity and specificity are poor if nontraumatic vascular processes are being considered.

III.52. Answer c.
A significant component of magnetic resonance imaging findings showing dark T2 hypointensity and T1 hyperintensity suggests hemorrhage. Further confirmation can be sought with additional sequences such as gradient echo–weighted imaging. Longitudinally extensive T2-hyperintense signal is not specific. Assessing for gadolinium enhancement could be helpful in looking for an underlying mass or other possible process but is otherwise minimally valuable in this scenario. Although T1 hypointensity may be seen late after a hemorrhage, it is not as valuable in making the diagnosis more acutely. Although flow voids may be seen in underlying arteriovenous malformation, they cannot identify recent bleeding.

III.53. Answer a.
Although cavernous malformations and arteriovenous malformations are generally the most common causes of nontraumatic cases of hematomyelia, trauma is overall the most common cause. Dural arteriovenous fistulas cause cord edema rather than hemorrhage.

III.54. Answer c.

A transverse band or flat pancakelike appearance of enhancement on sagittal images, in which the width is greater than or equal to the height, is highly suggestive of cervical spondylosis. Dorsal subpial enhancement is associated with spinal cord sarcoidosis. The rim and flame enhancement pattern is suggestive of intramedullary spinal cord metastasis. The missing piece of enhancement sign is encountered in dural arteriovenous fistula, whereas a ring of enhancement can be seen with multiple sclerosis or aquaporin-4–immunoglobulin G–seropositive neuromyelitis optica spectrum disorder.

III.55. Answer d.

The enhancement accompanying cervical spondylotic myelopathy resolves slowly over time after successful surgical decompression (1-2 years), which can sometimes lead to diagnostic confusion. However, in the absence of clinical or radiologic worsening, slow resolution of enhancement should not rule out this diagnosis.

III.56. Answer e.

Both vitamin B_{12} deficiency and copper deficiency can cause subacute combined degeneration. A history of bariatric surgery is a risk factor for both. HIV infection is associated with derangements in the transmethylation pathways, and direct HIV infection is often not responsible for the myeloneuropathy. Nitrous oxide oxidizes the cobalt core of vitamin B_{12} and causes functional vitamin B_{12} deficiency. Pyridoxine deficiency can cause a peripheral neuropathy but not a myelopathy.

III.57. Answer a.

Both methylmalonic acid (MMA) and homocysteine levels may be increased with metabolically significant vitamin B_{12} deficiency; MMA is more specific than homocysteine for vitamin B_{12} deficiency. Increased gastrin levels and parietal cell antibodies are sensitive but not specific markers for pernicious anemia. Intrinsic factor antibodies are the most specific but are relatively insensitive.

III.58. Answer c.

Patients with myelin oligodendrocyte glycoprotein or aquaporin-4 autoimmunity can have subacute onset of myelitis symptoms. Patients with chronic adhesive arachnoiditis typically have insidious onset and progression of myelopathic symptoms after spine surgery in which dural injury has occurred. Paraplegia is not specific to any myelopathic diagnosis. Prominent spinal dural veins (flow voids) on magnetic resonance imaging can indicate a dural arteriovenous fistula. A longitudinally extensive T2-signal abnormality on spinal sagittal imaging can be encountered in all of these diagnoses.

III.59. Answer d.

Neuromyelitis optica spectrum disorders cause longitudinally extensive transverse myelitis. The others are risk factors for chronic adhesive arachnoiditis.

III.60. Answer b.

The patient has pneumonia and encephalitis. The subacute onset and the association of symptoms, together with cerebrospinal fluid signs of inflammation, are suggestive of *Legionella pneumoniae* or severe acute respiratory syndrome coronavirus 2 infection.

III.61. Answer a.

Autoimmune encephalitis is characterized by subacute onset (rapid progression, <3 months) of short-term memory deficit, altered mental status, or psychiatric symptoms. Seizures, cerebrospinal fluid pleocytosis, focal central nervous system signs, and radiologic features suggestive of encephalitis are also characteristic findings.

SECTION III (CASES 53-83) SUGGESTED READING

Anderson TL, Morris JM, Wald JT, Kotsenas AL. Imaging appearance of advanced chronic adhesive arachnoiditis: a retrospective review. AJR Am J Roentgenol. 2017 Sep;209(3):648-55. Epub 2017 Jun 22.

Auriel E, Charidimou A, Gurol ME, Ni J, Van Etten ES, Martinez-Ramirez S, et al. Validation of clinicoradiological criteria for the diagnosis of cerebral amyloid angiopathy-related inflammation. JAMA Neurol. 2016 Feb;73(2):197–202.

Bartleson JD, Swanson JW, Whisnant JP. A migrainous syndrome with cerebrospinal fluid pleocytosis. Neurology. 1981 Oct;31(10):1257–62.

Bhatia KD, Krishnan P, Kortman H, Klostranec J, Krings T. Acute cortical lesions in MELAS syndrome: anatomic distribution, symmetry, and evolution. AJNR Am J Neuroradiol. 2020 Jan;41(1):167-73. Epub 2019 Dec 5.

Biousse V, Newman NJ. Diagnosis and clinical features of common optic neuropathies. Lancet Neurol. 2016 Dec;15(13):1355–67.

Bower RS, Burrus TM, Giannini C, Erickson BJ, Meyer FB, Pirko I, et al. Teaching NeuroImages: demyelinating disease mimicking butterfly high-grade glioma. Neurology. 2010 Jul 13;75(2):e4–5.

Burkholder BM. Vogt-Koyanagi-Harada disease. Curr Opin Ophthalmol. 2015 Nov;26(6):506–11.

Byram K, Hajj-Ali RA, Calabrese L. CNS vasculitis: an approach to differential diagnosis and management. Curr Rheumatol Rep. 2018 May 30;20(7):37.

Calabrese LH, Mallek JA. Primary angiitis of the central nervous system: report of 8 new cases, review of the literature, and proposal for diagnostic criteria. Medicine (Baltimore). 1988 Jan;67(1):20–39.

Chiavazza C, Pellerino A, Ferrio F, Cistaro A, Soffietti R, Ruda R. Primary CNS lymphomas: challenges in diagnosis and monitoring. Biomed Res Int. 2018 Jun 21;2018:3606970.

Chung KK, Anderson NE, Hutchinson D, Synek B, Barber PA. Cerebral amyloid angiopathy related inflammation: three case reports and a review. J Neurol Neurosurg Psychiatry. 2011 Jan;82(1):20-6. Epub 2010 Oct 9.

Conway BL, Clarke MJ, Kaufmann TJ, Flanagan EP. Utility of extension views in spondylotic myelopathy mimicking transverse myelitis. Mult Scler Relat Disord. 2017 Jan;11:62-4. Epub 2016 Dec 9.

Cunningham ET Jr, Rathinam SR, Tugal-Tutkun I, Muccioli C, Zierhut M. Vogt-Koyanagi-Harada disease. Ocul Immunol Inflamm. 2014 Aug;22(4):249–52.

Egan RA. Diagnostic criteria and treatment algorithm for Susac syndrome. J Neuroophthalmol. 2019 Mar;39(1):60–7.

Ehlers S. Tumor necrosis factor and its blockade in granulomatous infections: differential modes of action of infliximab and etanercept? Clin Infect Dis. 2005 Aug 1;41 Suppl 3:S199–203.

Flanagan EP, Kaufmann TJ, Krecke KN, Aksamit AJ, Pittock SJ, Keegan BM, et al. Discriminating long myelitis of neuromyelitis optica from sarcoidosis. Ann Neurol. 2016 Mar;79(3):437-47. Epub 2016 Feb 12.

Flanagan EP, Krecke KN, Marsh RW, Giannini C, Keegan BM, Weinshenker BG. Specific pattern of gadolinium enhancement in spondylotic myelopathy. Ann Neurol. 2014 Jul;76(1):54-65. Epub 2014 Jun 14.

Foutz A, Appleby BS, Hamlin C, Liu X, Yang S, Cohen Y, et al. Diagnostic and prognostic value of human prion detection in cerebrospinal fluid. Ann Neurol. 2017 Jan;81(1):79–92.

Gelfand JM, Genrich G, Green AJ, Tihan T, Cree BA. Encephalitis of unclear origin diagnosed by brain biopsy: a diagnostic challenge. JAMA Neurol. 2015 Jan;72(1):66–72.

Geschwind MD. Rapidly progressive dementia. Continuum (Minneap Minn). 2016 Apr;22(2, Dementia):510–37.

Gorman GS, Schaefer AM, Ng Y, Gomez N, Blakely EL, Alston CL, et al. Prevalence of nuclear and mitochondrial DNA mutations related to adult mitochondrial disease. Ann Neurol. 2015 May;77(5):753-9. Epub 2015 Mar 28.

Goyal G, Young JR, Koster MJ, Tobin WO, Vassallo R, Ryu JH, et al; Mayo Clinic Histiocytosis Working Group. The Mayo Clinic Histiocytosis Working Group Consensus Statement for the Diagnosis and Evaluation of Adult Patients With Histiocytic Neoplasms: Erdheim-Chester disease, Langerhans cell histiocytosis, and Rosai-Dorfman disease. Mayo Clin Proc. 2019 Oct;94(10):2054-71. Epub 2019 Aug 28.

Greco A, De Virgilio A, Gallo A, Fusconi M, Turchetta R, Tombolini M, et al. Susac's syndrome: pathogenesis, clinical variants and treatment approaches. Autoimmun Rev. 2014 Aug;13(8):814-21. Epub 2014 Apr 12.

Grommes C, DeAngelis LM. Primary CNS lymphoma. J Clin Oncol. 2017 Jul 20;35(21):2410-8. Epub 2017 Jun 22.

Hajj-Ali RA, Calabrese LH. Diagnosis and classification of central nervous system vasculitis. J Autoimmun. 2014 Feb-Mar;48-49:149-52. Epub 2014 Feb 1.

Han CH, Batchelor TT. Diagnosis and management of primary central nervous system lymphoma. Cancer. 2017 Nov 15;123(22):4314-24. Epub 2017 Sep 26.

Headache Classification Committee of the International Headache Society (IHS). The International Classification of Headache Disorders, 3rd edition (beta version). Cephalalgia. 2013 Jul;33(9):629–808.

Huang C, Wang Y, Li X, Ren L, Zhao J, Hu Y, et al. Clinical features of patients infected with 2019 novel coronavirus in Wuhan, China. Lancet. 2020 Feb 15;395(10223):497-506. Epub 2020 Jan 24. Erratum in: Lancet. 2020 Jan 30.

Ishido T, Horita N, Takeuchi M, Kawagoe T, Shibuya E, Yamane T, et al. Clinical manifestations of Behçet's disease depending on sex and age: results from Japanese nationwide registration. Rheumatology (Oxford). 2017 Nov 1;56(11):1918–27.

Keegan BM, Giannini C, Parisi JE, Lucchinetti CF, Boeve BF, Josephs KA. Sporadic adult-onset leukoencephalopathy with neuroaxonal spheroids mimicking cerebral MS. Neurology. 2008 Mar 25;70(13 Pt 2):1128-33. Epub 2008 Feb 20.

Kelley BP, Patel SC, Marin HL, Corrigan JJ, Mitsias PD, Griffith B. Autoimmune encephalitis: pathophysiology and imaging review of an overlooked diagnosis. AJNR Am J Neuroradiol. 2017 Jun;38(6):1070-8. Epub 2017 Feb 9.

Kidd DP, Burton BJ, Graham EM, Plant GT. Optic neuropathy associated with systemic sarcoidosis. Neurol Neuroimmunol Neuroinflamm. 2016 Aug 2;3(5):e270.

Konno T, Broderick DF, Mezaki N, Isami A, Kaneda D, Tashiro Y, et al. Diagnostic value of brain calcifications in adult-onset leukoencephalopathy with axonal spheroids and pigmented glia. AJNR Am J Neuroradiol. 2017 Jan;38(1):77-83. Epub 2016 Sep 15.

Kramer CL. Vascular disorders of the spinal cord. Continuum (Minneap Minn). 2018 Apr;24(2, Spinal Cord Disorders):407–26.

Kumar N. Metabolic and toxic myelopathies. Semin Neurol. 2012 Apr;32(2):123-36. Epub 2012 Sep 8.

Kumar N. Neurologic aspects of cobalamin (B$_{12}$) deficiency. Handb Clin Neurol. 2014;120:915–26.

Kunchok A, Aksamit AJ Jr, Davis JM 3rd, Kantarci OH, Keegan BM, Pittock SJ, et al. Association between tumor necrosis factor inhibitor exposure and inflammatory central nervous system events. JAMA Neurol. 2020 Aug 1;77(8):937–46.

Law LY, Riminton DS, Nguyen M, Barnett MH, Reddel SW, Hardy TA. The spectrum of immune-mediated and inflammatory lesions of the brainstem: clues to diagnosis. Neurology. 2019 Aug 27;93(9):390–405.

Lorentzen AO, Nome T, Bakke SJ, Scheie D, Stenset V, Aamodt AH. Cerebral foreign body reaction after carotid aneurysm stenting. Interv Neuroradiol. 2016 Feb;22(1):53-7. Epub 2015 Oct 28.

Low S, Han CH, Batchelor TT. Primary central nervous system lymphoma. Ther Adv Neurol Disord. 2018 Oct 5;11:1756286418793562.

Lu VM, Alvi MA, McDonald KL, Daniels DJ. Impact of the H3K27M mutation on survival in pediatric high-grade glioma: a systematic review and meta-analysis. J Neurosurg Pediatr. 2018 Nov 30;23(3):308–16.

Mao L, Jin H, Wang M, Hu Y, Chen S, He Q, et al. Neurologic manifestations of hospitalized patients with coronavirus disease 2019 in Wuhan, China. JAMA Neurol. 2020 Jun 1;77(6):683–90.

McKeon A. Immunotherapeutics for autoimmune encephalopathies and dementias. Curr Treat Options Neurol. 2013 Dec;15(6):723–37.

Mehta RI, Mehta RI, Solis OE, Jahan R, Salamon N, Tobis JM, et al. Hydrophilic polymer emboli: an under-recognized iatrogenic cause of ischemia and infarct. Mod Pathol. 2010 Jul;23(7):921-30. Epub 2010 Mar 19.

Mont'Alverne AR, Yamakami LY, Goncalves CR, Baracat EC, Bonfa E, Silva CA. Diminished ovarian reserve in Behçet's disease patients. Clin Rheumatol. 2015 Jan;34(1):179-83. Epub 2014 May 31.

Moriguchi T, Harii N, Goto J, Harada D, Sugawara H, Takamino J, et al. A first case of meningitis/encephalitis associated with SARS-coronavirus-2. Int J Infect Dis. 2020 May;94:55-8. Epub 2020 Apr 3.

Nouh A, Borys E, Gierut AK, Biller J. Amyloid-Beta related angiitis of the central nervous system: case report and topic review. Front Neurol. 2014 Feb 4;5:13.

Ozdal P, Ozdamar Y, Yazici A, Teke MY, Ozturk F. Vogt-Koyanagi-Harada disease: clinical and demographic characteristics of patients in a specialized eye hospital in Turkey. Ocul Immunol Inflamm. 2014 Aug;22(4):277-86. Epub 2013 Dec 11.

Petzold GC, Bohner G, Klingebiel R, Amberger N, van der Knaap MS, Zschenderlein R. Adult onset leucoencephalopathy with brain stem and spinal cord involvement and normal lactate. J Neurol Neurosurg Psychiatry. 2006 Jul;77(7):889–91.

Pilotto A, Masciocchi S, Volonghi I, De Giuli V, Caprioli F, Mariotto S, et al. SARS-CoV-2 encephalitis is a cytokine release syndrome: evidences from cerebrospinal fluid analyses. Clin Infect Dis. 2021 Jan 4:ciaa1933. Epub ahead of print.

Pilotto A, Odolini S, Masciocchi S, Comelli A, Volonghi I, Gazzina S, et al. Steroid-responsive encephalitis in coronavirus disease 2019. Ann Neurol. 2020 Aug;88(2):423-7. Epub 2020 Jun 9.

Ponzoni M, Campo E, Nakamura S. Intravascular large B-cell lymphoma: a chameleon with multiple faces and many masks. Blood. 2018 Oct 11;132(15):1561-7. Epub 2018 Aug 15.

Rabinstein AA. Vascular myelopathies. Continuum (Minneap Minn). 2015 Feb;21(1, Spinal Cord Disorders):67–83.

Rademakers R, Baker M, Nicholson AM, Rutherford NJ, Finch N, Soto-Ortolaza A, et al. Mutations in the colony stimulating factor 1 receptor (CSF1R) gene cause hereditary diffuse leukoencephalopathy with spheroids. Nat Genet. 2011 Dec 25;44(2):200–5.

Resende LL, de Paiva ARB, Kok F, da Costa Leite C, Lucato LT. Adult leukodystrophies: a step-by-step diagnostic approach. Radiographics. 2019 Jan-Feb;39(1):153–68.

Salvarani C, Brown RD Jr, Hunder GG. Adult primary central nervous system vasculitis. Lancet. 2012 Aug 25;380(9843):767-77. Epub 2012 May 9.

Salvarani C, Brown RD Jr, Muratore F, Christianson TJH, Galli E, Pipitone N, et al. Rituximab therapy for primary central nervous system vasculitis: a 6 patient experience and review of the literature. Autoimmun Rev. 2019 Apr;18(4):399-405. Epub 2019 Feb 10.

Salvarani C, Hunder GG, Morris JM, Brown RD Jr, Christianson T, Giannini C. Aβ-related angiitis: comparison with CAA without inflammation and primary CNS vasculitis. Neurology. 2013 Oct 29;81(18):1596-603. Epub 2013 Sep 27.

Scheper GC, van der Klok T, van Andel RJ, van Berkel CG, Sissler M, Smet J, et al. Mitochondrial aspartyl-tRNA synthetase deficiency causes leukoencephalopathy with brain stem and spinal cord involvement and lactate elevation. Nat Genet. 2007 Apr;39(4):534-9. Epub 2007 Mar 25.

Schwendimann RN. Metabolic and toxic myelopathies. Continuum (Minneap Minn). 2018 Apr;24(2, Spinal Cord Disorders):427–40.

Scolding NJ, Joseph F, Kirby PA, Mazanti I, Gray F, Mikol J, et al. Abeta-related angiitis: primary angiitis of the central nervous system associated with cerebral amyloid angiopathy. Brain. 2005 Mar;128(Pt 3):500-15. Epub 2005 Jan 19.

Shaban A, Moritani T, Al Kasab S, Sheharyar A, Limaye KS, Adams HP Jr. Spinal cord hemorrhage. J Stroke Cerebrovasc Dis. 2018 Jun;27(6):1435-46. Epub 2018 Mar 16.

Siva A, Kantarci OH, Saip S, Altintas A, Hamuryudan V, Islak C, et al. Behçet's disease: diagnostic and prognostic aspects of neurological involvement. J Neurol. 2001 Feb;248(2):95–103.

Stern BJ, Royal W 3rd, Gelfand JM, Clifford DB, Tavee J, Pawate S, et al. Definition and consensus diagnostic criteria for neurosarcoidosis: from the Neurosarcoidosis Consortium Consensus Group. JAMA Neurol. 2018 Dec 1;75(12):1546–53.

Susac JO, Murtagh FR, Egan RA, Berger JR, Bakshi R, Lincoff N, et al. MRI findings in Susac's syndrome. Neurology. 2003 Dec 23;61(12):1783–7.

Tobin WO, Guo Y, Krecke KN, Parisi JE, Lucchinetti CF, Pittock SJ, et al. Diagnostic criteria for chronic lymphocytic inflammation with pontine perivascular enhancement responsive to steroids (CLIPPERS). Brain. 2017 Sep 1;140(9):2415–25.

Toledano M, Davies NWS. Infectious encephalitis: mimics and chameleons. Pract Neurol. 2019 Jun;19(3):225-37. Epub 2019 Mar 16.

Vanderver A. Genetic leukoencephalopathies in adults. Continuum (Minneap Minn). 2016 Jun;22(3):916–42.

Venkatesan A, Michael BD, Probasco JC, Geocadin RG, Solomon T. Acute encephalitis in immunocompetent adults. Lancet. 2019 Feb 16;393(10172):702-16. Epub 2019 Feb 14.

Vilela P, Rowley HA. Brain ischemia: CT and MRI techniques in acute ischemic stroke. Eur J Radiol. 2017 Nov;96:162-72. Epub 2017 Aug 24.

Weidauer S, Nichtweiss M, Hattingen E. Differential diagnosis of white matter lesions: nonvascular causes-Part II. Clin Neuroradiol. 2014 Jun;24(2):93-110. Epub 2014 Feb 12.

Weinshenker BG. Tumefactive demyelinating lesions: characteristics of individual lesions, individual patients, or a unique disease entity? Mult Scler. 2015 Nov;21(13):1746-7. Epub 2015 Sep 11.

WHO classification of tumours of the central nervous system: International Agency for Research on Cancer (IARC). In: Louis DN, Ohgaki H, Wiestler OD, Cavenee WK, editors. Revised 4th ed. Lyon: International Agency for Research on Cancer. c2016. 408 p. (T1 hypointensity.)

Zalewski NL, Flanagan EP, Keegan BM. Evaluation of idiopathic transverse myelitis revealing specific myelopathy diagnoses. Neurology. 2018 Jan 9;90(2):e96-e102. Epub 2017 Dec 15.

Zalewski NL, Krecke KN, Weinshenker BG, Aksamit AJ, Conway BL, McKeon A, et al. Central canal enhancement and the trident sign in spinal cord sarcoidosis. Neurology. 2016 Aug 16;87(7):743–4.

Zalewski NL, Rabinstein AA, Brinjikji W, Kaufmann TJ, Nasr D, Ruff MW, et al. Unique gadolinium enhancement pattern in spinal dural arteriovenous fistulas. JAMA Neurol. 2018 Dec 1;75(12):1542–5.

Zalewski NL, Rabinstein AA, Krecke KN, Brown RD Jr, Wijdicks EFM, Weinshenker BG, et al. Characteristics of spontaneous spinal cord infarction and proposed diagnostic criteria. JAMA Neurol. 2019 Jan 1;76(1):56–63.

Zalewski NL, Rabinstein AA, Krecke KN, Brown RD, Wijdicks EFM, Weinshenker BG, et al. Spinal cord infarction: clinical and imaging insights from the periprocedural setting. J Neurol Sci. 2018 May 15;388:162-7. Epub 2018 Mar 17.

Zeydan B, Uygunoglu U, Saip S, Demirci ON, Seyahi E, Ugurlu S, et al. Infliximab is a plausible alternative for neurologic complications of Behçet disease. Neurol Neuroimmunol Neuroinflamm. 2016 Jul 8;3(5):e258.

INDEX

CPSIA information can be obtained
at www.ICGtesting.com
Printed in the USA
BVHW012020180723
667441BV00002B/2